OCULAR EXAMINATION

basis and technique

OCULAR EXAMINATION

basis and technique

ARTHUR H. KEENEY, M.D., D.Sc.

Ophthalmologist-in-Chief, Wills Eye Hospital and Research Institute;
Professor and Chairman, Department of Ophthalmology,
Temple University School of Medicine,
Philadelphia, Pennsylvania

With 161 illustrations

Saint Louis
THE C. V. MOSBY COMPANY
1970

Contributors

Ben P. Houser, Jr., M.D.

Wills Eye Hospital and Research Institute, Philadelphia, Pennsylvania

Arnold B. Popkin, M.D.

Assistant Surgeon and Director of Electroretinography Laboratory, Wills Eye Hospital and Research Institute, Philadelphia, Pennsylvania

Joel Porter, M.D.

Senior Resident Surgeon and NINDS Trainee in Visual Physiology, Wills Eye Hospital and Research Institute, Philadelphia, Pennsylvania

Lov K. Sarin, M.B.B.S.

Senior Assistant Surgeon, Retina Service, Wills Eye Hospital and Research Institute; Clinical Associate Professor of Ophthalmology, Temple University School of Medicine, Philadelphia, Pennsylvania

Joseph U. Toglia, M.D.

Associate Professor of Neurology and Otorhinology, Temple University School of Medicine, Philadelphia, Pennsylvania

Terrance L. Tomer

Director, Retinal Photographic Laboratory, Wills Eye Hospital and Research Institute; Assistant Instructor of Ophthalmology, Temple University School of Medicine, Philadelphia, Pennsylvania

Wayne W. Wong, M.D.

Staff Ophthalmologist, Queen's Medical Center, Honolulu, Hawaii

Preface

This book has two major areas of address. The first is to the initial ophthalmic examination by the primary eye examiner—the front line practitioner and his assistants or the resident physician in training who must master and learn to efficiently perform each technique. The second address is to the subspecialty or consultation examinations by ophthalmologists who make a "pet" of particular disease groups or who limit their work entirely to one subject area.

In every case, the philosophy of approach is to achieve the optimal number of examining procedures in the minimum number of patient visits and with the least movement of the patient within the examining offices. Professional workers can move more rapidly and without issuance of instructions than can perplexed and uncertain patients. Chapter 1 is therefore devoted to the lay-out, organization, and equipment of the examining office.

Awareness by both the profession and the U. S. Public Health Service of the need to achieve fuller distribution of eye services obviously catalyzed long dormant and floundering interest in the role of ophthalmic aides, assistants, or technologists. Traditionally the American ophthalmologist has relied on four basic sources of help in his profession.

1. His intelligent and attractive Girl Friday, who most commonly is not a registered nurse

2. His operating-room scrub assistant, who now more commonly is a scrub technologist rather than a nurse

3. The optician, as the skilled professional in spectacles, contact lenses, low vision aids, and prosthetic design; more recently the ocularist, who has evolved from this group as a unique artist-craftsman devoting his entire energies to design and fabrication of artificial eyes, orbital replacements, and special ocular prosthetics

4. Least commonly, the orthoptists, who number about 350 in the United States

Federal enactment in 1966 of the Allied Health Professions legislation was followed by slow movement over the next 2 years to define, outline training of, and establish career tracks for ophthalmic aides, ophthalmic assistants, optometric assistants, and optometric technologists. The underlying philosophy that every health procedure should be performed by individuals with the minimum skill level has not been completely attractive even to senior ocular surgeons who may enjoy adroitly removing —as any druggist might also do—a broken cilium from its painful lodgement in a lacrimal punctum or prescribing a proper residual vertical prism to wipe out the last symptom in an adult who has had long overdue vertical muscle surgery. Nonetheless, increasing formalized assistance and aid to the harried practitioner is evolving, as are constructively conjoint programs between ophthalmologists and optometrists.

Examinations covered in this book represent practical working techniques. The book does not purport to be encyclopedic in listing every eponymic variation of instrument or technique, nor historically replete in presenting prototypes. My personal preferences and biases—as for my own Near Vision Test Card—reflect 25 years of active practice and are by design part of this volume. Hopefully these are leavened, here and there, in sections authored by associates who have plowed their single furrows to exquisite excellence.

The eye is a unique and matchless organ of inquiry. In its naked and unaided outward range to inquire of man's environment it resolves the craters of the recently perambulated moon and the minimal separable intervals between stars that are millions of light years away. To the unaided examiner inquiring inwardly, ocular motility, pupillary action, even the color and composition of its outer coats display the story of half the cranial nerves, index the occurrence of jaundice, anemia, or polycythemia, and differentiate many variations in disturbances of the pituitary and thyroid systems. Relatively simple optic tools of the past century enormously multiply the fruits of these inquiries. Seemingly sophisticated instruments of the moment uncover many more subtleties and commensurately extend the examiner's responsibilities for early detection of disorder and avoidance of visual catastrophe.

This book is primarily centered upon instrumental techniques that increase the examiner's clinically significant penetration of the visual system. In most sections, some outline of normalcy and normal variation in structure and function is included as a base line from which pathologic deviations are measured. To the reader having working familiarity in this area, terseness of presentation is offered to make more palatable the inherent value of orderly review.

Retinoscopy and refraction, though in-

herent components of ocular examination, are treated extensively in many other separate publications and are therefore not detailed here. Similarly, bacteriology, virology, and radiology, which must frequently be brought into full-scale study of the visual system, are reserved to their detailed expositions elsewhere. The initial steps and the detailed extensions that the examiner must accomplish in his clinical setting are the core of this volume.

The trustees of any institution fundamentally provide the basis and orientation within which professional staff members develop their interests, their skills, and their responsibilities to patients. Conversely, by inattention or preoccupation, they may tolerate major abrogations of professional growth and obligation. To the Board of Directors of the Wills Eye Hospital and Research Institute, I express sincere appreciation for providing and maintaining the matrix upon which patient care, research, and efforts such as this evolve. Particularly, I thank Mr. Donald C. Rubel, Mr. William P. Cairo, and Dr. Max M. Leon for their many hours devoted to the professional aspects of the Wills, with no tangible compensation other than personal satisfaction.

My indebtedness to many members of the Wills Hospital family is both specific and continuing. Every individual within my own office has labored in manuscript production, editing, and typing. Mrs. Anthony Kidawa, Mrs. Patricia Upham, and Mrs. Richard Haberkost more tangibly emerge from these pages also as models. Mrs. Marie Moore and Mrs. Frederick Colvin have contributed many hours of personal assistance, typing, and refinement.

My closest companion both in creativity and confinement through this work has, of course, been Dr. Virginia Keeney, whose decades of rapid alternation between wife, mother, and civic worker on one hand, and physician, counselor, and critic on the other, have been of enormous value.

I also wish to acknowledge the professional photographic assistance of Mr. Paul

Axler, of the Visual Education Service of Wills Eye Hospital, who has made most of the photographic illustrations.

The stimulation and excitement of the large corps of resident physicians has certainly contributed both to genesis and detail. Many individual residents have assisted in specific areas, particularly Dr. Joel Porter, Dr. Joseph Calhoun, and Dr. James Copeland. Also, individual manufacturers and distributors of equipment have been particularly cooperative in supplying materials on request. The help of Mr. Al Hart in multiple personal ways has also freed many hours for the development of these materials.

The assistance of several staff members in preparing sections representing their intense personal interests has been of great value. I wish to thank Dr. Lov K. Sarin of the Retina Service for his section on indirect ophthalmoscopy; Dr. Ben P. Houser, Jr., recent Chief Resident, for his section on the pupil; Terrance L. Tomer, Retinal Photographer, for his section on fundus photography and angiography; Dr. Joseph U. Toglia, neurootologist, for his section on nystagmography; and Dr. Arnold B. Popkin of the Electrophysiology Service for his section on electroretinography.

Arthur H. Keeney

Contents

xii   *Contents*

Part one

Basic principles

Chapter 1

Basic preparation for the examination

THE EXAMINER

"A misleading symptom is misleading only to one able to be misled."

SIR HENEAGE OGILVIE

The most important basic preparation to examination is thorough understanding of normal variations and disease processes. Well-organized knowledge, analytic curiosity, probing skills, consideration, and ingenuity can circumvent a lack of equipment and devices. Instruments are merely extensions of the neurosensory capability of the examiner and, like the finest electron microscope, are worthless without the interpretations of a perceptive eye and intelligent brain. The optimal formal education of the examiner is not an end in itself but merely a base line of provisional data on which must be built a lifetime of further refinement, increasing knowledge, and seasoned judgment. No instrument or group of instruments can exceed the inherent abilities of the examiner.

SPACE FOR THE EXAMINING AREA
General examining room

Ophthalmic examining space should be inviting and gracious to help make the patient feel at ease. Tiny rooms cluttered with equipment and optic mirrors are dehumanizing and mechanical; narrow pie-shaped rooms compressing to projection chart width at the far end are oppressive.

The examining room should ideally be 24 ft. long. This distance may be measured diagonally within shorter walls or lengthwise in a room no narrower than 9 ft. This allows the examiner to move behind the examining chair or to lower the chair back for recumbent procedures. The available "lane length" of 20 ft. from the patient's eye to the projection screen is minimal for standardization of acuity notations, motility notations, and the practical simulation of ocular resolving power at infinity. This distance is distinctly inadequate for eliciting divergence excess types of intermittent exotropia, and therefore the space must include a window where binocularity under remote fixation (preferably a block or more away and under bright illumination) can be assessed.

Equipment in the examining room must necessarily be extensive to achieve maximum efficiency of one-stop service, in terms of both minimum number of visits to the office and movement within the office. For optic reasons, equipment surfaces should be dull or matte and of black, dark gray, or subdued dark tones. This reduces annoying light reflections and distractions to both patient and examiner. Nothing could be more optically illogical and bedazzling than to attempt intraocular examinations near a large picture window with polished, gay coral instruments, as shown in some manufacturer's catalogs. Also, for patient

3

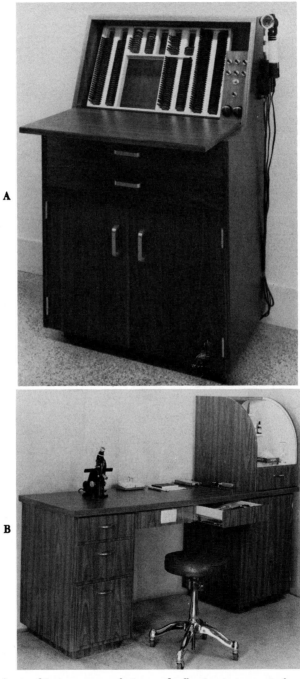

Fig. 1-1. Solid front cabinetry removes knives and offensive instruments from immediate view. **A,** Jenkel-Davidson cabinet (Jenkel-Davidson Optical Co., San Francisco, California 94119); **B,** Benson desk (Benson Optical Co., Minneapolis, Minnesota 55440).

reassurance and relaxation, cold chrome and hospital pastels should be avoided.

Small instruments, knives, scissors, and syringes should be stored in solid-door cabinets. Neither children nor adults are made happy by the display of punctum dilators or chalazion curettes in military columns (Fig. 1-1). These should be appropriately grouped, wrapped, labeled, sterilized, and then stored in the cabinets.

The use of woods such as walnut, mahogany, ash, or chestnut with upholstering colors such as tan, deep red, gray, umber, or muted greens minimizes the sometimes painful suggestion of shots and sutures. Also, this affords an attractive method of designating examining rooms by woods or colors. (Though an esthete might make faint pause over being sent to the gray or the blue room, no one really wants to be consigned numerically to room two or geographically to the back room; however, almost everyone is satisfied to be escorted to the walnut room.)

Illumination in the examining room should be predominantly artificial, usually subdued, and under intensity control. It is essential, however, that the room be rendered quite dark for procedures such as indirect ophthalmoscopy; therefore, venetian blinds should be of the interlocking and light-proof type, supplemented by full-length lined drapes at each side of the window to eliminate light-streaking at the edges. Subdued light from an indirect source behind a cornice is less desirable than that from a table lamp with an opaque shade, because the latter is generally warmer and allows the patient or relative to read by its localized intensity while awaiting the examiner's entrance or for drops to take effect.

Access for the examiner and the patient is preferably by different doors. The patient should be able to enter and leave from a corridor or alcove off the reception area. This should be arranged so that others in the reception area do not look directly into the examining room when the door is opened. The examiner, on the other hand, should enter and leave by a back corridor or small interchange room where he can receive information about the next patient, calls, or other messages. Some doctors like to keep a dictating system in such in-between rooms so that notes may be promptly dictated after the patient is seen.

Seating in the examining room must not only provide full access to the patient in either the sitting or recumbent position but should also provide mobility space for the examiner, who generally uses a stool with large casters (small casters catch in rugs) with a back. (The back on the stool becomes increasingly comforting in latter hours of the day and with advancing years of practice.) There should also be pleasant adjacent seating for at least *three* relatives or attendants within each examining room. Here a medium-sized or three-cushion davenport is particularly appropriate because (1) a single patient or family unit is being served and (2) it affords a place for fainting or ill individuals to recline. The common pattern of several members of the family accompanying a youngster or an elderly patient often provides a quick index of hereditary problems in the family and saves repetition of explanation to different generations. Don't be trapped by letting a mate or grown sibling remain out in the reception area when a lengthy explanation must be given.

A small washbasin, such as a stainless steel "trailer sink," should be in every examining room so that the doctor may wash his hands in the presence of the patient. Its base can be attractively boxed to the floor, obscuring unsightly plumbing and giving storage space for paper towels, tissues, and so on.* A mirror should also be in every examining room so that ladies may adjust their hair or hats after the physician leaves.

Special examining room

Each patient care room in an office or clinic should be fitted for the accomplish-

---

*Franklin Optical Co., Instrument Division, Oakland, California 94612.

ment of as many procedures as possible. This also applies to minor surgical undertakings and to those procedures that can well be delegated to a technologist. Thus neither patient nor staff time is lost in moving people from room to room. Exceptions are needed, however, such as in the employment of large or complex equipment (dark adaptometers, Tubinger perimeters, and ultrasound) or of instruments that must be electrically shielded (for electroretinography or electroencephalography); where technologists will spend relatively long periods with patients (orthoptic studies, electronic tonometry, fluorescein angiography, electrooculography, and contact lens fitting), or where patients may merely remain in the office for protracted periods (mydriatic instillations, water provocative tests, and subcutaneous Prostigmin tests).

It is not efficient planning to set aside a separate room for special study of strabismus, retinal detachment, or glaucoma. Even the special consultant in these fields should accomplish his investigations in a flexible and multiple-purpose room. He may consign some procedures, however, to other office areas where the technologist and patient are removed from distractions and disturbances. In large clinics with multiple examiners, it is generally advantageous to equip groups of separate rooms in which associated technologists do their work. This applies most immediately to contact lens fitting, tonography, fluorescein angiography, orthoptics, and electrophysiology.

NONEXAMINING SPACES IN THE SUITE
Reception area

Appurtenances and decor in the reception area should be inviting and domestic or club-like rather than sterile and professional. Reception room furniture should be covered with a good, fabric-backed, flexible plastic such as Naugahyde because it (1) harbors less dust and allergens than wool, (2) adds softness that wooden or molded furniture cannot give, (3) is less expensive than leather or wool upholstery, (4) will

last longer, and (5) cleans easily with only soap and water. Chrome-like furniture should not be used because of its cold and commercial feeling. Cane, though more artistic, is impractical because of frequent breaks and chronic need for recaning.

Seating is most commonly needed for singles or doubles, and the two-cushion settee or loveseat will reassuringly accommodate two adults plus an apprehensive child patient. There is little invitation to the larger davenport, particularly the three-seater, when strangers occupying each end block all access to side tables and the last man in is faced with elbow-rubbing center isolation.

A children's table, round (to reduce corner injuries and proprietary sides) and of solid hard wood, with four to six solid children's chairs should be placed in one corner of the reception area, perhaps semipartitioned off by a sturdy wrought-iron trellis or half-height book shelves. Several good youth magazines will earn you gratitude from the children and also younger mothers who want to get with it and sit on the children's chairs. (More mature mothers or grandmothers will appreciate a few adult-size chairs overlooking the children's unit.)

The number of reception spaces should be in a ratio of approximately seven to each examining chair. Thus the minimum should be about seven; with two examiners using four units, there should be nearly twenty-eight reception spaces, including the children's unit. Three to ten of the total should be in a separate "mydriatic room" if possible. This reduces any shock of a jammed waiting room for entering patients and gains semiprivacy for the occasional scene of a child resisting drops. In this mydriatic room where many patients are precluded from reading, a truly high-fidelity sound system may be an appreciated comfort and divertissement to the captives.

The reception desk should be in direct view from the patient's entrance door and afford surveillance of the entire reception area. It needs a slightly elevated, protective front "barrier" to keep small hands or the idly curious adult from delving into work materials. If the receptionist must also answer the telephone, as is often done, she should have a "hush booth" or recessed alcove so that every incoming call is not a matter for public display or reception room entertainment. The receptionist's telephone should be impossible to reach from the waiting area, to avoid preemption by patients.

The reception area is the nerve center of a busy office; here a gracious nonprofessional must make semiprofessional decisions regarding the urgency of calls that would interrupt work in progress, problems that must be meshed into crowded schedules, and complaints that can safely be postponed for decision. She must be schooled in the separation of *true emergencies* (chemical burns, acute glaucoma, lacerated eyes, vascular occlusions), *urgencies*, both medical and social (retinal detachments, uveitis, lacrimal infections, departures for Africa, out-of-state grandmothers of patient families who will only be in town for 10 days but who have chronic glaucoma plus cataracts), and *elective problems* (periodic change in spectacles, blepharochalasis, cataract rechecks, involution of the macula, old ptosis).

The appointment book should be large and open and lie completely flat on the secretary's desk. It should show at least a whole day on one page or at most the entire week on the total open pages in direct view. Time intervals are preferably printed in units of 15 minutes. Minimal information listed should be the patient's full name, the nature of the visit (new examination, follow-up visit, glasses recheck, postoperative sutures), and the telephone number where the patient could be reached in case it is necessary to cancel or to reschedule appointments. Entries should always be made with a pencil, which is preferably tied or chained to the book. Though the receptionist should not be trapped with a small or crowded appointment book page, she should keep for the doctor's reference a

vest-pocket counterpart of this book indicating surgical schedules, hospital admissions, luncheon commitments, and out-of-town schedules. She should steal this from his pocket at least twice a week to be sure it is up-to-date.

Though good commercial reception and appointment books may be purchased from many suppliers, after a few years in practice it will be preferable for the physician to design, with his receptionists, an appointment book geared to his particular demands.

Lighting in the reception area should be slightly subdued because many patients may have irritable eyes or dilated pupils. This also affords a gentle transition into the further subdued light of the examining room. Windows with glass curtains or partially turned (not light-tight) venetian blinds preserve some relief from claustrophobia and yet reduce brightness. A few table lamps with opaque shades facilitate reading for those who want to browse through the fresh and unusual magazines.

Piped-in music of low fidelity is often resented by intelligent persons rendered captive to another individual's preselection. Such obligate aural salads are less appropriate to the professional office than to the commercial world, and the expense might more productively be directed to interesting and current literature.

All hats, overcoats, and extra garments that the patient may wish to remove should be handled *before* the patient is seated in the examining chair and *before* the physician enters the room. The most practical place is an alcove with hat shelves between the reception room and the corridor entrance to the examining area. Coats and raingear should never be permitted to take up reception seats for both esthetic and economic reasons. Women must always be reminded to keep their purses with them, and patients insisting on taking outer gear back into the examining areas should be accommodated rather than debated. There should be a closet for the doctor and the staff away from the reception area.

Bookkeeping

Though an accounting firm, office management service, or, in recent years, some banks should ultimately, properly, and with conservation of the doctor's time supervise all fiscal procedures, it is essential to have some bookkeeping resource immediately available. Here routine charges can be posted and explained, cash payments can be received and receipted, status of accounts can be updated and revised, minor problems can be answered and corrected. This area should be available along the path of the departing patient, but not in the open reception area where frank and clear discussion of finances, essential to the well-being of most patients, might be embarrassing. Courtesy here is essential, and, in the event of questioning, the accounting aide should immediately express the possibility of an office error that she will be pleased to check. Though a small chair may be moved from nearby, no chairs should be placed at this desk, as they encourage lingering and unneeded conversation both by the staff and patients.

Lavatories

Facilities for patients should be available within the building, preferably on the same floor, but *not* within the suite. An office lavatory is essential to conserve the time of the office staff, for the occasionally ill patient with nausea and vomiting of angle-closure glaucoma, or following Prostigmin testing. The lavatory should be small, contain an adequate wall mirror, and preferably be painted throughout in a uniform and unattractive shade of red or purple. This has remarkable value in discouraging staff members from lingering.

Typing and correspondence

The doctor should never economize on professional height and properly designed desks and seating for secretarial help. Whether time-efficiency is best served by dictating notes after seeing a patient or by writing notes with many abbreviations during the examination, there will continue to be increasing numbers of forms, letters, and patient reports to prepare. Every referring practitioner, resident, intern, or other professional colleague deserves a brief (preferably one page, single-spaced) understandable report of the findings, recommendations, and reasons therefore. A few excellent secretaries can be taught to formulate such letters from examination notes —this has danger, however, of uncomplimentary routinism being detected by those who refer patients repeatedly. In most cases these letters should be dictated personally, and thus a progressive load of typing evolves. Efficiency is best served not by direct dictation to a secretary but by the use of identical dictating equipment on the examiner's desk, between examining rooms, in his car, and at home. Both written materials and instructions thus accumulated on a catch-as-catch-can basis wherever the doctor is reach the typist without interrupting either person.

The typing space should be isolated from phone calls but accessible by intercom. Often the best location for this space is off the corridor between examining rooms or adjacent to the mydriatic room. The typist may double to attend the mydriatic room and relieve others in the office. It is valuable to have some flexible person such as this to fill in when other members of the staff are absent.

Intercommunications

Each inner room—excluding the lavatory and mydriatic room—should be equipped with a station of a separate intercom system. Squawk boxes and loud-speaker systems, no matter how subdued, are not appropriate to the private and confidential nature of activities in the office. The instrument should be of one-piece or French phone design to be completely controlled with one hand or caught easily between the ear and shoulder.

The use of telephone circuitry for intercom purposes seems simple and frugal. Actually, it is complicated and perpetually expensive. Whenever telephone circuits are used for intercommunications, this precludes use of the telephones for their outside purposes and prevents office staff members from delivering confidential spoken messages simultaneously while the doctor is talking on an outside line. With separate intercom instruments, it is possible to hold one to each ear in order to receive comments or information from the aide while handling a problem via the telephone. Of course, with either separate intercoms or intercom circuits on the telephone, it is possible to get the often-needed assistance of the appointment secretary or office aide on the same line with a major call. Remember also, the monthly charge for each button and each light goes on forever, whereas I have had the satisfaction of using substantial office intercom phones without a penny of maintenance for more than a decade.

The telephone extension in each office where patients are received should be without a dial. The doctor's own calls will be dialed by his secretary, and the available dial in a room where a patient is waiting his arrival is often an inducement to initiate a nonoffice call that ties up the office line and often has to be terminated with loss of the examiner's time on entering the room or with some embarrassment on the part of the patient.

Both the telephone and the separate intercommunication phone should be located where they can be reached from the examining chair without rising or moving.

BASIC EXAMINING EQUIPMENT

Certain basic examining equipment needs to be present in any examining room for either initial ophthalmic examination or subspecialty and consultation examination. Selecting, modifying, or designing equipment is part of the fun and a manifestation of the individual's penetration. As early as possible in training years, the young practitioner should initiate appraisal of portable

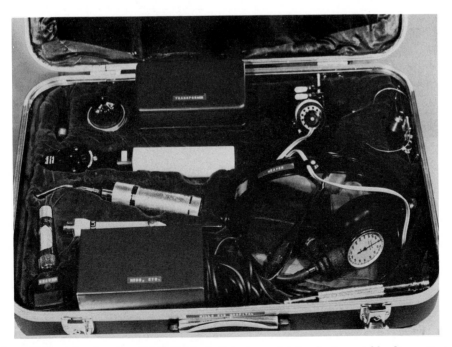

Fig. 1-2. Example of custom-fitted, hard plastic case containing basic portable diagnostic instruments, transformer, and small assortment of drugs. At left from bottom upward are: retinoscope, ophthalmodynamometer, transilluminator, direct ophthalmoscope, +30-diopter lens, and three-mirror contact lens. At right are power handle for retinoscope, sphygmomanometer, percussion hammer, binocular indirect ophthalmoscope, and loupe. (Designed by John H. Weaver, M.D.)

instruments and begin their purchase. He thus becomes familiar with performance and design limitations of major hand equipment. He works more readily and easily with his own instruments and learns their care and repair. These common items essential for every resident include (1) a giant (hand) ophthalmoscope, (2) an indirect binocular ophthalmoscope, (3) a multiple-mirrored contact lens for examining the angle and fundus, (4) a Schiøtz tonometer, (5) a surgical loupe, (6) a good retinoscope, (7) a simple exophthalmometer, and (8), as the British say, a splendid inspection torch. Before completion of training he should add (1) his first, simple external camera, (2) an ophthalmodynamometer, (3) an electric keratoscope or Placido's disc, (4) a hand rotary prism or prism bars, and (5) possibly a Lancaster transilluminator. He should also be using and evaluating major examining units such as slit lamps, refractors, and lensometers from various manufacturers so that well-reasoned orders can be placed several months before intended use. Thus the basic hand tools to equip the first of minimally two and ultimately three or more complete examining units in an office are familiar acquisitions or the components of a portable case (Fig. 1-2) early in professional life.

The initial as well as each subsequently fitted examining room should have not only as full equipment as possible for "one-stop service" but should also have compact grouping of the maximum amount of equipment to minimize movement by the examiner and to avoid movement by the patient. This generally necessitates stand-mounted (Figs. 1-3 and 1-4) (hydraulic or electric) instruments, with the second choice being wall-mounted (spring-counterbalanced) instruments. Wall-mounted projectors and cabinetry are desirable to conserve valuable floor space and to reduce floor clutter; however, wall-mounted refractors and slit lamps tie the examining chair and the patient so close to the wall that the chair rotation (90 degrees) for 1-meter tangent screen examination is not practical. Similarly, these restrict the desirable arc of access when the chair back is dropped to place the patient horizontal for indirect ophthalmoscopy.

The examining chair should be relatively narrow, with only short, elbowrest type armpieces. This allows the doctor to roll quite near, as is necessary for direct ophthalmoscopy, lacrimal irrigations, and similar close control maneuvers. Since the chair is narrow, the elbowrests or any sidepieces must be hinged to turn away from the occasional broad beam of alimentary overindulgence. The chair should be comfortably padded and without an extending footrest, or at most with an inconspicuous folded rest to be turned out only when obligatory. Furniture projections such as footrests may easily trip the unwary patient, just as com-

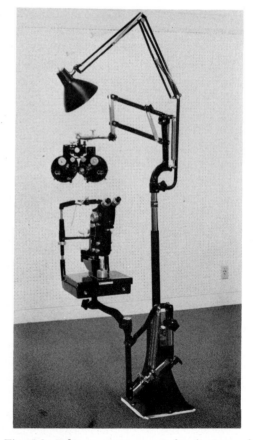

Fig. 1-3. Reliance spring-mounted refractor and slit lamp on floor stand, which must be bolted to floor. (Reliance Koenigkramer Co., Cincinnati, Ohio 45216.)

fortably long armrests traumatize the examiner's abdomen. A headrest, usually adjustable, is indispensable for indentation tonometry, orbital tonometry, esthesiometry, and even the ocasional psychologic retreater apprehensive about fingers or instruments approaching his eyes. Both the chair and the space must allow full reclining range of the back. The chair's height also must be adjustable, preferably by a footpump hydraulic system rather than electrically. This is not only healthy for the sedentary examiner but also reduces service costs and interruptions as well as capital outlay.

Closely grouped to the examining chair are the obligate, heavy items: refractor, trial case, lensometer, slit lamp, and tangent screen. In spite of the obvious efficiency and facility of modern refractors, the trial case —and less often the trial frame—continues to be indispensable for retinoscopy of small

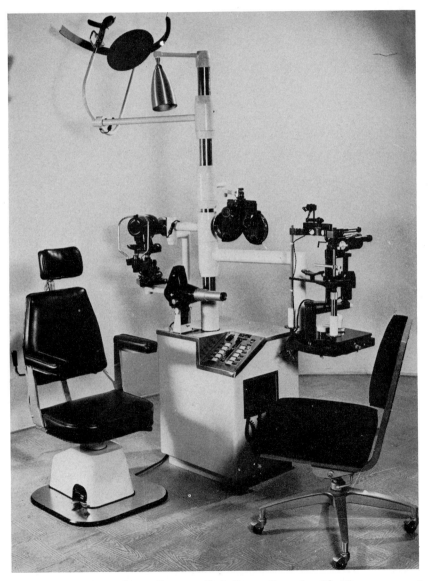

Fig. 1-4. Guyton-Carlson electrically controlled diagnostic unit with 33-cm. arc perimeter swung upward from patient. (Carlson Manufacturing Co., Royal Oaks, Michigan 48067.)

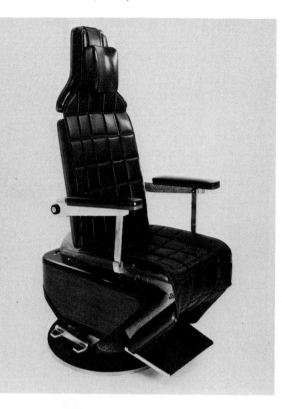

Fig. 1-5. Compact examining chair (SMR Maxi Chair G-1, 1969) may be adjusted from lowest seat position 18 in. above floor to a maximum elevation of 38 in. Chair is fully reclining to the semi-Fowler position. Footrest is retracted in low position as illustrated but extends outward when chair is elevated or reclined. Loose upholstery cushioning slides over structural elements of the chair during adjustment to avoid disturbing patient's clothing. Chair rotates 360 degrees. Headrest is adjusted forward and backward. (Produced by Surgical, Mechanical, Research Inc., Newport Beach, California 92663.)

children, handling the patient with spinal deformity, and refining high dioptric corrections (such as in the aphakic patient) over his spectacles. The trial case should not be a compromise economy kit but should provide a full range of lenses with compensated base curves, to simulate as closely as possible what the patient will finally wear.

Small items for the examining desk such as punctum dilators, lacrimal cannulas, sterile fluorescein paper strips, individually packaged sterile cotton-tipped applicators, a nasal speculum, and opaque and red clip-on lenses are built up in keeping with the examiner's preference and practice. Similarly, a selection of minor surgical instruments for chalazia, suture removal, and biopsy must be accumulated in accordance with individual needs.

Chapter 2

Indications for diagnostic examination steps

THE PATIENT'S HISTORY

Proper examination requires the systematic application of successive diagnostic maneuvers or steps. From the hundreds of possible and variously productive tests that can be catalogued, it is essential to select efficiently the germane and needed procedures. Two things enable the clinician to do this appropriately and with significant security. The first is the patient's *history,* properly evoked and verified, if necessary, internally, by cross questions to elicit corroborating details, or externally, by obtaining old records, hospital summaries, or slides of previous tissue specimens. (Copies of pathology reports should be received with suspicion as secondary evidence because they (1) may come from nonrepresentative sections of a lesion, (2) are subject to differences in interpretation by various pathologists, (3) sometimes are precast by interpretations no longer consonant with better understanding of the process, and (4) may be plagued by even more clerical errors than appear between lensometer readings from a pair of spectacles and a crumpled old copy of a prescription that the patient carries.) The second is that sense of correlation known as *clinical judgment,* which grows in proportion to a practitioner's years of self-critical diagnostics, periodically refined by review of his data and accomplishments.

> "A clinician is complex. He is part craftsman, part practical scientist, and part historian."
> THOMAS ADDIS

Obtaining the history

Chief complaints are the first subjective leads obtained in the diagnostic examination. The clinician should note several items of objective information as he crosses the examining room to the patient—or, with less conservation of his time, as the patient comes to the examining position. For example, searching movements of the patient's eye and head in scrutinizing the doctor immediately suggest impairment of central vision, whereas failure of the patient to recognize the examiner's outstretched hand in greeting is a tip-off to major field loss. Both for mental analysis and for commitment to record, complaints should be reduced to succinct and compressed expressions, refined in specific details such as severity, intermittency, or character and dated as to onset. Thus no patient may state his complaints as "painless progressive impairment of vision for 4 years, more marked o.d. than o.s." but this capsules the salient features for differential diagnosis of senile nuclear cataracts; "intermittent painful blurring of vision o.d. with redness and watery discharge for 4 years" aims the studies toward recurrent uveitis.

To weigh both accuracy and significance, it is often best if the patient—whether young child or aged grandparent—describes his own symptoms rather than having them interpreted and edited by a hopefully helpful adult. Similarly, undue influence on the independence of the diagnosis is often avoided by tactfully turning the patient's narrative away from recounts of previous professional advice. Where the name of an earlier examiner is volunteered, it may expedite obtaining desired details later and should therefore be quietly recorded. If the name is not volunteered, do not probe, because the patient may consider this a violation of confidence or prejudicial to the examiner's own thinking. Innocuously noting where previous care was rendered may serve fully to obtain old records with less suggestion of prying.

History of the present illness should add specific details in relation to each chief complaint. If the chief complaint is "dull, bioccipital, and bifrontal headaches intermittently for 2 years," the further details should specify the severity in some degree, the presence or absence of aura, the duration of episodes and periods of relief, any association with use of the eyes either for near or far, complications such as nausea and vomiting, and concomitants such as nasal stuffiness or allergy. Lack of clear characterization of the complaint or lack of interference with usual activities is important in indicating less significance or a more functional than organic base.

Previous operations, surgical complications, and specific drugs with dosage and frequency should be noted in sufficient detail and date to evaluate past efficiency and to relate to future therapy.

Past history should outline any other or unrelated eye injuries or disturbances. The age and circumstances of wearing glasses should be recorded. Recently worn and unwearable spectacles should be verified on the lensometer with particular attention to prismatic elements (prescribed or inadvertent). They should also be checked on the face, particularly for fit on the bridge, centration of the visual axis with the optic center, and characteristics of any segments.

Medical history should particularly annotate systemic disease relating to vision, such as diabetes, thyroid disturbances, tumors, or vascular alterations. Medications

being taken and any drug idiosyncrasy should always be noted.

Family history should stress heritable ocular diseases (such as macular disturbances, color blindness, congenital defects, retinal detachments, cataract, or strabismus) and familial systemic diseases (such as diabetes, hypertension, and the like). Where serious visual defects are incompletely understood in remotely located siblings or cousins, it is helpful family counseling as well as assistance in diagnosis to request follow-through correspondence.

METHODOLOGY OF HISTORY INTERVIEW

Most productive clinicians prefer to have an intelligent and courteous aide record not only identifying vital statistics (never asking a lady's age in earshot of a public area) or fixed-field information, but also the previously discussed details of complaints, present illness, and past, medical, and family histories. The aide may check any medications with the patient and phone R numbers to druggists for verification of unlabeled prescriptions. Any alert high school student can be trained to neutralize spectacles or, if they should be lost or broken, to phone for recent prescriptions. She may also check visual acuity with and without glasses if so trained and instructed.

By virtue of intimate knowledge of disease, the skilled examiner can elicit most pertinent details of disease quite directly. He may prefer to invest additional time this way rather than to delegate the preliminary chores. Even with delegation, he must verify and amplify some details of the history as developed.

Short and complex ophthalmic record forms requiring more than seven pages may be found in other eye texts or obtained from commercial record companies. Printers and business form manufacturers are eager to sell forms printed to individual preference. In many cases, allocated record spaces will be insufficient for complex aspects or unneeded by the astute clinician. For initial and less complicated ophthalmic examination, plain white record forms, preferably 5 × 8 in. or 8½ × 11 in. (standard correspondence paper size), give the best flexibility of space and conservation of storage needs. Specific components of the examination may be conspicuously identified, where indicated, by a series of rubber stamps (refraction, fundus outline, lid sketch, muscle diagram, and so on) available commercially or on individual design (Fig. 2-1). Preprinted record forms, preferably in identifying colors, are desirable for the more structured subspecialty or consultation examinations such as strabismus, retinal detachment, glaucoma, uveitis, corneal disease, and plastic work. Records lightly shaded in various colors are also expeditious in identifying different members in a group practice.

The technique of having an accompanying secretary make shorthand notes from observations during the examination is recommended for cold efficiency. The secretary and her note pad conspicuously disrupt the confidentiality of patient relations though safeguarding the male examiner who is otherwise often alone with patients. Where anterooms or alcoves are available just outside of examination areas, it is preferable that the doctor use a dictating unit there between patients. A few hand-recorded notes, dates, and numbers such as tension, refraction, or exophthalmometry tend to ensure better accuracy of the ultimate record.

A valuable safeguard against confusion of right and left is the well-established convention of examining and recording details of the *right* eye first. Even if this eye is gone, the first notation should be a description of the socket or postsurgical site.

Study should be given by the individual starting practice to the use of computer-compatible information forms. Several types have had considerable trial, as the old Hollerith IBM cards, which can accommodate up to 250 bits of information per card and

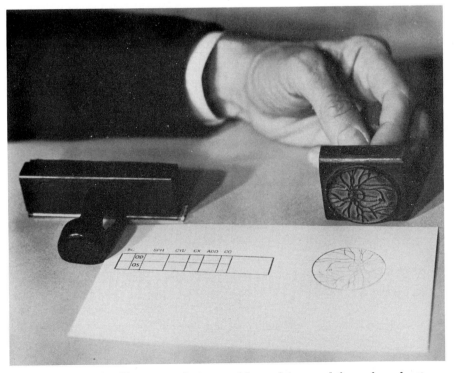

Fig. 2-1. Examples of rubber stamp devices useful on plain record forms for refraction and posterior pole fundus findings. Other types are available commercially and on individual design.

which have been used by the Lovelace Foundation° with twelve separate cards for history, external examination, fundus, glaucoma, refraction, and so forth. Other mark-sense devices may represent even more voluminous check lists. Large information scoring sheets inevitably present a forbidding specter of boxes to be checked, but they can be completed in a few minutes by one who has gained familiarity with the alternatives, and they commit diagnostic efforts and data to the ultimate potential of machine reading efficiency. Color coding of individual forms again aids identification in preparation and in manual handling of small numbers of forms. System developments are available to reduce or to eliminate the time-consuming and expensive handling of laborious checklists and key punch recording of data (fixed field length methods). Special typewriters (costing $2,000 to $3,000) based on standard keyboards have been available for several years to type out hard copy on usual paper for routine use and at the same time prepare punch paper tape in machine language. This variable field length technique imposes essentially no restrictions on the amount or type of verbal or numerical data that may be included. The paper tape, after necessary editing or correcting from the hard copy, is then used to place the information on magnetic tape for computer storage, analysis, and retrieval. Several thousand reports or about 4,000 pages of narrative can be placed on a single reel of magnetic tape ($35) and retained indefinitely.

SEMANTIC AWARENESS IN VISUAL EXAMINATIONS
WAYNE W. WONG, M.D.

> "I know that you believe you understand what you think I said, but I'm not sure you realize that what you heard is not what I meant."
> ANONYMOUS, 1969

Ocular examination provides rich opportunity for both objective determinations and subjective verifications. Frequently in

---
°Albuquerque, New Mexico.

visual components of examination, the subjective elements are vitally important to ultimate patient comfort and tolerance. Assessing subjective complaints and subjective responses requires acute penetration and deciphering of the sematics involved. Both objective analysis (such as external inspection, ophthalmoscopy, and retinoscopy) and subjective responses (such as optotypes, Maddox rod, stereoacuity, "better or worse" comparison of two lenses, duochrome, cross cylinder, and Simultantest) should be related. They are pivotal to medical records, proceeding to additionally indicated steps and securing ultimate visual comfort. The vital help and inherent hindrance of language during subjective procedures are replete with frustrating and even humorous reactions. These have provided an experiential lore for most mature examiners. The beginner must be aware of psycholinguistic factors, their potential for misleading, and the most efficient phrases to minimize semantic obstacles.

Obtaining a history

Before any words are spoken, an interaction between patient and examiner—a nonverbal phase of communication—occurs that plays an important part in decisions to be made about the patient and his problems. The manner of the patient's entrance, his facial expression, and even his mode of attire initiate both an informative and a reactive process. A counterpart reaction occurs in the patient, but at this time his reaction is of secondary importance since he is seeking help and has placed himself in a submissive role.

The history-taking begins as the patient starts verbalizing the reasons for his visit. It expands, for better or for worse, as the patient searches for words to express his feelings or adds small stories or phrases that enter his mind. The examiner should be attuned to both appropriateness and relevancy of such extensions or else he may abruptly frustrate the patient's attempted delineations by impatience or by an omnipotent attitude (Lee, 1941). He further must remember that any word may have a list of uses and meanings, and he must be aware that what is being said may not represent what he assumes it does. Transmitting an "all-knowing" attitude makes the patient either disdain or feel no need to elaborate further details such as the relative degree of pain or discomfort he has experienced. Patient No. 1 is not the same as patient No. 2 nor patient No. 3, either medically or according to indexing principles of general semantics (Johnson, 1946; Korzybski, 1950).

Many patients who come for visual examination do not identify visual deficiency as the reason for their visit; rather they relate their visit to a list of symptoms of discomfort about the eyes or head that they think to be of ocular origin. The examiner, therefore, must *scan* the patient's problems as the patient believes he sees them. The real reason for the visit may be consciously or inadvertently submerged in a host of less relevant descriptions. The manner, more than the order, in which the patient's complaints are enumerated often gives the direction in which diagnostic steps must proceed, if one but takes time to listen actively and applies the effort to listen analytically.

Korzybski (1950) coined a term to characterize communications as "time-binders" in which the understanding of words bridges the gap of time. Through long training we enter an environment of words used so often that we fail to realize how a simple isolated word from a particular patient refers to a moving complex of events involving people and things. When a patient says "pain," he is thinking of a specific kind of pain in his experience; we cannot feel the identical "pain." Too often we become bracketed by linguistic conditioning and listen to a patient in terms of premature generalizations, such as "a poor historian," "a perfectionist," "a chronic complainer," "a low I.Q.," or "a nut." Once a patient's complaint is classified so subjectively, listening is impaired and induced deafness becomes a barrier to better understanding.

Labels for human beings should be avoided.

Obtaining a visual record

Determining uncorrected vision on the Snellen chart requires a subjective response, which must receive critical analysis. The mere request to read the letters evokes a host of semantic reactions that vary with each individual. The poor question, "Can you see the letters in the bottom line?" often results in a mere affirmative answer. Similarly, when asked to read the letters on the bottom line, many patients will answer that they "can see the letters but can't read them." A perfectionist whose life and interest require attention to small details tends to concentrate and linger silently on a particular letter until positive that he is absolutely correct before verbalizing the letter. Others decline to guess or hazard a "mistake" in reading the letters, and if there is the slightest question that they might be "wrong," they will remain silent while mentally trying to identify the letters correctly. Such patients, when asked "What do you *think* the letters look like?" or "Let's see how well you can *guess*," will often read the entire row correctly.

This response occurs because anything we see is in part independent of what is being seen and in part determined by the characteristics of stored past experiences. For example, the rows of letters in some projector slides end with a code number. Many patients cannot conceive of a row of letters that may have a numeral for the last symbol; consequently, they try to make the terminal numeral into a letter, such as calling "2" a "backward s" or "z." If several rows of letters or an entire chart must be presented, it is often most efficient to say "Please read aloud the smallest letters you *can* see." It is better to expose only one line of letters at a time, beginning if possible with sufficiently large stimuli to afford the encouragement of success before proceeding rapidly to letters approaching the limits of resolution.

Some fatiguing patients fail to grasp that

the purpose of the Snellen chart is to determine the smallest symbols that *can* be read. Such patients often wish to waste effort in reading entire lines or, under test of the second eye, may insist on reading the entire chart again, beginning with the largest letter. These mental attitudes and rigidities reveal not only personality patterns but barriers that must be overcome in order to record visual acuity.

To encourage and elicit maximal acuity in an elderly individual or the new aphakic patient or following ocular disease, we should patiently prod the patient onto "the next line" or through isolated rather than crowded lines of letters. For Federal Aviation Administration examination of flyers or even for driver licensing, however, we should identify the level of immediate or definitive and prompt response. If a patient must be cajoled, pushed, and laboriously brought to read a smaller line to qualify for transport vision, both he and the examiner are failing to recognize the responsibility of *prompt* visual decision.

Determination of central acuity is so subject to variables that it is helpful to seek specificity not only in the fractions recorded but in the type of symbols used, that is, serif or nonserif letters, Louise Sloan (1959) equal difficulty letters, numbers, letters in isolation or row, and so on. This is particularly important in industrial injuries where vision as recorded before and after an accident plays a major role in the settlement. One must detect the low-grade myopic patient whose usual habit is to squint or frown ever so slightly to read the 20/70 line and then, with momentary glimpses of the smaller letters or figures through his temporary stenopeic eyelid–pupillary slit, quickly scan and read the 20/40 line. A similar situation occurs with a young hyperopic patient whose accommodative effort momentarily brings better reading. Such subtle maneuvers often are not involved following an eye injury because the patient is inescapably aware of possible compensatory settlement. Recorded vision

should be so noted that another examiner on another date may repeat the testing under essentially similar conditions.

Snellen's real contribution was to standardize the size and form of test letters with relation to the distance from the observer. When this standardization was accepted, examiners could communicate with colleagues in other parts of the world and know they were approaching comparable measures. This reduced confusion concerning acuity and its notation. However, all 20/20 visions are not equal. A person who correctly reads the 20/20 line letters with a normal rate and cadence distinctly exceeds a patient who also reads correctly the same line while laboriously picking out each letter with much ocular and cerebral effort.

Visual acuity notations often should be amplified by adjectives describing the manner in which "best" visual acuity is achieved. When the patient is unable to "read" an entire row of letters, the number read correctly out of the total on that row may be recorded. For instance, if there are ten letters on the 20/20 line and the patient with effort reads correctly only four, his acuity is more meaningfully recorded as "20/20, four out of ten with effort," rather than merely "20/20−." Since all charts do not have the same number of letters on each row, recording the total number of letters on the row adds exactness. Reading a Snellen line fully and in usual cadence and rhythm should be designated without modification as "20/20," "20/15," and so on; descriptions such as "slow," "hesitantly," "with great effort," or "poorly" will reveal for subsequent examination the functional level in which the patient responded on that day. Ideally, a different set of letters or numbers should be used for each eye, and traditionally the right eye is examined first. If different letters cannot be used for each eye, the poorer eye should be tested first so that the second eye will not have the benefit of visual recall from the first. Once the visual stimuli of a row of letters are consciously or subliminally recognized in the cerebral cortex, their influence cannot be removed.

The "dominance" of one eye in relation to the other is a confusing area because instrumental techniques for identifying the dominant or the controlling eye are numerous, and determination may be *subjective* or *objective*. In a binocular individual, there is commonly a favored or preferred eye, only crudely or roughly analogous to the preferred or stronger extremities. One sees this when recording uncorrected vision, for one eye may be able to read two or three lines or more on the Snellen chart than does the other, and yet both eyes end up with the identical prescription lenses. There may be *central* or *peripheral* suppression of vision in the nonpreferred eye or local pathology (either current or antecedent) responsible for reduced acuity of one eye.

Subjective phase of refraction

Objective refractometers* have not become popular because subjective response plays a more important part than do instrumental findings. For the final prescription, most examiners rely increasingly on subjective responses in proportion to the patient's maturity, intelligence, and analytic capacity.

This phase of ocular examination is also steeped in neurolinguistic reactions. If the examiner anticipates the alternative reactions, both accuracy and speed are gained while adverse reactions and fatigue are reduced. In a myopic patient at his final lens or end point of refraction, adding a −.25

---

*Refractometers or optometers such as the Hartinger Coincidence Refractionometer (Carl Zeiss) or the Eye Refractometer (Rodenstock) are still subjective to the extent of dependence upon personal interpretations by the examiner. The new (1970) infrared Ophthalmetron of Safir (Bausch and Lomb) is objective both from the point of view of the patient and the examiner. During the course of a 3-minute reading, it automatically prints out a continuous curve of refractive power through a rotation of 180 degrees. Dioptric values above and below zero are recorded on the abscissa, and axis notations are indicated on the ordinate.

sphere will often evoke the remark, "That is better." However, if the examiner specifically asks if the test letters appear "smaller and darker" or "more sharply outlined and farther away" (rather than bigger and easier to see), an affirmative answer is evidence of overcorrection.

Often a patient will find it seemingly impossible to determine which is the better lens when adding or subtracting as little as a .25 sphere, but he will respond definitively when questioned in the negative— "Does this make it worse?" Also, more accurate differential plus increased patient relaxation and confidence are obtained if the examiner states that the lenses are very close and briefly compliments the patient on making a differential. Empathy with the task must be shown promptly, and there is never reason to berate or chastise the patient for not reaching a decision. In the hyperopic adult, the final prescription should be the lens that is "comfortable" when reading the 20/20 or best line. The accommodative power of each hyperopic patient varies with age, energy, and previous lens wearing. The end point must be verified subjectively. This is best done quickly and by asking, after increasing the power by a .25 sphere, whether this makes the letters "more comfortable or bigger and easier to see." If it does, then he is a candidate for the greater strength.

Often in refinement of an "end point," when the patient is asked which of two lenses is "better," there is confusion, particularly if a long line of letters is exposed. The examiner should verbally direct the patient's attention to a particular *pair* of letters or narrow the projected test line, thus concentrating the area of resolution and yet providing a necessary shift in fixation to avoid retinal fatigue. If there is still some hesitation, attention may be briefly channeled to the vertical bars and the horizontal bar of the letter "H" so that comparison is reduced to horizontal and vertical components. This affords opportunity to compare this image of "H" with one stored in his brain. In such decisions it is best not to push to a line beyond practical resolution but to use a slightly larger letter that affords resolution with less effort.

Brighter eye phenomenon

After each eye has been corrected optimally to 20/20 or better, there normally is further improvement in acuity when the eyes are tested binocularly. The patient may be able to read an additional line or read with greater facility and cadence. Such performance automatically screens out significant heterophoria at that test distance. The patient may remark, however, that one eye "sees better" than the other. Time and fatigue are reduced if the examiner elicits the patient's meaning of "better." Difference of resolving power is not involved, because the patient has demonstrated ability to read 20/20 or better with each eye. However, if one eye is covered while the patient is reading the test chart and then the cover quickly changed to the opposite eye, the patient may be made aware that blackness of letters, brightness of the background, or overall field differs between the two eyes. He may even report a faint difference in color value between the two eyes so that the image from one seems slightly browner or muted. The "brighter eye" is usually the eye the patient calls the "better eye."

The patient, if need be, can be reassured then that the "brighter eye" phenomenon is a normal or physiologic variation and has nothing to do with visual acuity. This "brighter eye" phenomenon is a quantitative variable of the image that does not lend itself to clinical measurement but that can be studied under laboratory conditions. It is related to the variables called hue, saturation, and brightness (in terminology endorsed by the Optical Society of America) (Evans, 1948). It is a peripheral or "sensory dominance" (input) in contrast to "motor dominance" of an eye that is used for sighting a gun or similar aligning. This phenomenon is related to that which occurs when a person is suddenly exposed to bright lights and shows a preference for

"seeing" with one eye by closing the other, such as when walking from a dark room into bright sunlight or being suddenly roused out of a sound sleep with the room lights turned on. The child with divergence excess exotropia classically shows this by closing one eye in bright light.

Semantic reaction to the word "see"

The ability to "see" is both a peripheral optic accomplishment and a cerebral process of registration, classification, and association in Brodmann's areas 17, 18, and 19. We only "see" or perceive what we have learned to interpret. This requires functions of the angular gyrus and the surrounding temporoparietal lobe. Clinical refractive examination embraces many of these central nervous system elements, but refraction per se measures only the optic components on the visual or fixation axis of foveal vision.

Parafoveal, paramacular, perimacular, and peripheral vision, however, are more important end-organ and optic components for spatial orientation, travel, and nonreading activities. Some patients having "old shoe" familiarity with 20/200 uncorrected binocular vision prefer to go about their daily duties and even driving without refractive correction, because they "need glasses only for reading." The word "see" has different meanings to different people. It is important that the patient be enabled to convey, and the examiner be alert to appreciate, the range of visual task relations for that specific patient to his "seeing." Though the 20/200 uncorrected patient may be safe and comfortable at a party, he certainly cannot resolve freeway control signs quickly enough or at sufficient distance to avoid initiating a chain of rear-end crashes.

Contact lens patients with only 20/30 or even 20/40 vision resulting from residual posterior corneal or lenticular astigmatism often feel they "see better" with their contact lenses than when enjoying 20/20+ vision with spectacles. This may be related in part to the wider field, size difference, or relief from spectacle frame scotomas afforded by contact lenses. It may also result from motivation and the fact that 20/20 by itself is far from the only criterion for routine or casual "seeing." Sloane (1962) brought this out in his editorial "Visual Function is not a Number." Twenty/twenty aphakic vision may be crippling or very restrictive and disturbing to the spatial relations of an elderly person who was mobile and well-adjusted to his broader and less magnified visual world with 20/70 phakic vision.

An individual's total "seeing" relates to several components of optic and also cerebral patterns to which he has adapted and familiarized himself. Though words will always be inadequate, one must earnestly seek to explain and interpret aphakic vision to a patient before cataract surgery. Based specifically on his previous refractive status, this must be in terms of differences in size, brightness, nearness, color, and prism displacement. Even brief forewarning prior to surgery will help to reduce postoperative

disturbances but can never replace the actual experience of being aphakic.

Responsibility of the examiner

The examiner's responsibility extends until the patient has stabilized and optimized himself in a visual world and is adapted to a set of glasses that he uses with real functional advantage, with protection to his eyes, and without discomfort. The patient also tends to hold him responsible for any error induced by the optician. Any discomfiture related to new spectacles must be heard with an unprejudiced mind and without fear of bruising one's ego. It is necessary to be sure that the prescription was (1) correctly derived, (2) properly related to previously correct or incorrect spectacles, (3) accurately written, and (4) precisely rendered into spectacles. The examiner must verify power, interpupillary distance, base curve (Fig. 2-2), and prescribed or induced imbalance. The patient's description of the circumstances under which his symptoms occur often will pinpoint the

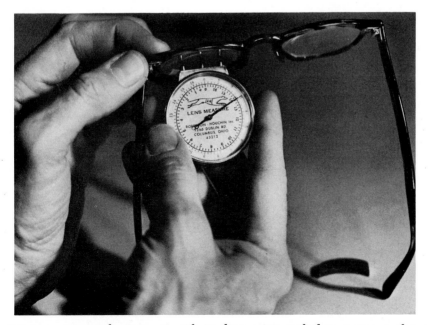

Fig. 2-2. Lens measure shown in use with its three points applied to concave surface of a lens measuring nearly −3 diopters in its horizontal axis. With contact established in this fashion, lens measure is rotated through 180 degrees to check for consistency of spherical surface or to measure variations in diopterage that would indicate cylindric component.

causes of discomfort—if the physician listens with discriminatory discernment.

Importance of listening to patients' complaints

Bifocals must never be insisted upon by the examiner but the reasons for considering them should be explained. The patient should be given a choice of buying such pairs of glasses as he wants, but the advantages and disadvantages must be *understood* by him. The word "bifocals" often causes a strong psycholinguistic reaction; some patients will even refuse to try to understand their described benefits. Such patients, often women who associate bifocals with aging, may pleasantly accept a separate pair of "reading glasses" or demiglasses and less easily adapt to "invisible bifocals" such as the "Younger," "Varilux," "Progressor," and "Omnifocal" lenses.

On the other hand, when intermediate viewing becomes a problem, the word "trifocals" may bring a reaction of utter despair to such patients. If "bifocals" sound troublesome, "trifocals" must be three times worse. Complaints associated with multifocals may be lessened by proper instruction when the patient is handed his first prescription. Often a patient has difficulty in verbalizing his problems of intermediate distance viewing but can readily demonstrate this when asked to recount his visual demands when this discomfort occurs. It is often informative if he will dramatize what he does in his office with letters, adding machine tape, people in the room, at the piano, and so on.

When a patient complains of reading discomfort with bifocals, it is important to inspect the glasses as the patient wears them. Top edges of the bifocals must be horizontal and a pantoscopic tilt of at least 15 degrees should be present to bring the lower edges of the eyepieces close to the zygomatic eminences. The presbyopic patient often cannot see that he is looking through the bifocals for distance viewing or through only one segment if the frames are not seated correctly on the face. Vague complaints that are difficult to verbalize may be caused by a change in either base curve or the shape of the bifocals. If a patient has been using a Ful-vue, flat-top bifocal for years and his new lenses are Kryptok, he will have complaints because of the "image jump" from distance to near viewing. The use of minus cylinders in one pair of spectacles and plus cylinders in another will often cause symptoms that are difficult for the patient to describe, as it is a novel experience for which he has neither linguistic equipment nor standard of comparison to describe the "different" visual sensation. The lensometer is of no help here, but a lens measure (Fig. 2-2) applied to the old lens and the new lens may clearly reveal different base curves as the cause of distress.

In myopia, a change of lens to a higher power may create sensations of smallness or the floors appearing to "float" and objects appearing to "move" quickly with each head movement. These sensations usually disappear in a few days as the brain becomes adapted to the altered image schemes created by the new lenses. If these symptoms persist, then we should compare the base curves of the old lens with the new one; if there is a significant difference, the new lens should be reground as closely to the old base curve as possible. Such a difference may be encountered when plastic lenses are used because the various manufacturers of plastic lenses each have varying base curves for different power ranges. For example, if a patient has become accustomed to the Armolite plastic lens and his new pair is American Optical Company's AOlite plastic lens, even though he is able to read the 20/20 line without difficulty he may complain of discomfort because of the difference in base curves used in molding. The brain, being accustomed to the perceived image through one set of base curves or plus cylinder lenses, finds it difficult to adapt to another set of base curves or minus cylinders. If the examiner is unaware of this and the patient is unable to describe this sensation with other than vague or everyday words, a label of psychoneurosis is easily and erroneously attached to the patient. This produces dissatisfaction for patient, examiner, and optician.

Another situation difficult for the patient to describe is the vague discomfort, particularly noted by a hyperopic patient, when reading or looking at near objects. In such cases the eyepieces may be fitted perpendicular to the ground; and as the eyes rotate downward to read, there is an induced oblique astigmatism. This will disappear immediately if the bottom of the lenses is tilted (pantoscoped) closer to the cheeks so that the visual axis strikes the glasses near the theoretically desirable perpendicular for all lines of gaze.

After one has eliminated each mechanical and optic source of discomfort, it is still necessary to listen to the patient to rule out psychologic factors. It is not uncommon for a patient, particularly a woman, to be dissatisfied with the type, style, or color of frame she has selected. The patient may be reluctant or unable to verbalize this directly and hence may be unhappy with her "glasses." Occasionally a patient may have a deeply rooted or near pathologic fixation in search of "one pair of glasses" that will resolve all problems. Such a patient may refuse to accept the reality of other ocular or central nervous system disease to the degree that she has seen half a dozen eye examiners and with fanatic zeal is continuing her search for the elusive "one pair of glasses." Such a patient requires a psychiatrist.

Summary

Those of us entrusted with the eyesight of fellow humans must be constantly aware that each patient differs in his past experiences and will respond in a different manner. Because of such different personal make-up, each will react differently to a given situation. We must also become aware of our own reactions to the patient, the significance of the manner in which the patient presents his problems, and the variables in his verbalization. Visual acuity notations should use short descriptive terms in addition to the usual Snellen fraction for a more exacting appraisal. When both examiner and examinee have an approximately common image of the problem, both the establishment of visual acuity and identification of correction can be interesting, pleasant, efficient, and rewarding.

Chapter 3

The initial examination

Much is learned in the immediate confrontation with the patient, in far less time than it can be described, simply by the Sherlock Holmes technique of critical observation plus clinical judgment. The ocular apparatus, being located accessibly on a surface area of the body and being transparent in much of its structure, lends itself to accurate verification or cross-checking of diagnostic findings by subjective and objective techniques. The fact that the eyes and orbits are also in a frontal area in the upper portion of the body makes for easy examining access in a conventional chair and with minimum social concerns of disrobing. By the same token, this may lull the examiner into omitting necessary physical steps such as looking at the axillary skin folds in the presence of angioid streaks, holding a youngster upside down when evaluating a deep hemangioma, or having the patient recumbent with at least 270 degrees of access about the head for indirect ophthalmoscopy.

A general impression of the patient's development, health, and mental ability is attained both by observation and by his manner and accuracy in responding to examining procedures. Often a fairly good estimate of the intelligence quotient and even occupation is derived in the course of ocular examination. General body posture and particular head position (such as face turning, elevation, or depression of the chin) give clues to neuromuscular disturbances and to imbalances of the extraocular muscles. Noting scars of previous injuries or surgery will tell more about

what can be improved in the future than will most patients' prolonged narrative of what happened in the past. Similarly, skin disturbances, enlargement of glands, and even subtle disturbances in form or functions of facial components serve as guideposts to increase the directness of historic questions and diagnostic steps.

PRELIMINARY INSPECTION

After reading the notes previously recorded by the aide, brief introductory exchanges, and verification of seemingly salient points, directness is served by a preliminary but systematic examination of the adnexa and anterior segments with the aid of a bright focal penlight or "inspection torch." Whether this takes place in the office with available high-intensity bracket magnifiers (Luxo, Dazor, Fresnel-Burton) or in an emergency room with small surgical lights (Rene, Castle, American Sterilizer), these diffuse sources should be avoided because they produce photophobic responses, lid closure, avoidance movements of the head, and temporary dazzling impairment of retinal sensitivity. The small professional pocketlight (Welch-Allyn, Oculus, Mite-T-Light, Keeler Pen Torch) or the more cumbersome (and expensive) transformer-based units such as the Barkan hammer light, Ortho-Lite, Mayou focal illuminator, and Rayner Premier Hand Lamp have the important advantage of providing narrowly concentrated light beams with almost no dazzling effect except when particularly directed into the pupil to test pupillary reactions. (The thick-handled rechargeable pocketlights generally take up too much desk space and are awkward pocket stretchers.) Small diameter tips such as the Finnoff nosepiece, National curved, straight, and angulated metal extensions, or Mayou curved and straight tips have usefulness for transilluminating possible cystoid masses on the lid or iris and even for checking an occasional paranasal sinus for cloudiness that may be causing orbital symptoms. As an alternative, a hand ophthalmoscope may be used for this inspection. By rotating the +20-diopter lens into position, localized magnification of 5× is obtained when the instrument and the examiner's eye are brought to 1 in. from the ocular surface. Magnification of 2× to 3× with a clip-on loupe (Telesight, Keeler), a headband, or spectacle-mounted aid (May, Oculus, Beebe Binocular loupe, Bausch and Lomb DuaLoupe, Dana) helps this survey but should not be used under 2× because of limited value nor much over 3× because of limited range (Fig. 3-1).

The lightweight, flat, foldable, metal-frame Zeiss or Cameron 2× loupe with an 8-in. working distance may be slipped on with or without conventional spectacles. It has a real working asset of pocket portability in most hard spectacle cases. The physician's habit of keeping one of these and a penlight in his suit jacket is an advantage for neighborhood foreign body problems, anterior segment problems on rounds, and even splinter assistance for the children.

The heavy but inexpensive hair crumplers with padded headbands and side shields (Berger Magni-Focuser, Donegan OptiVisor, Donegan Optiloupe) are better suited to industrial inspection lines than intermittent office use. A heavier (13.5 oz.) and expensive exception to the head-mounted units is the 8× "Beckerscope" (1969) with 8-in. working distance, as designed by Stanley C. Becker; this is suitable as a mobile, miniature surgical microscope.

The old technique of a condensing lens for illumination in one hand and a magnifying glass (Ukaim, Hastings, Coddington) in the other precludes most opportunities for manipulations and is not recommended. Similarly most of the old, hand, monocular slit lamps Bausch and Lomb 7.5×, Bishop-Harman 12×, Krimsky 10× "feather weight," Bettman and McNair 8-25×, Zeiss Jena 6×) afford neither good slit characteristics nor use flexibility. (One recent exception for mobile clinic work is the Kowa portable slit lamp with power supply and

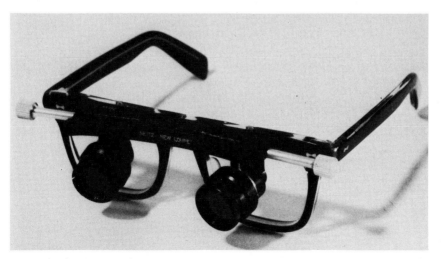

Fig. 3-1. Example of spectacle-mounted loupe with adjustable interpupillary distance. (Neitz Instruments Co., Ltd., Tokyo, Japan.)

carrying case, which is a $600 to $900 investment; see p. 73.)

The preliminary inspection—which can be accomplished while talking to the patient—should grossly survey:

1. Symmetry and mobility of the face, especially about the orbits
2. Condition of the skin, particularly the lids
3. Condition of the brows and lashes (for movement, loss, scaling, color, malposition)
4. Position and action of the lids (without touching them)
5. Position of the lacrimal puncta and evidence of lacrimal disturbances
6. Condition of the conjunctiva (for congestion, edema, masses)
7. Preauricular nodes (if the face must be steadied or elevated, the examiner can do this with the fingers of each hand palpating these nodes for enlargement and tenderness at the same time)
8. Position and movement of the globes (for exophthalmos and muscle action)
9. Condition of the cornea (for brightness, irregularity, scars)
10. Gross characteristics of the anterior chamber (for obliteration, hemorrhage, masses)
11. Condition of the lens (for dislocation, opacity, and partial or complete absence)

The alterations of pathologic disturbances in the eye, as elsewhere in the body, present almost limitless variations, degrees of severity, and stages of activity. For basic simplification, however, all biologic disorders can be reduced to nine types. The examiner must always be ready to recount these groups when faced with a lesion of unidentified cause. The nine basic disorders include:

1. Congenital defects
2. Infections
3. Allergies
4. Injuries
5. Vascular defects
6. Neoplasms
7. Degenerations
8. Endocrine disturbances
9. Vitamin deficiencies

The ocular examiner has one additional aspect of physiology beyond the preceding nine classifications; this is the special area of optic or visual disturbance. Each of the above mechanisms can affect optic and visual function of the eyes. Therefore the examiner must recognize their roles as well as the unique ocular elements of the visual system.

Negative findings should not be recorded. Positive findings, which may be noted tersely if desired, bracket subsequent questions to significant areas and indicate the examining procedures apt to be productive. Thus noting active tearing or epiphora eliminates a rose bengal test for lacrimal deficiency, noting acute allergic lid edema contraindicates refractive procedures, or noting a dark limbal mass obligates transillumination.

VISUAL ACUITY
Basic concepts

Immediately following amplification of notes in the history and the simultaneous completion of preliminary inspection, visual acuity should be checked (if this was not previously done by the aide). This should precede any manipulation of the globe (which the patient might later claim as related to his visual loss) or intraocular examination (where the dazzle of lights might affect attempts to establish visual acuity shortly thereafter).

On a parity with though usually less urgent than pain, loss of vision is the demanding concern of the patient. Therefore it is essential to record acuity in detail on the initial examination and as part of every general physical examination. This should be done first without the spectacle correction (*sc*) and then with correction (*cc*), always approaching the *right* eye first. On each follow-up examination acuity is usually checked, but it is done primarily for distance and with the appropriate distance spectacle correction in place. Distance acuity is more significant and reproducible than near acuity and is less subject to the variables that alter near acuity (illumination, pupillary size, refraction, accommodation).

Basis of measuring acuity

Clinical measurements of visual acuity are based on historic convention and utility, recognizing from astronomic observations in the mid-1700's that the minimum separable capability of a healthy human eye is approximately 1 minute of arc. Under exquisite laboratory conditions this may range downward to 15 or 30 seconds of arc; study of interconal distance at the fovea generally would support such a functional ability. The aligning power or ability of the eye to detect a break in a contour, however, is about five times finer or accurate within 3 seconds of arc. This aligning power is used to make readings on vernier scales.

Utilizing the average and commonplace minimum separable distance of 1 minute of arc, test letters such as E's are constructed in which each of the total five horizontal strokes and spaces subtend 1 minute, and the overall letter subtends 5 minutes. Commonly the largest letters used in office testing are sized to subtend 5 minutes at a distance of 200 ft., and the smallest subtend 5 minutes at 10 ft. To test the eye in a position of focal rest or without accommodative muscle effort, the test distance should simulate infinity. For practicality and again by historic convention, this is commonly taken to be a test distance of 20 ft.

Using the Snellen notation, acuity is expressed by first recording the test distance (commonly 20 ft.) and then recording the distance at which the smallest letter seen should be read by an average normal eye. Thus at a test distance of 20 ft., if the patient can see only the letter that should be seen at 200 ft., his Snellen notation is 20/200. (In the metric system this would be 6/60.) If he reads at 20 ft. the size letters

that the average person can see, the Snellen notation is 20/20 (or 6/6). If he sees considerably better than average and can recognize letters that the average person must approach within 10 ft. to recognize, his Snellen notation is 20/10 (6/3).

Notation of visual levels below 20/200

If the patient cannot recognize the largest letter available (commonly the 20/200 letter), it is helpful to walk the patient slowly toward the chart, noting the distance at which he first recognizes the letter. If this is at 8 ft., the Snellen notation is 8/200. When the patient cannot see the largest letter at any distance, the examiner may spread his fingers in good light and estimate the most remote distance at which the patient counts fingers (such as, C.F. at 3 ft.). Failing this, the patient is asked to detect hand movements, usually horizontal or vertical, and note is made of the maximum distance at which this is possible (for instance, H.M. at 2 ft.).

The next lowest quality of vision is the preservation of *light projection* or localization of light in space. This may be noted as "accurate light projection" or "temporal light projection only." The final and minimal visual response is *light perception* only and may be expressed as "L.P. only" or its absence as "no L.P." If a patient with markedly limited acuity can localize doorways, tell where windows and bright lights are located, doesn't stumble over major objects of furniture, and by aligning power can tell curbs and sidewaks, it is a significant functional guide to note "travel vision." This is far more valuable than retention of mere light perception and projection.

Illiterate and preschool techniques

For a patient who is illiterate or competent only in another language, a size series of so-called "illiterate E's" may be used, asking the patient to indicate in which direction the fingers or openings point. This can also be done with children down to the age of 3 or 3½ if they are bright and cooperative, or by the age of 4 if somewhat dull or reluctant. Charts and individual cards with schematized pictures (Henry Allen, 1961) are advantageously designed for the 2½- to 3½-year-old at the attention range of 30 to 200 in. but are influenced by family cultural patterns and are slightly less accurate than illiterate E's. Sjögren's hand test (1939) made of simplified block prints of the hand with fingers outstretched on each of six cards are graduated in levels from 20/120 to 20/20 for use at 20 ft., but patients tend to lose attention at this more remote range and the cards again are slightly less accurate than the E's.

Equipment for distance visual acuity measurements

Countless distance test devices (Ives, Wall and Ochs, Cardsell), wall charts (Dennett, Cowan, Sloan, Ewing, A.M.A., Landolt, Berens, and Beach), and illuminated cabinets (Green, Black, Rogers, Da-Laur Good-Lite, Graham Field) are still catalogued for measuring distance acuity. All, however, were superseded by a first generation of complex projection devices (Clason, Ferree-Rand). Now a second generation of Project-O-Charts (American Optical), Compact Acuity Projectors (Bausch and Lomb), Rodavist (Rodenstock), or T/O-Matic (Titmus) make all of the previous devices truly obsolete.

Easily washable metal projection screens no longer carry exploring children's fingerprints. Projection slides are available in any combination of letters, numbers, illiterate E's, Allen figures, Landolt C's, Sjögren's hands, duochrome, astigmatic tests, and astigmatic dials. Lens quality and projection clarity exceed the definition previously attained in variously smudged, yellowed, or dirty test cards. It would no longer be possible for the late Walter Lancaster (1952) to write that projectors "will please those who are satisfied with mediocrity, and place convenience first." Indeed remarkable convenience and reduction in time-fatigue for the patient are served by availability of projector mountings for wall, desk, and floor or incorporation in major diagnostic

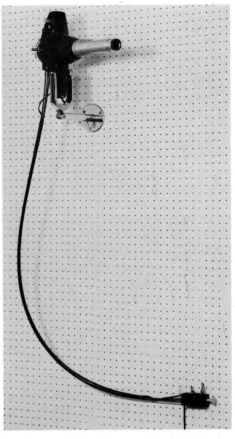

Fig. 3-2. Jenkel-Davidson remote control Selectachart with 5-ft. range.

ensembles. Where these still may not be in easy reach (Fig. 3-2) of the examiner, electric remote controls are available to regulate vertical movement of the projector slide, vertical width of the line aperture, and horizontal width of the frame for single or multiple characters.*

Inherent advantages of the projector over the wall chart include (1) avoidance of the chart being exposed for inadvertent memorization, (2) complete control of the optotypes without leaving the examining position, (3) essentially limitless combinations of optotypes, polarized stereopsis tests, polarized phoria tests, color tests, fixation

---

*Jenkel-Davidson Selectachart, 5-ft. range; House of Vision Projector Command, 5-ft. range; T/O-Matic, 12-ft. range; Benso-Matic Visual Acuity Projector Control, 15-ft. range.

or attention devices, and other tests, (4) display of single test figures, which often aid the senescent and hesitant, or (5) display of full lines for the vigorous performer or to bring out the "crowding phenomenon" (von Noorden), which may reveal subtle amblyopia in children who perform better or even normally with isolated symbols.

Louise Sloan (1959) has shown that non-serif or Gothic letters, particularly when arranged in groups of similar complexity, give more consistent and accurate results, though they are 5% to 10% easier to recognize than the original serif capitals used by Snellen. Letters and numbers in the patient's own language most closely relate to his daily seeing requirements and therefore are the most practical optotypes. Clearly some letters such as I, L, and T are much easier to recognize, whereas W, M, and X are much more difficult. The Sloan recommendation to use only the ten letters—D, K, R, H, V, C, N, Z, S, O—makes for better uniformity of difficulty in successive test lines or type sizes.

Because visual resolving power increases with light intensity (within limits), some effort should be made to standardize the level of test screen illumination between 20 and 80 footcandles. The importance of precision in such illumination is largely outweighed by (1) the enormous light adaptation capacity of the healthy human retina, which under laboratory conditions may reach 100,000-fold, and (2) age-linked changes in retinal sensitivity, which essentially require doubled intensity for visual recognition under dim illumination for each 13 years of adult life. Any planned changes in screen illumination, however, should be accomplished with an iris diaphragm in the projector and not by rheostat. Reducing current to the bulb changes its temperature and color emission characteristics, thus introducing a chromatic variable.

Several screening charts such as the line of transilluminated charts by Good-Lite Company* or their more recent Insta-Line

Chart with remote control linear illumination, similar to the old Green's Illuminated Vision charts, are suitable for presenting any one of several preset lines at a time.

Near visual acuity

Measurements of near acuity are functionally important not only for quantitation of bifocal strength but also because many occupational and educational demands are primarily for near, because low vision aids are more frequently needed for near than for distance, and because calculations of visual impairment for compensation and insurance purposes weigh both distance and near acuity (A.M.A., 1958). Measurements of near acuity are less reproducible (coefficient of reliability, 0.75 to 0.78) and are affected more than measurements simulating infinity (coefficient of reliability, 0.95 to 0.97) by pupillary size, illumination levels, accommodative requirements, refractive errors and type of distance correction, and the impairments of presbyopia. These variables negate somewhat even the most precise size reduction of the 5-minute distance optotype to correspond with the same visual angle at a near reading distance. Dozens of proper names* obfuscate both literature and catalogues to such a degree that the proper numbering of type sizes from *one* as the smallest appears on some cards completely reversed and on others supplanted by metric distances or Snellen-like designation in inches such as 14/14. Near test confusion was particularly eponymized by the 1854 "Schriftscalen" of Eduard Jaeger, which was merely a series of variously sized type selected from materials on hand at the convenience of Jaeger's printer.

Near acuity notations should be based on the Snellen principle of a 1-minute arc of minimal resolution and, for practical comparison to reading needs, should pre-

---

*Forest Park, Illinois 60130.

*Landolt, Reid, E. Fuchs, Kuchler, Smee, Striedingen, Birkhauser, Golvin, Miller, Friedman, Evans, Schweigger, Benjamin Franklin, Boettcher, Berens, Hutchinson, Fink, Lebensohn, Guibor, Sloan, Studt-Abel, Good-Lite, Keeler, Stimson, and so on.

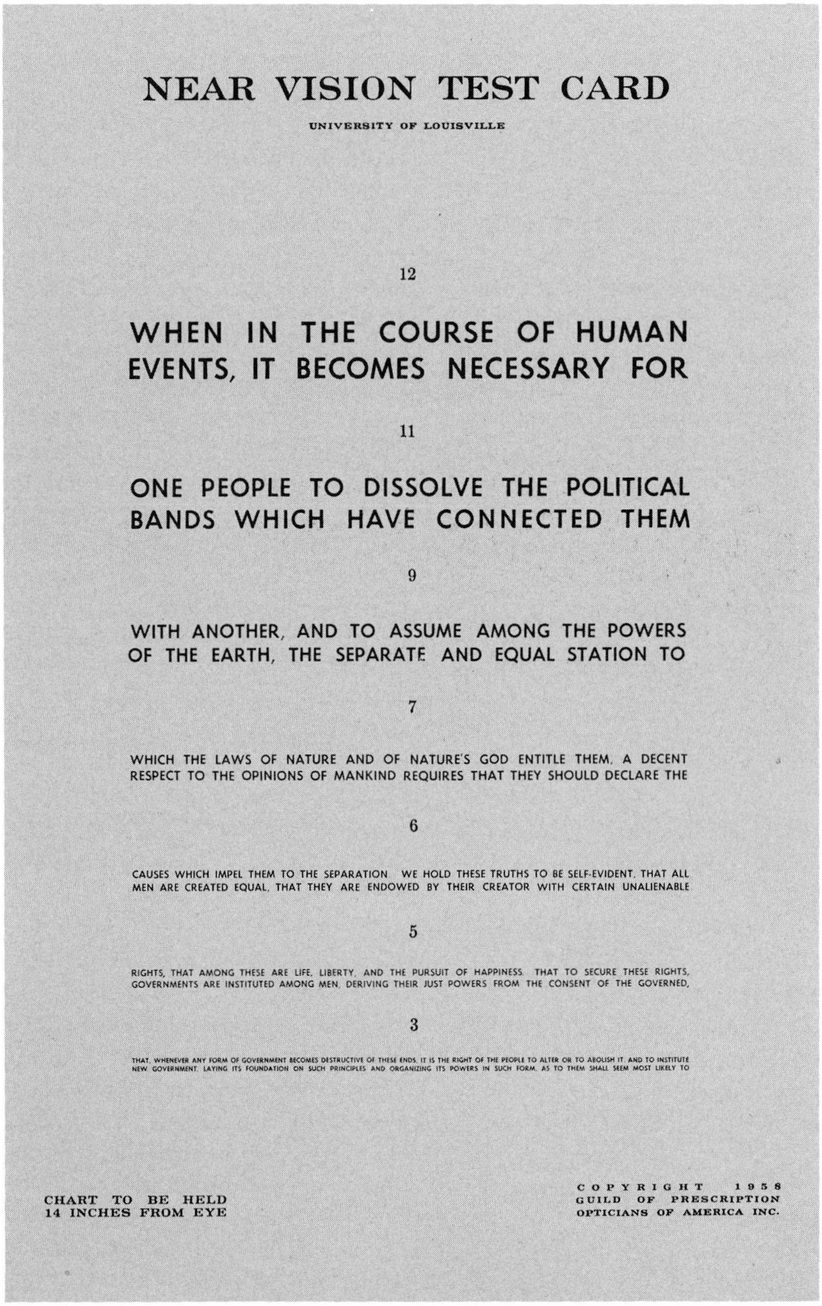

NEAR VISION TEST CARD

UNIVERSITY OF LOUISVILLE

12

WHEN IN THE COURSE OF HUMAN EVENTS, IT BECOMES NECESSARY FOR

11

ONE PEOPLE TO DISSOLVE THE POLITICAL BANDS WHICH HAVE CONNECTED THEM

9

WITH ANOTHER, AND TO ASSUME AMONG THE POWERS OF THE EARTH, THE SEPARATE AND EQUAL STATION TO

7

WHICH THE LAWS OF NATURE AND OF NATURE'S GOD ENTITLE THEM, A DECENT
RESPECT TO THE OPINIONS OF MANKIND REQUIRES THAT THEY SHOULD DECLARE THE

6

CAUSES WHICH IMPEL THEM TO THE SEPARATION. WE HOLD THESE TRUTHS TO BE SELF-EVIDENT, THAT ALL
MEN ARE CREATED EQUAL, THAT THEY ARE ENDOWED BY THEIR CREATOR WITH CERTAIN UNALIENABLE

5

RIGHTS, THAT AMONG THESE ARE LIFE, LIBERTY, AND THE PURSUIT OF HAPPINESS. THAT TO SECURE THESE RIGHTS,
GOVERNMENTS ARE INSTITUTED AMONG MEN, DERIVING THEIR JUST POWERS FROM THE CONSENT OF THE GOVERNED,

3

THAT, WHENEVER ANY FORM OF GOVERNMENT BECOMES DESTRUCTIVE OF THESE ENDS, IT IS THE RIGHT OF THE PEOPLE TO ALTER OR TO ABOLISH IT, AND TO INSTITUTE
NEW GOVERNMENT, LAYING ITS FOUNDATION ON SUCH PRINCIPLES AND ORGANIZING ITS POWERS IN SUCH FORM, AS TO THEM SHALL SEEM MOST LIKELY TO

CHART TO BE HELD
14 INCHES FROM EYE

COPYRIGHT 1958
GUILD OF PRESCRIPTION
OPTICIANS OF AMERICA INC.

Front

Fig. 3-3. Front and reverse sides of author's disposable near vision test card with matte finish (reduced one-fifth). (Distributed by Guild of Prescription Opticians of America, Washington, D. C.)

NEAR VISION TEST CARD

UNIVERSITY OF LOUISVILLE

REVISED JAEGER STANDARD	NEAR SNELLEN NOTATION	METRIC DISTANCE	DISTANCE SNELLEN APPROXIMATION	DECIMAL NOTATION	A. M. A. 1955 NEAR VISUAL EFFICIENCY
12	14/89 (in.)	2.25 M.	20/130 (ft.)	0.15	10%

WHEN IN THE COURSE OF HUMAN EVENTS, IT BECOMES NECESSARY FOR

11	14/79	2.0	20/120	0.2	13%

ONE PEOPLE TO DISSOLVE THE POLITICAL BANDS WHICH HAVE CONNECTED THEM

9	14/60	1.5	20/85	0.22	20%

WITH ANOTHER, AND TO ASSUME AMONG THE POWERS OF THE EARTH, THE SEPARATE AND EQUAL STATION TO

7	14/42	1.05	20/60	0.35	40%

WHICH THE LAWS OF NATURE AND OF NATURE'S GOD ENTITLE THEM. A DECENT RESPECT TO THE OPINIONS OF MANKIND REQUIRES THAT THEY SHOULD DECLARE THE

6	14/35	.82	20/50	0.4	50%

CAUSES WHICH IMPEL THEM TO THE SEPARATION. WE HOLD THESE TRUTHS TO BE SELF-EVIDENT, THAT ALL MEN ARE CREATED EQUAL, THAT THEY ARE ENDOWED BY THEIR CREATOR WITH CERTAIN UNALIENABLE

5	14/28	.75	20/40	0.5	90%

RIGHTS, THAT AMONG THESE ARE LIFE, LIBERTY, AND THE PURSUIT OF HAPPINESS. THAT TO SECURE THESE RIGHTS, GOVERNMENTS ARE INSTITUTED AMONG MEN, DERIVING THEIR JUST POWERS FROM THE CONSENT OF THE GOVERNED,

3	14/21	.53	20/30	0.6	95%

THAT, WHENEVER ANY FORM OF GOVERNMENT BECOMES DESTRUCTIVE OF THESE ENDS, IT IS THE RIGHT OF THE PEOPLE TO ALTER OR TO ABOLISH IT, AND TO INSTITUTE NEW GOVERNMENT, LAYING ITS FOUNDATION ON SUCH PRINCIPLES AND ORGANIZING ITS POWERS IN SUCH FORM, AS TO THEM SHALL SEEM MOST LIKELY TO

1	14/14	.37	20/20	1.0	100%

EFFECT THEIR SAFETY AND HAPPINESS. PRUDENCE, INDEED, WILL DICTATE THAT GOVERNMENTS LONG ESTABLISHED SHOULD NOT BE CHANGED FOR LIGHT AND TRANSIENT CAUSES AND ACCORDINGLY ALL EXPERIENCE HATH SHOWN, THAT MANKIND ARE MORE DISPOSED TO SUFFER, WHILE EVILS ARE SUFFERABLE, THAN TO RIGHT THEMSELVES BY ABOLISHING THE FORMS TO WHICH THEY ARE ACCUSTOMED. BUT WHEN A LONG TRAIN OF ABUSES AND USURPATIONS

CHART TO BE HELD
14 INCHES FROM EYE

COPYRIGHT 1958
GUILD OF PRESCRIPTION
OPTICIANS OF AMERICA INC.

ENGINEERED AND PRODUCED BY
COURIER-JOURNAL LITHO CO., LOUISVILLE 18, KY.

Back

Fig. 3-3, cont'd. For legend see opposite page.

sent sentence structure and word arangements simulating conventional near tasks. The examiner should also be freed from need to look with the patient at the card for verification, thus avoiding time loss or awkward repositioning of either patient or examiner. The card should have a matte finish or minimal glare surface (though dull surfaces commonly predispose to ink spreading, which is intolerable in the small type sizes). My inexpensive card (Fig. 3-3) meets these essentials, provides a revised Jaeger Standard of notation, gives physiologic approximations for near or distance notations, and includes a rounded-off version of Visual Efficiency (A.M.A.).

Near testing should be done immediately after recording uncorrected distance acuity and before creating the near point disturbances that accompany dilation of the pupils. Excellent near acuity with poor distance acuity at any age suggests myopia and very little astigmatism. Contrariwise, good distance acuity and poor near acuity suggests moderate hyperopia (with little or no astigmatism), presbyopia (usually beginning in the forties), or accommodative (nerve III) impairment. Comparably poor acuity at both near and distance suggests significant astigmatism or significant pathology. Thus the near determination may verify the distance acuity or immediately yield further diagnostic leads.

In near examinations, care must be taken to provide comfortable reading light on the test material, usually in a ratio about threefold greater than the room light. Within moderate limits, resolving power or clinical manifestation of acuity is proportional to increasing illumination. Added light often helps the maturing patient with early involutional disease of the macula but may distinctly handicap the more mature patient with nuclear (axial) lens opacities.

The most definitive examination of near acuity comes after optimal distance correction has been determined and with such correction in place. Once the patient has been properly rendered emmetropic for distance—and there are no cycloplegic ef-

fects—a relatively precise, age-correlated near point (punctum proximum) can be measured and the indicated dioptric power of lens adds determined for near working distances. If the near test card is mounted on an "accommodation arm" or extension of a refractor, it is necessary to check adequate focal light on the test card when it is changed from the right (first) to the left (second) eye or when the card must be brought closer than the usual reading distance of 13 to 15 in. to assist subnormal vision by magnification or added dioptric power.

As a valuable check on the accuracy of distance refraction correction, the monocular near blur point should be at almost identical distances in front of each eye. For the average presbyopic patient on monocular testing, this should be set at 14 in.; when both eyes are uncovered (binocular verification) the patient will usually demonstrate a closer blur point by about an inch. If the monocular near blur points are unequal, this first suggests reexamination of the distance correction and only secondarily suggests unequal accommodative power. The latter should be further evidenced by cataractous changes, unequal pupils, or other finding of third nerve impairment.

The position for measuring near acuity has been overemphasized by traditional examiners who are oriented exclusively to trial frame techniques rather than refractors *and* trial frames. Aside from motility problems, particularly those associated with V, A, or X phenomena, there is neither theoretic nor practical necessity to make near measurements in vertically altered lines of gaze rather than through a properly positioned refractor. It is essential to know the patient's occupational near range requirements; rarely these will be *upward* in certain control engineers or electronic specialists actually working at times inside equipment with overhead elements. Measurements through a refractor generally give more precise linear control than can be secured with a trial frame. Additionally, the frame with two or three lenses slipped in place and often with insufficient pantoscopic tilt of the eyepiece produces misleading marginal aberrations that underestimate the final near acuity achievable with a single lens having its lower edge properly tilted almost into contact with the malar eminences.

PRELIMINARY EXAMINATION OF BROWS, LIDS, CONJUNCTIVA, AND ADNEXA
Brows

Configuration of the brow is normally symmetric and should be observed for loss of hair, particularly from the temporal ends. Hypothyroidism is often responsible for such loss and is further indicated by roughness or puffiness of the skin. In areas where leprosy is endemic, it is frequent to find loss of the eyebrows as one of the early and classic manifestations of the disease.

Seborrhea of the brows is often a concomitant of similar disturbances producing oily scales throughout the scalp and along the cilia of the lids. This is a frequent cause of chronic marginal blepharitis.

Movement of the brows should be noted for evidence of integrity of the upper divisions of the facial nerve, which also supply the orbicularis oculi muscle, which is responsible for closing the lids. Unilateral impairment of brow movement indicates peripheral rather than central impairment of nerve VII because the brows receive bilateral central innervation.

Lids
Lid structure

The lids participate in essentially all of the dermatologic disturbances that plague the body. The skin of the lids is the thinnest and most delicate of any skin surface and therefore some dermatologic diseases present here with greater functional disturbance than similar processes elsewhere. The chronic dry scaling of atopic dermatitis or neurodermatitis produces darkening and inelasticity of the lids, which is also prog-

nostically related to the development of dermatogenic cataracts.

Mechanical disturbances involving relaxation and redundancy must be noted for their weight, unattractive appearance, and, particularly in the upper lids, their awning-like restriction of upward field. When this is a relaxation of the skin alone, it is commonly called *dermatochalasis*. When it relates to recurrent lid edema or is compounded by two or three pockets of fat herniation forward through defects in the septum orbitale (or rarely when it is related to systemic trichinosis), it is referred to as *blepharochalasis*. The weight of these disturbances in the lower lid may pull the lid border from the globe, causing a mechanical ectropion. If the lower tear punctum is also dragged forward, this is marked by epiphora over the lid border onto the cheek. Correct diagnosis of cause may eliminate disturbances producing intermittent edema, but the most frequent varieties are related to maturity. Here correct diagnosis, followed by appropriate excision and septal repair if needed, usually leads to major cosmetic and significant functional improvement.

Redness and parchment-like consistency of the lid skin with minor swelling and moderate itching suggest an allergic or sensitivity reaction. This may be accompanied by pale edema (chemosis) of the conjunctiva. Such findings call for diagnostic elimination of all possible skin allergens including soaps and cosmetics, search for environmental allergens, and, often, skin testing for hypersensitivity.

Any skin tumor or cancer that develops elsewhere may also appear in the lids, and the lower lid is particularly susceptible to basal cell carcinoma. All painless circumscribed areas of skin thickening without discoloration should be considered to be possible malignancies until proved otherwise. The yellowish infiltration of xanthelasma, particularly radiating from the inner canthal area, may be associated with elevated serum lipid fractions. Any such circumscribed yellowish or lipid-type deposition calls for careful study of serum cholesterol and other lipids in order to decide whether medical therapy or surgical excision is needed.

Painful, tender, and inflamed masses in the lid suggest infections or possibly occult foreign bodies. Palpation of fluid-filled or fluctuant masses without pulsation suggests incision for drainage and possible culturing of released material if it appears purulent.

Chronic redness and irritation is often overlooked when resulting from low-grade chronic inflammation in the lash follicles or the meibomian (tarsal) glands. All such irritable eyes and lids should have careful inspection of the lashes for scaly or seborrheic debris about their bases. This is related rarely to pediculosis of the lashes or commonly to *Demodex* mites in the follicles, which may be evidenced by excreta on the cilia. In doubtful cases of chronic lid border irritation a few lashes may be pulled individually and their bulbs inspected under the high power of the slit lamp (30× to 40×) to reveal the *Demodex*, which has a body diameter slightly less than the diameter of the cilia.

Lumpiness or thickening in the vertical patterns of the meibomian glands as seen through the tarsal conjunctiva or secretions localized over their orifices on the lid borders suggests chronic inflammation of these glands and indicates a need for mechanical expression. This is easiest done by the examiner's thumbnails bringing the conjunctival surfaces of the upper and lower lids together. Gentle pressure, though somewhat uncomfortable to the patient, will often deliver through the lid border orifices offending and inspissated secretions that must be eliminated before clearing of low-grade infections can be expected. Bacteriologic culturing and testing of colonies for antibiotic sensitivity is not obligatory in initial therapy. If adequate response is not achieved in a few weeks of treatment, however, then careful bacteriologic and sensitivity studies are indicated.

Lid function

Following evaluation of the appearance, structure, and abnormalities of the lid substance, it is essential to evaluate the closing and opening mechanisms. Impairments of closing predispose the cornea to drying, ulceration, and secondary infection, whereas impairments of opening may render the eye visually useless.

Orbicularis function and lid closure. Facial (nerve VII) paralysis or Bell's palsy is usually a peripheral interruption in the nerve interfering with brow motion as well as orbicularis closure. Physiologically, the lid borders should come into smooth apposition without forceful exertion. When there is poor closure some corneal protection is afforded by the physiologic Bell's phenomenon of upward rotation of the eye on attempted closure.

Ectropion and lid relaxation from other than facial nerve impairment should be evaluated for senile (atonic) or other causative mechanisms. Sometimes cicatricial scarring below the lid border actively pulls the lid away from the globe with the similar disruptive effect of causing lacrimal punctal eversion. This leads to epiphora. Cicatricial scarring may follow lacerations, thermal or chemical burns, or postradiation atrophy, which is usually accompanied by epilation and depigmentation.

Exaggerated closure may be unilateral or bilateral and, at times, very incapacitating. Protective *ptosis* or *lid closure* may be initiated by corneal ulceration and chronic or acute injuries to the epithelium. This appears bilateral following epithelium damage from ultraviolet exposure. It is diagnosed by fluorescein staining, which shows punctate destruction of the epithelium, particularly in the exposed interpalpebral area. Acute extraocular muscle paralysis often produces voluntary unilateral protective closure. This is diagnosed by the patient's ability to open the eye on request, thus revealing an ocular deviation and a subjective complaint of diplopia.

Severe photophobic disturbances usually relate to active disease involvement of the cornea. Classically, the extreme photophobia of childhood or youth that causes a youngster to crawl under the bed or to bury his face in a pillow relates to bilateral interstitial keratitis of congenital syphilis, phlyctenular keratitis with round cell infiltrations of the limbus or cornea, or congenital glaucoma with stretching of the globe. The diagnosis of one of these three conditions can almost be guaranteed on the basis of history from the parents and the avoidance behavior of the child. In areas where acute trachoma is endemic, this process may also create similar, though slightly less, photophobia in its initial stages.

Blepharospasm may result from acute trigeminal nerve irritation by foreign bodies or abrasions, but under these circumstances it is unilateral and relieved by diagnostic instillation of topical anesthetics. Essential or functional blepharospasm is usually a severe bilateral problem of psychiatric origin causing great withdrawal and distress by the patient and those around him. The patient often affects digital elevation of his lids but, on quiet discussion, may be shown to have voluntary opening power. In more entrenched blepharospasms (sometimes referrred to as conversion hysteria) there is total inability to open the lids. A local anesthetic block of the facial nerve or brief general anesthesia is necessary to gain visualization of the globe in order to rule out pathology in it. The individual with advanced parkinsonism may also be plagued by bilateral blepharospasm.

Levator function and lid opening

Ptosis. Elevation of the upper lid is normally carried out by the levator muscle, which has common embryologic origin with the superior rectus muscle and also shares with it common innervation by the superior division of the oculomotor or third cranial nerve. Examination of the ptotic individual requires careful estimation of residual levator function, which must be differentiated from frontalis muscle assistance. It is usually necessary for the examiner to hold the soft tissues in the brow region firmly

against the underlying bone of the skull in order to eliminate frontalis muscle activity in a patient who has resorted to this in compensation for a levator impairment. Localized muscular dystrophy is often suggested when the superior rectus muscle is impaired concurrently with the levator and a hypotropia exists.

Evaluation of ptosis also requires careful examination of downward rotations, because localized levator dystrophies and fibrous replacements of the elastic muscle tissue often limit the downward excursion of the lid during depressed gaze. This is called lagophthalmos. Such lid limitation in downward gaze accompanying ptosis will restrict the amount of surgical resection of the levator that can be done in planning for improvement of the primary position.

It is helpful to measure the vertical width of the interpalpebral fissure at its midpoint in the (1) primary position, (2) maximally depressed gaze, and (3) maximally elevated gaze, in order to quantitate in millimeters the amount of ptosis and lid lag in each eye.

Though congenital (bilateral or unilateral) and often hereditary ptosis is the most common anomaly of the lids, differential consideration must always be given to neurogenic and myasthenic mechanisms. Congenital ptosis remains throughout life, is affected only slightly by fatigue, and may become worse in late adult years. Testing for myasthenia gravis should be done particularly in older males and younger females having a history indicating increasing ptosis with fatigue. Usually the disease is acquired rather than congenital. One of the simplest tests in the partially ptotic individual is to open and close the lids rapidly twenty or thirty times. This usually increases the ptosis in myasthenia gravis. Variable diplopia (caused by involvement of extraocular muscles), jaw weakness, and difficulty in swallowing are further diagnostic signs of myasthenia.

The most specific test is intravenous injection of edrophonium chloride (Ten-

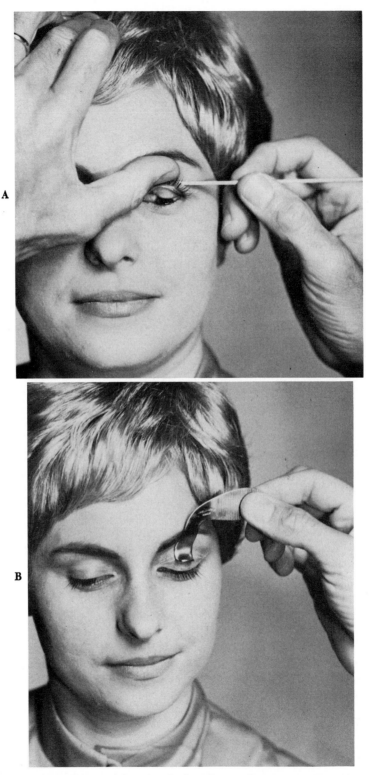

Fig. 3-4. A, Eversion of upper lid with aid of applicator directing pressure at upper edge of tarsal plate. **B,** Walker lid everter for left upper lid. **C,** Double eversion of upper lid exposing conjunctiva of the cul-de-sac over curved tip of Walker everter.

silon,* 10 mg./ml.) in dosages of 1 to 10 mg. For adults, the entire 1-ml. test dose (10 mg.) is taken into a tuberculin syringe and the needle inserted into an antecubital vein. Two milligrams is given and the needle is left in place. A positive improvement in ptosis should be noted within 45 seconds; if this is not seen, then the remaining 8 mg. is injected. Failure to attain distinct improvement in the ptosis after this second injection is a valid negative test. Dosage should be reduced by weight for children, administering 1 mg. for a weight of 75 pounds. All effects are usually over within a few minutes.

A less pleasant and more time-consuming alternate test is the long established (M. B. Walker, 1934) use of neostigmine bromide (Prostigmin,* 1-ml. vials of 1:1,000, 1:2,000, and 1:4,000) by subcutaneous or intramuscular injection. One or two milligrams in an adult usually pro-

_____
*Roche Laboratories, Nutley, New Jersey 07110.

duces improvement in 15 to 30 minutes. Children may at times require the full adult dose, but the amount may be scaled down to 1/50 mg. in the newborn. All effects are usually over in 45 to 60 minutes.

Side effects of nausea, vomiting, intestinal peristalsis, urinary evacuation, bradycardia, and bronchial secretions are infrequent but more marked with Prostigmin than with Tensilon. A syringe containing 1 mg. atropine sulfate ready for intravenous or subcutaneous injection should be available whenever such cholinergic agents are injected.

Upper lid tucking or lid retraction. As the reverse of blepharoptosis, some patients present with tucking of the upper lids and deepening of the upper lid folds. This is usually bilateral, though frequently asymmetric, and classically is associated with hyperophthalmic Graves' disease (thyrotoxic exophthalmos) and its concomitants of tachycardia, nervousness, heat intolerance, and weight loss. With nystagmus,

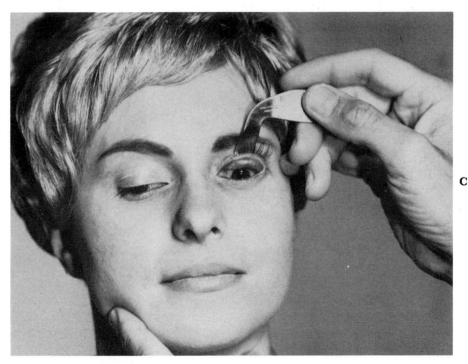

C

Fig. 3-4, cont'd. For legend see opposite page.

paralysis of upward gaze, or multiple sclerosis, such lid retraction may be evidence of major pathology in the brainstem.

Conjunctiva

The conjunctiva, normally a smooth, glistening, and essentially transparent mucosal layer, flexibly unites the lids and globes with well-moistened appositional surfaces. It extends from tight apposition on the inner surface of the lids (palpebral portion), through loose folds in the fornices (cul-de-sac portion), to an intermediate degree of attachment to the anterior globe (bulbar portion). In the circumferential area extending 2 or 3 mm. from the limbus, it becomes firmly attached to the globe.

In the bulbar and lower lid portions it is easily accessible to direct inspection by instructed rotation of the globe and gentle downward traction of the lower lid. Inspection of the upper palpebral and cul-de-sac portions is slightly more difficult because of the protective reflexes and the presence of the levator structures blending with the upper tarsal plate. In sensitive individuals, those with some lid spasm, or those harboring acute pathology behind the lid, it is often necessary to instill a topical anesthetic before everting the lid.

Eversion is done while asking the patient to look downward. The examiner grasps the upper cilia between the thumb and forefinger of one hand and "flips" the upper lid with finger pressure directed downward against the upper edge of the tarsal plate. Often this pressure can be directed more precisely or more effectively with the end of a cotton-tipped applicator or match stem (Fig. 3-4, *A*). This eversion still does not expose the upper cul-de-sac, which may harbor foreign bodies as large as a BB. For such exposure a lid everter such as the Walker (Fig. 3-4, *B*, right and left) or a lid retractor such as the Desmarres must be pressed gently above the upper edge of the tarsal plate (Fig. 3-4, *C*) and the lid pulled upward over the instrument. The curved end of the instrument then will press forward the cul-de-sac tissues, permitting identification and removal of foreign debris or study of the characteristics of this area where lymphomatous masses and chronic viral inflammations may be manifest.

The conjunctiva is the portion of the eye most frequently involved in bacterial and viral inflammations. Fortunately, these inflammations tend to be contained and generally accessible to microbiologic diagnosis; they endanger vision only by corneal extension. Unfortunately, most conjunctival infections produce very little immune reaction and tend to involve the similar epithelium of the cornea, but the process here is commonly mild. At times, however, it can be rapidly destructive and resistant to most antibiotic therapy. Practically every pathogen that attacks the body can be harbored in or infect the conjunctiva. In addition a few pathogens, particularly viruses such as the large trachoma virus, seem to appear almost exclusively in the conjunctiva or cornea.

The spectrum of neoplastic disease in the conjunctiva is also similar to that of tumors affecting epithelial membranes elsewhere. Fortunately, the conjunctiva is easily available for excisional biopsy of suspect lesions. This may be done rather widely because of the easy mobility of bulbar and cul-de-sac conjunctiva to cover defects. In melanotic changes possibly indicating malignancy, almost half of the bulbar conjunctiva may be excised and still afford easy repair by sliding to cover the defect.

Adnexa

Lacrimal glands. Normally the lacrimal glands are inconspicuous in their location at the superior temporal portion of the orbital rim. The upper lid configuration, which commonly gives an S-shaped curve to the upper lid with downward depression in the outer third of the border, should be noted for swellings in this area. Ordinarily, on eversion of the upper lids, with the gaze directed straight down, the lacrimal glands do not herniate. If the gaze, however, is directed down and to the opposite side and the upper lid retracted temporarily while it is everted, it is usually possible to visualize the palpebral lobe of the gland. In advanced years, there is a physiologic tendency for the gland to drop downward and be visualized more easily. As in many other ocular evaluations, it is most important to compare the appearance of the right and left structures.

In young people, the gland may be involved in congenital, benign tumors. In mid- and later life, the glands may be symmetrically enlarged with blood dyscrasias. The lacrimal glands are histologically almost identical to the salivary glands and generally may show any pathologic process or malignancy that the salivary glands can develop. Such local malignancies are most often unilateral, and the highly lethal mixed cell tumor is one of the more common. Tender, red, and painful swelling of localized infection or abscess occurs but is unusual.

Preauricular gland. The preauricular gland, a lymph node, is generally located anterior to the tragus of the ear or over the condyle of the mandible. It is the first interceptor station of lymphatic drainage from the lids, conjunctiva, and associated superficial adnexal structures. Thus both acute and chronic infections of the lids or conjunctiva may cause enlargement, low-grade pain, moderate tenderness, and rarely redness at this site. The gland is ordinarily neither tender nor palpable unless involved by inflammatory disease. Its involvement is an index of the severity of the infectious process. It rarely participates in diffuse disturbances of the lymphatic system.

Orbit

The orbit is a complex, rigid, conic receptacle constituted by seven bones and primarily serving as a protective housing for the globe and its appendages. Its major anterior opening or "base" affords access to the globe plus suspension for the lids. Its major posterior opening or optic foramen at the orbital apex affords passage-

way for the optic nerve and its attendant supporting structures, connecting via the optic chiasm to the brain. Two further major openings, the superior orbital (sphenoidal) fissure and the inferior orbital (sphenomaxillary) fissure, are of diagnostic and x-ray importance. Several medium-sized openings (infraorbital canal, superior orbital foramen or notch, the nasolacrimal canal) may also be identified by special x-ray examinations, but numerous and more variable small openings for arteries, veins, and nerves are generally of obscure diagnostic identification.

Thickness of the orbital bones varies widely from the extremely thin lamina papyracea of the ethmoid bone, which may actually contain bony dehiscences, to the usually strong and massive superior orbital margin. With advancing years, there is thinning of the periosteum and also of the bone, particularly in the roof and lateral wall areas.

Angulations of the orbital bones vary widely (Keeney, 1957) from outward angulation in embryologic life and early childhood to various final positions that may be measured on submentovertex x-rays. This varies not only among individuals but also among races. The mechanical position or angulation of the orbits appears to have a positional influence on the globes in about one-fourth of nonparalytic and nonaccommodative horizontal strabismus patients.

Because the orbit has common boundaries with paranasal sinuses above (frontal), medially (ethmoids), and below (maxillary), it is vulnerable to the transmission of infection or neoplasm from these structures.

Diagnostic examination of the orbit (see also pp. 208-212) primarily involves the following:
A. Preliminary inspection for:
1. Lid swelling and distortion: this may be secondary or collateral edema from deep orbital cellulitis, paranasal sinus infection, or mechanical stretching of the lids by a tumor mass.
2. Secretions and discharge from the

conjunctiva or from the homolateral nasal passage: the latter may represent primary nasal disease extending into the orbit or, less commonly, drainage from lacrimal infection into the nose.

3. Exophthalmic displacement of the globe: this may be directly forward, such as from a mass within the muscle cone, or obliquely, in relation to masses localized elsewhere in the orbit.

4. Disturbances of the rim contours: these may be from traumatic fracture displacement, neoplastic erosion (better seen on x-ray), or, rarely, inflammatory thickening of the periosteum.

5. Congestion and edema of the conjunctiva: this may be caused by superficial and local infection or by deeper infection that has extended across the conjunctival barrier.

6. Vascular anomalies evident in the lids or conjunctiva: these may be histo-logically benign hemangiomas or serious distensions of deep vessels following carotid artery–cavernous sinus fistula.

7. Impaired rotation of the globe in any direction: orbital tumors and inflammatory disturbances may directly invade and limit these muscles or by their mass may inhibit rotation in their direction. At other times, inflammation, trauma, or neoplasm may interrupt the nerve supply to given extraocular muscles without mechanical restrictions; in these cases, passive or forced ductions by the examiner are usually free.

B. Palpation of the orbit for:

1. Any masses accessible to the exploring fingertip applied through the lids.

2. Comparison of retrobulbar resistance in the two orbits: this is easily done by simultaneous thumb pressure against each globe through the closed lids (Fig. 3-5).

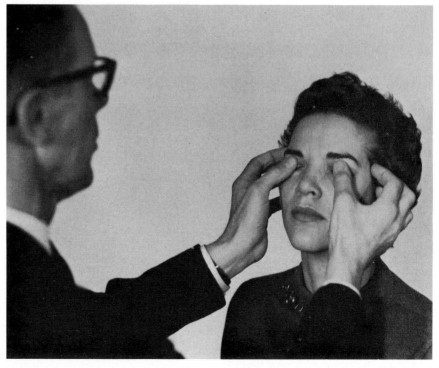

Fig. 3-5. Tactile comparison of retrobulbar resistance in the two orbits by simultaneous direct thumb pressure against each globe through the closed lids.

3. Tactile evaluation of the orbital rims: rarely a linear fracture or bone mobility resulting from fracture will be revealed by careful palpation and comparison of right and left orbital rims, even when such defects do not appear on x-ray films.

C. Ophthalmoscopy for:

1. Venous congestion indicating impairment of return blood flow from the globe.

2. Arterial pulsations or arterial insufficiency indicating compression of the arterial supply by increased intra-orbital pressure or secondarily increased intraocular pressure (compression glaucoma).

3. Striations, usually horizontal, at the posterior pole, as evidence of compression against the back curve of the globe.

D. Auscultation for vascular sounds or bruits

E. Roentgenographic examination: standard skull views, special projections, laminography, contrast studies

F. Ultrasound examination

TRANSILLUMINATION AND CONTACT ILLUMINATION

The transillumination and contact illumination methods of diagnosing structural changes in the visual apparatus have been rendered less essential by improvements in (1) binocular indirect ophthalmoscopy, especially of the peripheral fundus, (2) direct and indirect gonioscopy of the anterior chamber angle, (3) slit lamp examination of both the posterior pole and peripheral fundus with the aid of contact lenses, (4) bone-free x-rays of the lids and anterior segment using dental film, and (5) ultrasonography with its ability to penetrate opaque media and to differentiate solid from cystic lesions.

Almost any small light of medium to moderate intensity can be used if it is fitted with an opaque collar or tubular shield to reduce the distraction of lateral light scattering. The Finnoff transilluminator, supplied in straight, angular, and extended length heads by various manufacturers (Welch Allyn; Propper; National), is a standard item for lid and anterior bulbar transillumination and can also be used as a general inspection torch. The small, curved Lancaster-Boehm (1913) transilluminator of stainless steel has a greatly reduced diameter compared to the Finnoff and can be insinuated into the conjunctival cul-de-sac beyond the equator. The two types of minute, 1½-volt bulbs manufactured for this unit provide either end lighting or side lighting directed toward the concavity of the carrier shaft. The instrument may be sterilized for use through a conjunctival incision or for retrobulbar transillumination at surgery. Engraved markings encircle the shaft at 1-cm. intervals, so the position or depth of the bulb can be recorded during use. Both the very small diameter and the tendency for the lamps to heat render the Lancaster transilluminator unpleasant or painful when pressed deep into the conjunctival cul-de-sac. The MIRA High Intensity Transilluminator with straight and right angle probes is fitted to a 5-ft. long, flexible, fiber optic bundle and therefore yields cold light at its tip. The remote light source is 150 watts.

External transillumination is of differential value in examination of the *lids,* the *globe,* and the *orbit.* So-called transpupillary transillumination—a fundamental step in genesis of the ophthalmoscope—is of value in identifying opacities in the media. This is best done with a direct ophthalmoscope held a foot or two away from the pupil and facilitating coincidence of the examiner's line of vision with the line of illumination. By shifting the examiner's line of observation laterally, transpupillary transillumination is of some value in examining the coats of the eye anterior to the equator. This may reveal scleral thinning, pigment loss, cysts, staphylomas, ruptures, or intramural foreign bodies.

Intraoral or indirect light from a bright source within the mouth will, at times, transilluminate a clear cyst within the globe or orbit and differentiate it from opaque solid masses such as neoplasms or hematomata.

Contact illumination through the center of the anesthetized cornea may be done with the Finnoff illuminator or the end light-bulb of the Lancaster instrument. Drance (1963) refined corneal contact illumination and designed an illuminator with a concave face that fits the central or pars optica surface. This is helpful in identifying the elusive limbal area and the proximal limit of the anterior chamber angle, particularly following mobilization of a conjunctival flap at the time of anterior segment surgery.

Transillumination of the lids from the inner surface with the aid of topical anesthesia and the side lightbulb of the Lancaster transilluminator will usually resolve any question of solid versus cystic mass in the lid and may be pivotal in ruling out or localizing a radiolucent foreign body.

Transscleral transillumination generally requires topical anesthesia. This technique is particularly essential when a pigmented lesion of the iris, the limbus, or the ciliary body is under study. Benign cystic lesions in these areas usually appeared dark in focal illumination but bright in transillumination. Eyes have been needlessly removed under the impression that such masses are malignant melanomas (the latter are opaque). Anterior scleral transillumination may be of assistance in identifying iris pigment loss, configuration of the pupil in the presence of corneal opacity, or even opaque foreign bodies hidden within a cataract. Difficulties of light positioning and irregularities of scattering make transillumination progressively less accurate in more proximal portions of the globe. Observation through the pupil of such transillumination, however, may reveal opaque (solid) masses beneath a retinal detachment or clear cysts in more peripheral sites. An extension of this technique is the Osmond (1954) combination of 12-volt transilluminator and annular diathermy electrode. This is available as a separate

unit or adapted to fit major Keeler ophthalmoscopes. It may be employed at surgery to aid in localization of retinal holes during ophthalmoscopy. Similarly, for office indirect ophthalmoscopy, scleral depressors are available (Univis) with cool, fiber-optics illumination for the gadgeteer.

When there is gross reduction of vision to the level of poor light projection or questionable light perception, transscleral transillumination can elicit entoptic observation of the retinal blood vessels in the presence of a large hyphema, mature cataract, or dense blood staining the cornea. If retinal function is retained behind such opacities, the intelligent patient may describe a very helpful "map" of branching vascular shadows throughout his retinal area. This gives better geographic data with much less equipment and time than is involved in electroretinography.

INSTRUMENTAL VISUAL SCREENING

As yet there is no machine substitute for the direct questioning, the skill, and the penetrating analysis of a knowledgeable examiner in either preliminary or definitive examination. Such an individual may perform superbly with minimal or relatively primitive equipment such as a simple Snellen chart and an ophthalmoscope. On the other hand, economy and maximum distribution of care are often efficiently served by nonprofessional screening done by trained volunteers or school, industrial, and highway employees prepared exclusively for such work. A parallel is seen in the teams of x-ray technicians who take preliminary chest x-rays in tuberculosis detection campaigns or office assistants who perform urinalysis in diabetic screening.

Such public health visual screening should be organized and directed by professional personnel skilled in eye diseases and their detection. Very productive screening can be accomplished with quite simple accessories such as a Snellen chart and a flashlight. Instrument manufacturers, however, market a series of variously complex equipment particularly directed to school screening, industrial preemployment evaluations, and driver licensing. Increasing educational, insurance, and safety calls for such procedures, plus the growing population involved, have created significant personnel and instrument markets. At times such programs have yielded a series of instrumentally derived numbers without fully established significance or relation to seeing functions.

Most of these instruments are outgrowths of the simple stereoscopes (Brewster, 1838; Wheatstone, 1838) with their pairs of stereoscopic or disparate targets. In the second half of the nineteenth century pairs of disparate pictures or stereophotographs became very popular for home amusement viewing. Early students of visual physiology turned to mathematically and physiologically designed pairs of printed stereograms with which to study quantitative aspects of binocularity (Stereocomparator of Tourcade, 1900).

An element of automation by self-administration and self-pacing of the test steps has been introduced by Tracor Medical Instruments* in their P. W. Johnson Vision Screener (Model RA-116). This 15-pound table-model unit is based on the three basic requirements of the Massachusetts Vision Test. It screens (1) by use of the "tumbling Snellen E" for simulated distance acuity that may be switched for either 20/30 or 20/40 level, (2) for vertical and horiontal heterophoria by use of a red ball which, as presented to one eye, should be within a green field seen by the other eye, and (3) for hyperopia at the +1.75- or +2.25-diopter level, again by switch selection. The examiner explains the basic test procedure to the subject and then needs only to monitor the examination, which proceeds automatically at the rate established by the subject pressing "Yes" or "No" buttons for each test. In testing large numbers of subjects, the candidates may be identified by use of numbered

*Austin, Texas 78721.

tokens inserted in the Yes-No control box.

A Tracor model with a more extensive and complex series of targets including central acuity levels, stereoacuity, and fundamental color recognition is available for industrial use (Model RA-116A). Another model introduced in 1970 is specifically designed for driver testing programs. It has a horizontal form field attachment that may be inserted at the top of the ocular end of the screener.

The following instruments are currently marketed for visual screening programs or "battery tests" and are designed to be operated by nonprofessional workers after brief instruction.

1. American Automobile Association, N.W. Washington, D. C. 20006

   Driver Evaluator No. 3574 (Federal Stock No. 6910-597-9651)
   The Driver Evaluator is a rugged welded-steel, table-top unit requiring about 13 ft. of available room length to simulate a 20-ft. test distance with a mirror at 10 ft. It provides four tests:
   a. Letters for Snellen acuity notation from 20/100 to 20/13
   b. Near range depth judgment
   c. Horizontal form field
   d. Recognition testing of basic traffic control lights of red, amber, and green
   A fiber case is available for protection during transportation.

2. American Optical Company, Safety Products Division, Southbridge, Massachusetts 01550

   Sight Screener (Model 18010A)
   The first of this series was introduced in 1946 and its numerical findings adapted to Hollerith form reports. Though generally similar to other instruments for this purpose, the Sight Screener differs by using Polaroid double-printed vectographs for targets rather than relying entirely on the Brewster stereoscope principles of viewing horizontally juxtaposed stereograms through base-out prisms. Case is made of cast aluminum and total weight is 22 lbs.

3. Bausch and Lomb, Inc., Rochester, New York 14602
   Under the general trade name Ortho-Rater, Bausch and Lomb introduced its first screening instrument of this series in 1943. Three models are now produced.

Master Ortho-Rater

The Master Ortho-Rater is a self-contained unit with all target slides mounted internally on two manually controlled rotating drums, presenting seven far point tests on one drum and five near point tests on the other. Results of these twelve tests are hand-recorded on a Hollerith-style card, noting gross color screening, central acuity using right eye, left eye, and then both eyes at near and distance, and instrumental representations of vertical and horizontal phorias for near and simulated distance. A Perimeter attachment is available as an auxiliary mounting on the headrest to assess form recognition in the horizontal only. Table space of 10 × 25 in. is covered by the instrument and it easily adjusts from 23 to 30 in. in height to accommodate the test subject.

Modified Ortho-Rater

The Modified Ortho-Rater uses the same optic principles as the Master Ortho-Rater but has manually inserted slides and simplified internal construction and is less expensive.

School Vision Test Model

The School Vision Test Model is mechanically and optically the same as the Modified Ortho-Rater, but it has base measurements of only 10 × 21 in. and weighes 19 pounds. Findings are derived from slides providing six illiterate performance examinations including the +1.75-diopter lens test for hyperopia, as modified from the Massachusetts Vision Test (Sloan, 1940). Additional interchangeable slides are available and may be stored in the base.

4. Good-Lite Company, Forest Park, Illinois 60130
The Good-Lite Company, which has produced many durable, simple, and portable illuminated test charts, introduced in 1968 a modification of the remote-controlled Green's Illuminated Vision Charts, under the name Insta-Line Chart. This utilizes a 10-ft. space and can test acuity against crowded (linear) versus isolated optotypes. Standard phoria screening at 6 prism diopters in or out and 1.5 prism diopters up or down is included. This unit, like the A.A.A. Driver Evaluator, avoids the instrumental or proximity factor inherent in completely contained table-top devices.

5. Keystone View Company, Meadville, Pennsylvania 16335
Keystone, in conjunction with E. A. Betts (1933), introduced a pioneer line of screening equipment for school use under the name Telebinocular. In the mid- and late 1930's this was modified for industrial use and made more durable. All Telebinoculars are of open construction between the oculars and the stereo-gram targets. This enables the examiner to monitor the tests under his direct view and to point out areas on the target when he wishes the examinee's attention at a particular point. All models avoid mirrors and have completely interchangeable targets that are produced in a large and varied series. Simple design permits essentially no possibility for internal mechanical jamming or failure. Four models are available:

a. Ophthalmic Telebinocular: most versatile and complex of the line
b. Keystone Orthoscope: lighter and simpler but affording similar measurements as Ophthalmic Telebinocular
c. School Visual Survey Telebinocular: all plastic and less complex than the preceding models
d. Driver–Visual Survey Telebinocular: plastic and of same basic design as others but supplied with highway-type targets and horizontal form field attachment

6. G. Rodenstock Optische Werke, Munich, Germany

Rodenstock Vision Screener R5 for Children

The Rodenstock Screener is a small, light, and plastic-encased instrument of simple Brewster stereoscope principles. It was designed in close cooperation with Dr. C. Cuppers of Giessen. Target pairs are printed on flat discs inserted at the base of the machine at the back. Illiterate E's are used for visual acuity measurement in five gradations. The phoria test is a dot within a rectangle allowing 1 prism diopter of vertical imbalance up or down and 3 prism diopters of exophoria or 1 of esophoria within the established screening limits. Stereoacuity is tested with groups of three Punch and Judy figures: three test settings present one figure out of plane with the other two by 360, 240, and 120 seconds of arc.

Rodenstock Vision Tester Rodatest

The Rodenstock Rodatest was developed in the mid-1950's by Dr. H. Schober from the basic stereoscope design. Nine pairs of targets are mounted on one drum and viewing conditions may be modified by interposing varying lenses and diaphragms on a second drum. Visual acuity is evaluated by modified Goldmann optotypes (squares subdivided into four smaller squares composed of dots of two different diameters) through ten gradations. Dissimilar targets presented to each eye in the form of a modified Maddox wing are used for rough quantitation of phorias at near and simulated distance. Six sets of stereograms are designed to quantitate stereoacuity from 720 to 22 seconds of arc. Color testing is specifically excluded in favor of more consistent targets that can be made from pigments rather than by transmitted light. The unit is suitable for industrial screening.

7. Titmus Optical Company, Petersburg, Virginia 23803

T/O Vision Tester

The T/O Vision Tester is a lightweight (17 pounds), high impact resistant plastic unit of stereoscopic design with a relatively large drum carrying twelve sets of test slides or stereograms. These may be presented by manual rotation or by push-button controlled electric motor drive. A large number of additional test slides are optional (stereoacuity, color, subnormal vision, peripheral fusion, Massachusetts Vision Test, Michigan Pre-School Test, Driver's License and Traffic Signal Recognition). A horizontal form field perimeter with scale (Model 67) attaches to the top of the Tester.

Titmus Biopter Visual Skills Testing Instrument (Model 130Z)

Model 130Z is a minimally expensive, simplified, open construction stereoscope. It utilizes only nine hand-inserted stereograms. A simple scoring sheet presents easily noted findings at a glance. It is probably the least expensive of all screening devices and carries the same accuracy achieved with basic printing of any stereogram.

Titmus Bioptor No. 2 (N 109Y)

Titmus Biopter No. 2 is a slightly more substantial version of the simple Bioptor with clips to hold auxiliary lenses.

8. Carl Zeiss, Jena, German Democratic Republic (East Germany)

Rapid Vision Tester

The Rapid Vision Tester is a heavy, electric motor–driven unit. Stereograms are presented on a drum. Acuity is measured by checkered square patterns. Phorias are measured at 40 cm. and at simulated distance.

Zeiss Stereoscope

The Zeiss Stereoscope is an extremely simple, open-construction instrument without an illuminating system. Stereograms are designed for children and adults. The instrument is also usable orthoptically as a home training instrument.

All of these screening devices must be considered as auxiliary and yielding only partial information that necessitates interpretation and assessment of significance. An intelligent secretary, clerk, or nonprofessional operator, however, can obtain with such equipment preliminary leads that are of value, particularly in mass surveys of industry where thousands of individuals may be involved or in driver licensing programs where millions of people are examined. The nature of patient performance in this test situation is such that overestimation of ability tends not to occur. An inherent source of distress, however, lies in overdetailed numeric findings or instrumental suggestion of deficiency when no significant abnormality exists. A problem of overreferral that tends to discredit the best intentioned surveys or public health programs may be created. Therefore screeners must be used within predetermined ranges of reporting and with planned retesting in borderline cases or uncertain results before considering that such subjects have valid need for more detailed consultation.

No reassurance can be given concerning glaucoma, which is one of the most serious and frequent causes of progressive visual loss in our more mature population.

Table-top compactness, portability, generally self-contained design, potential for multifaceted testing, and results presented in seemingly specific numbers lend attractiveness to these units, particularly for public health workers and mass survey planners. They do not, however, establish ocular diagnosis and can, in the absence of proper patient explanation, be permitted to give a false sense of security to individuals passing the tests.

"The resolution of visual acuity in terms of geometry is to ascribe an unjustified simplicity to a complex and obscure psychological problem."

W. STEWART DUKE-ELDER, 1944

Chapter 4

Examination of the pupils

Ben P. Houser, Jr., M.D.

GENERAL PRINCIPLES

Examination of the pupils is not difficult, but attention to detail is imperative. Fundamentally, the pupils constrict (c) in light or in near regard and dilate (d) in darkness or in remote fixation, but subtle variations of these basic responses often aid in neuro-ophthalmic diagnosis. As in all physical examinations, normal ranges must be appreciated in order to identify pathologic variations. Responses of the normal pupil vary with basic room illumination, degree of accommodation, age, refractive state, and other factors.

Evaluation of pupillary responses requires a small flashlight as the basic instrument and in some cases a slit lamp for the fine beam to elicit hemianopic pupillary responses. For the practitioner, the large, expensive, and time-consuming infrared pupillography equipment is not necessary. Most pupillary diagnoses can be made with light and an occluder, plus a few topical drugs.

The most important of the reflexes of the pupil are outlined in Table 1. The light and near reflexes must be preliminary parts of every eye examination.

ANATOMY

Both the sympathetic and parasympathetic divisions of the autonomic nervous system exercise efferent influences on the pupils. In general, parasympathetic stimuli constrict the pupils by contracting the

Table 1. Summary of basic pupillary reflexes

Reflex	Stimulus	Reaction
Light	Light	Bilateral miosis
Near	Accommodation, convergence	Bilateral miosis
Orbicularis (Westphal-Piltz)	Forced closure of lid	Unilateral miosis
Vestibular	Caloric stimulation	Bilateral mydriasis (hippus)
Cochlear	Tuning fork	Mydriasis following brief miosis
Trigeminus	Touching cornea	Miosis following brief mydriasis
Psychosensory	Psychic and stimulation of any sensory nerve	Bilateral mydriasis
Vagotonic	Inspiration, expiration	Mydriasis, miosis

sphincter muscle in response to light and accommodation. Sympathetic stimuli dilate the pupils by contracting the radial dilator muscle of the iris. Both the sympathetic and parasympathetic systems are in constantly shifting balance. Thus the "resting" size of the normal pupil is never absolutely static but fluctuates continuously by a small, minute amount of physiologic hippus or alternate dilatation and constriction.

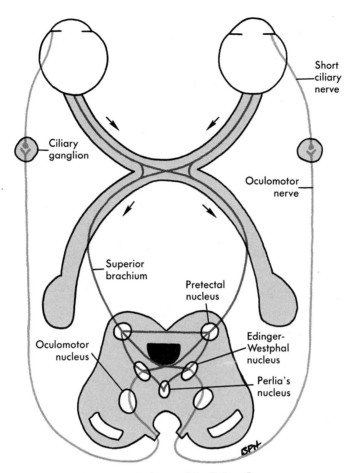

Fig. 4-1. Pathway of the light reflex.

Anatomy of the light reflex pathways

The anatomic pathway of the light reflex (Fig. 4-1) begins in the percipient cells of the retina where apparently specialized rods and cones absorb the light stimulus and initiate electrochemical impulses along the neural path. In the optic nerve these afferent fibers are geographically located in the peripheral or outer aspect. The fibers originating from the nasal hemiretina cross in the chiasm in a distribution similar to related visual fibers. Fibers from the temporal hemiretina traverse the chiasm uncrossed. All these fibers continue in the outer layers of the optic tract. Slightly anterior to the lateral geniculate bodies, they leave the tract and reach the tectum of the midbrain by way of the superior branchium conjunctivum. Synapse occurs in the pretectal nucleus. The fibers then proceed to the Edinger-Westphal nuclei of both sides through the posterior commissure and anterior to the aqueduct of Sylvius. The efferent arc begins at synapses in the Edinger-Westphal nuclei. The efferent fibers then continue posteriorly through the oculomotor nuclei to join the oculomoter nerve. These pupillomotor fibers synapse in the ciliary ganglion and then proceed as postganglionic fibers via the short ciliary nerves to the sphincter muscle of the iris.

Anatomy of the near reflex pathway

The near reflex pathway (Fig. 4-2), though parasympathetic, is controversial.

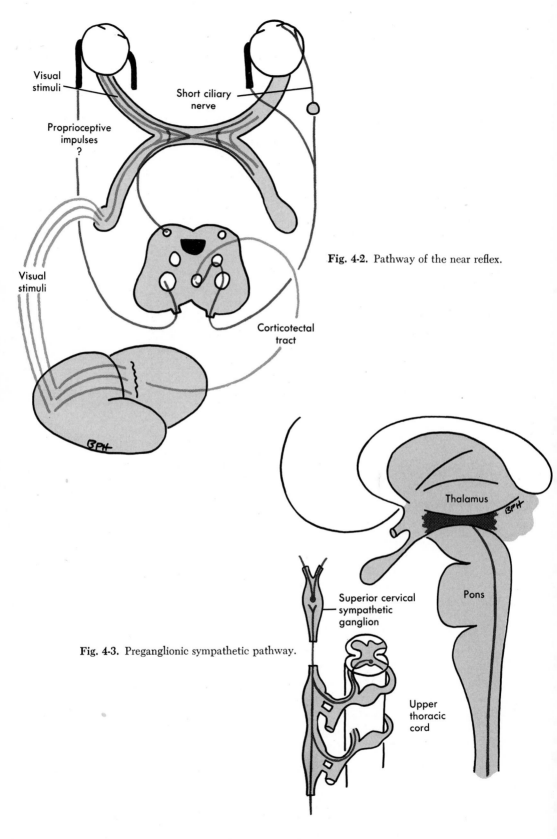

Fig. 4-2. Pathway of the near reflex.

Fig. 4-3. Preganglionic sympathetic pathway.

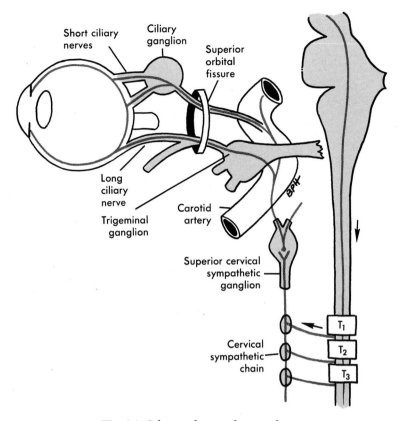

Fig. 4-4. Schema of sympathetic pathway.

The reflex is an inseparable triad of convergence, accommodation, and miosis. The most probable origin of the near reflex is in the visual cells of the retina, and the pathway is similar to the light reflex path back to the posterior third of the optic tract where the light reflex fibers leave. The near reflex fibers continue with the visual fibers along the geniculostriate radiation from the lateral geniculate body to the occipital cortex. The near reflex fibers then radiate to the frontal oculomotor centers, where they become part of a mass reflex that is mediated through the corticotectal tracts to the oculomotor nucleus.

The portion of the nucleus concerned with the near pupillary response is unknown. Perlia's nucleus apparently controls the convergence aspect of the reflex. The near reflex efferent fibers then share a common path with the light reflex fibers along the oculomotor nerve. Probably the fibers destined for the pupillary sphincter first synapse in the ciliary ganglion, or there may be a discrete path separate from the light reflex. This assumption is based on the preservation of the near pupillary reflex after ciliary ganglionectomy. The final common path is along the short ciliary nerves to the sphincter and the ciliary muscle.

Anatomy of the sympathetic pathway

The anatomy of the *sympathetic* pathway (Fig. 4-3) is fairly well established. The afferent impulses come from many sites, notably the cochlea, the skin, and the higher cortical centers of emotion. These arcs are complicated but seem to end in the hypothalamus, which apparently is the highest brain center involved in sympathetic control. The preganglionic fibers from the hypothalamus collect as a tract passing through the pons and medulla into

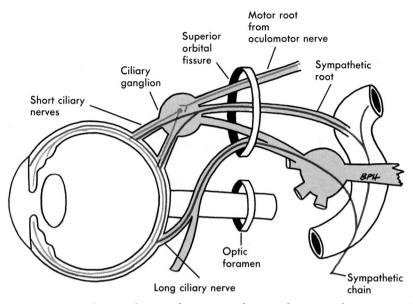

Fig. 4-5. Convergence of sympathetic and parasympathetic pathways at the superior orbital fissure.

the intermediolateral bundle of the spinal cord. The fibers controlling pupillary dilation leave the cord levels T_1, T_2, and T_3 (designated as Budge's area). The fibers collect into the thoracocervical sympathetic trunk and proceed to the superior cervical sympathetic ganglion where the first synapse occurs. Postganglionic fibers (Fig. 4-4) travel along the branches of the carotid artery to enter the globe with the long ciliary nerves to the dilator muscle of the iris. Some fibers pass through the ciliary ganglion without synapsing and enter the globe in the short ciliary nerves with the parasympathetic fibers. Both the sympathetic and parasympathetic fibers converge at the area of the superior orbital fissure (Fig. 4-5), through which they pass as the final common pathway of the efferent pupillary system. Lesions at the orbital apex may produce confusing pupillomotor signs by interfering with both systems in their close proximity. For this reason, disease of the eye itself sometimes has an unpredictable effect on the pupil, depending upon balance of the sympathetic and parasympathetic input to the iris muscles.

PUPILLOMOTOR VALENCE OR POWER

The concept of pupillomotor "valence" or "power" helps to evaluate pupillary responses. Each eye has a given pupillomotor power. The size of both pupils in the resting state is determined by the eye that exerts the greater pupillomotor power, providing the motor or efferent pupillary pathways are intact. For example, a lesion of the optic nerve will decrease the pupillomotor power of the involved eye. In the resting state, however, the pupils of both eyes will be equal since the uninvolved eye produces a pupillomotor power that floods the midbrain and is equally distributed and returned to both eyes by way of the efferent pathway. Therefore pupillary inequality in the resting state usually suggests a lesion of the efferent pupillary pathway.

Interestingly, a pupillomotor "valence" also exists in the retina (Fig. 4-6). The macular and perimacular areas have the strongest valence. The nasal hemiretina has a stronger pupillomotor valence than the temporal hemiretina. The practical

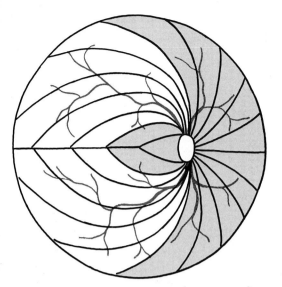

Fig. 4-6. The macular and perimacular areas have the strongest pupillomotor "valence." The nasal hemiretina has a stronger valence than the temporal hemiretina.

corollary is that similar retinal areas should be stimulated by the test light if the eyes are to be compared. If the nasal retina of one eye receives a bright light and the temporal retina of the fellow eye is stimulated by the same light, the test situation is not bilaterally equal.

TECHNIQUE OF TESTING

Preliminary inspection of both pupils should be made in the resting state in normal room illumination. While the patient is fixating at distance, note the size, equality, regularity, color of irides, and the presence of synechiae. Light response should be elicited while having the patient fixate at distance in average room light. A dark room may be used if this is the examiner's normal testing situation. Standardization in testing is important for follow-up and comparisons at later dates.

A small columnated light should be moved from the periphery to shine upon the posterior pole of the eye at a distance of about 8 in. The patient should be advised not to fixate on the light but to maintain distance fixation. The direct response

is noted and the fellow eye observed for consensual response. The light is then shifted to stimulate the posterior pole of the fellow eye and the observations are repeated. The pupils should be checked for rapidity of response, magnitude of constriction, and ability to maintain constriction. Fatigue of constriction under direct light is a subtle sign of decreased pupillomotor power.

The light should be alternately moved from one eye to the other to compare the pupillomotor power of each eye. The direct and consensual constriction of the pupils should normally be of equal magnitude. If in the alternate light testing (often called the "swinging light" test) one pupil dilates slightly when the light is moved to it from the fellow eye, this eye has less pupillomotor power than the fellow and a lesion of the homolateral optic nerve should be suspected.

A fine beam of light such as from a slit lamp is needed for testing hemianopic pupillary responses. Even the narrowest slit beam is somewhat inaccurate since the ocular media disperse the light and all retinal areas receive some light. However, in frank lesions the results are positive and helpful in the diagnosis and localization of hemianopic pathology. The nasal and temporal hemiretinas are alternately stimulated by a fine beam of light. The magnitude of constriction is noted and the results are weighed in view of the fact that the nasal hemiretina normally produces more pupillomotor power than the temporal hemiretina. This test is of particular value in chiasmal hemianopia where the normally stronger nasal hemiretinal fibers are destroyed and have no pupillomotor effect.

The near response of the pupil is usually tested binocularly since convergence is part of the reflex. Accommodation is essential and is probably the initiating stimulus. The patient first fixates binocularly at a distance and pupillary diameter is noted. The patient then fixates on an accommodative target approximately 6 to 8 in. from the eyes; this should not be a light since the light reflex may be stimulated. Again, the pupils should be compared for diameter, equality, and ability to maintain miosis. The degree of convergence should also be noted. In monocular individuals the reflex is elicited in the same way despite the absence of convergence. It is often possible to elicit the reflex in blind patients or in those with very limited vision if the patient can be made aware of a near object such as his own finger or if the tip of the patient's nose is touched.

A comparison between the magnitude of the light and of the near responses of the pupil should always be made. Normally, the amount of miosis should be about the same or slightly more with the near reflex, particularly if there is forceful accommodation.

Patients presenting with a miotic, apparently fixed pupil should be observed after 1 hour in a dark room. The ability of a small pupil to dilate in the dark is a helpful, diagnostic sign, particularly in the differentiation of an Argyll Robertson pupil from an Adie's myotonic pupil. Adie's pupil will frequently dilate after a protracted period in the dark while the Argyll Robertson pupil will not.

The sympathetic system is not usually tested specifically in examination of the pupils. The patient should be observed for associated sympathetic signs such as a widened palpebral fissure, pupillary dilatation, appearance of exophthalmus, sweating, flushing, hair condition, and iris color. Abnormality in these areas suggests increased sympathetic activity.

Sympathetic stimulation will produce a large pupil on the same side as the lesion (see p. 69). Conversely, sympathetic loss will produce a homolateral miotic pupil and other classic signs of Horner's syndrome. Amphetamines, cocaine, and similar drugs dilate the pupil through action on the sympathetic system. Anxiety states, with autonomic imbalance, will also produce large pupils because of the sympathetic dominance.

SPECIFIC PUPILLARY REFLEXES NOT ASSOCIATED WITH LIGHT OR NEAR

The orbicularis reflex (c) (Westphal and Piltz, 1920) is a homolateral constriction of the pupil on attempted forced closure of the lids against resistance of the examiner's fingers. It is present in about 80% of people and demonstrates integrity of the peripheral efferent pupillary pathway. The mechanism of the reflex has not been determined but it is important in validating Argyll Robertson pupils. A normal orbicularis reflex eliminates the efferent path as a site of the lesion. A false positive orbicularis reflex may appear if the patient converges.

The vestibular (d→hippus) *and cochlear* (c→d) *reflexes* probably represent overflow of caloric, rotational, or acoustic stimuli from the vestibular area of the midbrain and pons into the sympathetic pupillary dilating system. They are of little significance in ophthalmic disease but may at times assist in examination of the efferent pathways.

The trigeminus reflex (d) can be of practical value in verifying questionable peripheral efferent pupillary pathways. Touching the cornea will produce prompt mydriasis followed by miosis. The path of the reflex is uncertain, but most evidence indicates that the afferent trigeminal fibers stimulate the oculomotor nucleus by connections in the midbrain.

The psychosensory reflex (d) is easily observed in patients in cases of anxiety, hysteria, or fright. The reaction probably represents generalized sympathetic overlay. Bumke (1904) described the pupillary dilation in catatonia, and Redlich (1922) described reaction with intense muscular effort. The reflex is sometimes tested by pricking the skin or forcefully flexing a joint.

The vagotonic reflex (c, d) has a direct relationship to respiration with a slight dilatation on inspiration and a slight constriction on expiration. This is accentuated in pathologic breathing of hyperventilation and Cheyne-Stokes respiration.

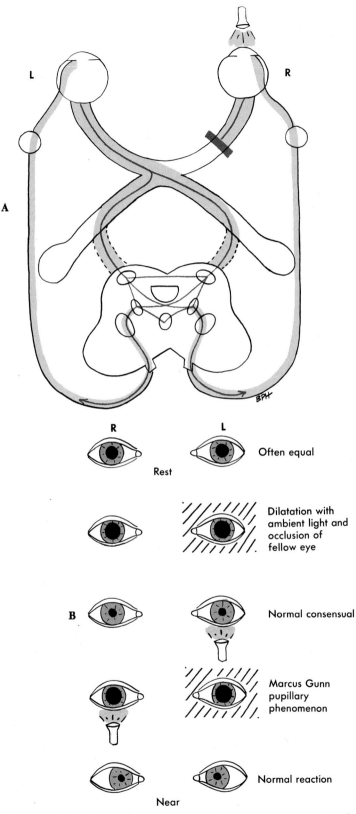

Fig. 4-7. Marcus Gunn pupil. **A,** The anatomy of the pupillary system as seen from behind. The impaired right optic nerve retards the direct pupillary reflex. Midbrain is bilaterally flooded with the stimuli, therefore the consensual response is normal. The typical clinical findings are seen in **B.**

PARASYMPATHETIC SYSTEM
Afferent tract

Optic nerve (Fig. 4-7). With a lesion of one optic nerve or of the nerve fiber layer of one retina there is a typical pupillary impairment. Both pupils exert specific pupillomotor power, and the size of both pupils is determined by the eye with the greatest pupillomotor power. In the resting state the pupils are usually equal since the normal eye is controlling pupillary size. In 1904, Marcus Gunn described an abnormal response of the pupil in a case of ipsilateral retrobulbar optic neuritis. With uniform ambient light, covering the normal fellow eye produces dilation of both pupils. Consensual response to light of the affected eye is normal. Direct light to the involved eye while the sound eye is covered, however, produces ipsilateral dilatation greater than in the resting state, indicating decreased pupillomotor power of the involved eye. The test may also be done without covering the fellow eye, but then the dilatation is of less magnitude since the normal eye is producing some pupillomotor effect. The reaction to near is normal. This type of response may occur with any lesion of the optic nerve such as:

1. Optic neuritis of any cause
2. Vascular accidents of the nerve
3. Tumors of the nerve and orbit
4. Trauma

Optic chiasm (Fig. 4-8). Sagittal division of the optic chiasm produces bitemporal hemianopia and similar interruption of the decussating nasal pupillary fibers. The hemianopic pupillary reactions are technically difficult to elicit because intraocular scatter of light stimulates the entire retina, particularly the macula. However, with a fine beam of light from a slit lamp, the bitemporal hemianopic pupillary response can often be observed. In each eye, light from the temporal field produces less pupillary constriction than light from the nasal field. When this test is positive it is often striking, but apparently normal pupillary responses do not rule out hemianopia.

Common causes of this pupillary response are the causes of interruption of the chiasm as outlined below:

A. Tumors
  1. Pituitary
  2. Meningioma
    a. Sphenoid
    b. Tuberculum sellae
    c. Olfactory groove
  3. Craniopharyngioma
  4. Third ventricle tumors
B. Aneurysms
  1. Internal carotid artery
  2. Junction of anterior cerebral and anterior communicating arteries
  3. Anterior cerebral
C. Infections
  1. Arachnoiditis
  2. Meningitis
    a. Syphilis
    b. Tuberculosis
    c. Others
D. Others
  1. Trauma
  2. Demyelinating disease (rare)

Anterior junctional syndromes (Fig. 4-9). The neurologic complex that constitutes the anterior junctional syndrome* often produces pupillary defects. Commonly, the lesion affects both decussating fibers of the optic chiasm and one of the optic nerves. In such cases the pupils are usually equal, and the eye ipsilateral to the involved nerve will show a Marcus Gunn response. Also, there is a poor pupillary reaction to light directed from the field of the hemianopia. The pupils react normally to near. These responses can often aid in localization of the cause of the hemianopic reaction.

The causes of this syndrome are similar to those that impinge upon the optic chiasm sagittally or posteriorly:

A. Tumors
  1. Pituitary
  2. Parasellar
    a. Meningioma of sphenoid
    b. Craniopharyngioma
  3. Third ventricle tumors
B. Aneurysms
  1. Internal carotid artery
  2. Junction of anterior cerebral and anterior communicating arteries

---

*Temporal hemianopic scotoma in one eye and superior temporal field defect in the other from lesions at the anterior edge of the chiasm.

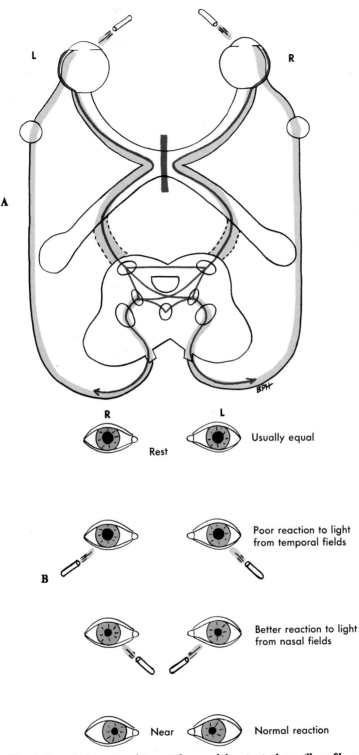

Fig. 4-8. Midline lesion of the optic chiasm. The nasal hemiretinal pupillary fibers are interrupted at the chiasm. Light directed from the temporal fields produces less pupillary constriction than light directed from the nasal fields.

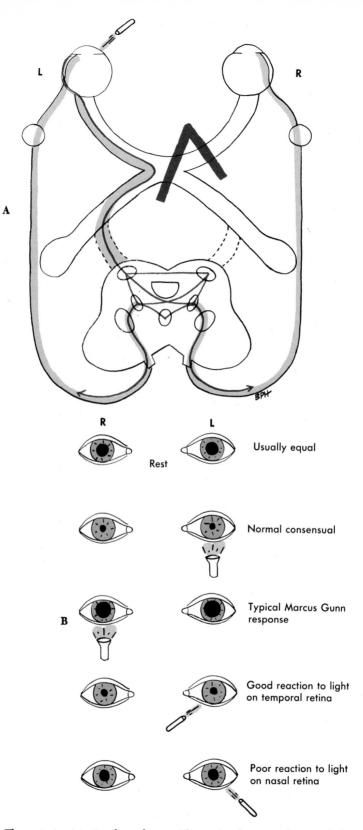

L

R

A

R   L   Usually equal

Rest

Normal consensual

B   Typical Marcus Gunn
response

Good reaction to light
on temporal retina

Poor reaction to light
on nasal retina

Fig. 4-9. The anterior junctional syndrome. The optic chiasm and one of the optic nerves are involved. The right eye shows a Marcus Gunn pupil. The left eye illustrates a chiasmatic hemianopic pupillary response.

Optic tract (Fig. 4-10). In 1872 Wernicke first described "hemianopic pupillary rigidity." Again, this may be a difficult response to elicit but in some cases it is quite apparent. The pupils are usually equal and light directed from the field of the hemianopia produces less pupillary constriction than light from the normal field. Wernicke believed that this response would differentiate anterior tract lesions from those posterior to the exit of the pupillary fibers. A more posterior lesion would not affect the pupils since the pupillary fibers exit from the tract via the superior branchium conjunctivum.

Disease of the optic tract is uncommon, is characterized by incongruous field defects, and may stem from:

1. Tumors: many types, especially of temporal horn
2. Vascular accidents: of anterior choroidal artery
3. Infections: temporal lobe abscesses
4. Degenerations: Schilder's disease

Superior brachium and pretectal areas (Fig. 4-11). The superior brachium and pretectal areas are uncommon sites of clinically recognizable disease but may be the site of pathology in Argyll Robertson pupils. A lesion in this area will have no effect on visual function since it is removed from the optic tracts and radiations, but the pupillomotor input to the midbrain is blocked. However, the pathways for the near reaction from the higher cortical centers, mediated through the oculomotor nucleus, are intact. The clinical picture of the pupil in light–near dissociation as classically described by Argyll Robertson (1869) is:

1. Miosis
2. No reaction to light
3. Normal reaction to accommodation
4. Irregularity of the pupil
5. Unilateral or bilateral with anisocoria
6. Iris atrophy—often sector atrophy, which may account for the irregularity
7. Heterochromia iridis—secondary to the prolonged miosis and iris atrophy
8. Orbicularis reflex often intact
9. Pupil dilates poorly with atropine

The literature shows that Argyll Robertson pupils may be associated with a variety of diseases. However, in over 90% of patients with true light rigidity of the pupil the correct causative diagnosis is syphilis.

Differential diagnosis of Argyll Robertson pupils

1. Syphilis	8. Diabetes mellitus
2. Multiple sclerosis	9. Trauma
3. Encephalitis	10. Herpes zoster
4. Brain tumors	11. Amyloidosis
5. Syringomyelia	12. Tuberculosis
6. Syringobulbia	13. Midbrain abscess
7. Alcoholism	14. Midbrain hemorrhage

Many cases of true unilateral Argyll Robertson pupil (Fig. 4-12) have been reported with characteristics identical to the bilateral disease. Again, the most common diagnosis is syphilis, but herpes zoster ophthalmicus has also been associated too frequently to be coincidental (Naquin, 1954). Some cases later become bilateral.

The site of the lesion has never been proved, but theoretically it would have to block all the pupillomotor input to one Edinger-Westphal nucleus.

The pathway for near is probably spared since it originates at higher levels and is only mediated through the oculomotor nucleus. Unfortunately pathologic data regarding this condition are lacking.

The failure of the pupil to react to near but its normal reaction to light may be called the *inverse Argyll Robertson pupil* (Fig. 4-13). This is very rare and is usually associated with a failure of convergence as well. Hypothetically, a lesion of Perlia's nucleus in the midbrain could produce this clinical picture. Because convergence is usually affected it is most likely caused by a cortical disease, and the failure of the near reaction of the pupil is secondary.

Efferent tract

Fixed pupil (Fig. 4-14). If the Edinger-Westphal nucleus and other portions of the oculomotor nucleus involved with the near

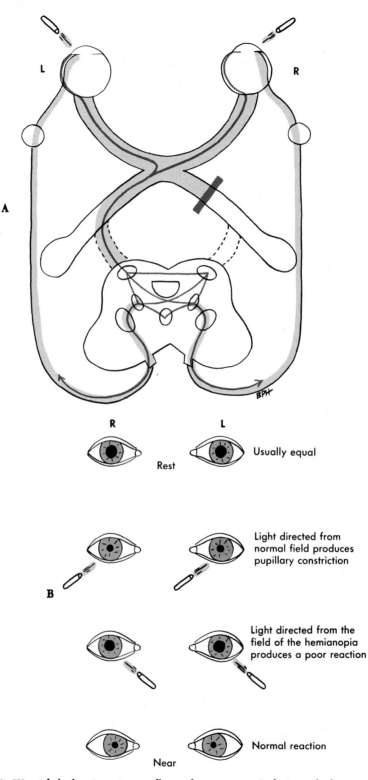

Fig. 4-10. Wernicke's hemianopic pupillary phenomenon. A lesion of the anterior optic tract will involve the pupillary fibers. Light directed from the field of the hemianopia will produce less pupillary constriction than light from the normal field (A and B). If the lesion is at the posterior limit of the optic tract the pupils will be normal (C).

reaction are both affected, a true internal ophthalmoplegia will develop. This is a failure of the pupil to react to light or to near and is accompanied by loss of accommodation. The condition may be unilateral or bilateral.

The local causes of internal ophthalmoplegia in the midbrain are varied:

1. Tumors: many types, primary and metastatic, including pineal tumors (Parinaud's)
2. Vascular accidents
3. Infections: encephalitis, abscess
4. Demyelinating disease: not uncommon (symptomatology in the midbrain is confusing)
5. Trauma

The pupils may also be fixed in other conditions. In midbrain lesions, the fixed pupil is usually dilated. There are other possible sites of pathology that will produce a dilated, fixed pupil.

1. Oculomotor nerve
2. Ciliary ganglion: Adie's pupil
3. Short ciliary nerves: trauma, pressure of acute glaucoma, after scleral surgery
4. Eyeball: trauma, posterior synechia, use of mydriatics and cycloplegics

Miotic fixed pupils are fairly rare but may occur in:

1. Lesions of afferent arc, superior branchium, or tectum
2. Ciliary ganglion (tonic pupil)
3. Eyeball (synechia following iritis or trauma)

In general, dilated fixed pupils occur with disease of the efferent path and miotic fixed pupils occur with disease of the afferent path.

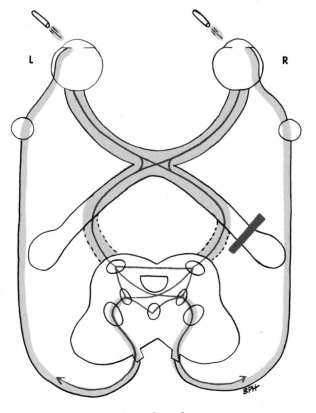

Fig. 4-10, cont'd. For legend see opposite page.

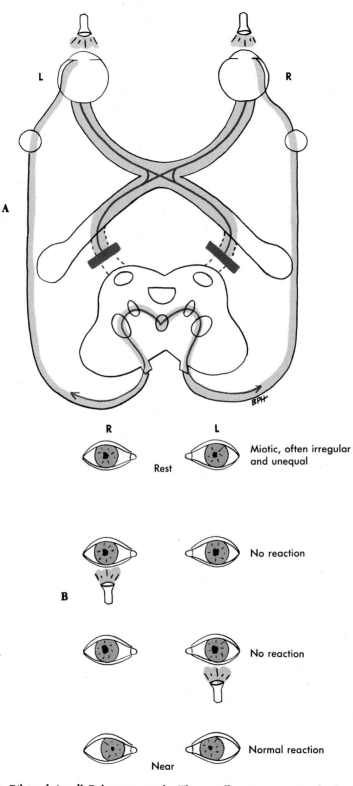

Fig. 4-11. Bilateral Argyll Robertson pupils. The pupillomotor input to the brain is blocked. The light reflex of the pupil is destroyed. The near reflex from higher cortical centers is intact.

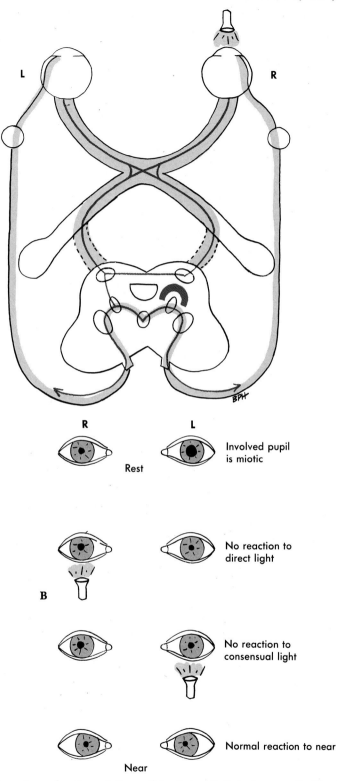

Fig. 4-12. The theoretic explanation of the unilateral Argyll Robertson pupil. The input to one Edinger-Westphal nucleus is blocked. The remainder of the pupillomotor system is intact.

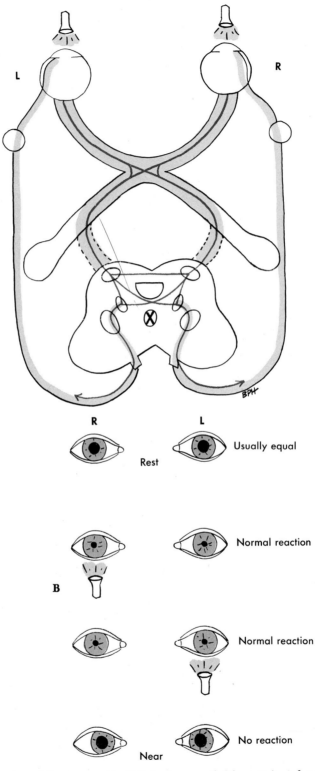

Fig. 4-13. Explanation of the inverse Argyll Robertson pupil (theoretic). A lesion of Perlia's nucleus in the midbrain could destroy the near response of the pupil and spare the light response.

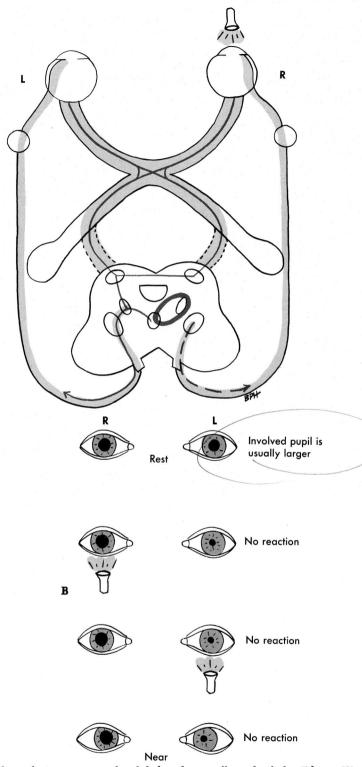

Fig. 4-14. Fixed pupil. A true internal ophthalmoplegia will result if the Edinger-Westphal nucleus and the other portions of the oculomotor nucleus, which are concerned with the near reactions, are affected. The lids and extraocular movements may be normal—as contrasted to third nerve palsy.

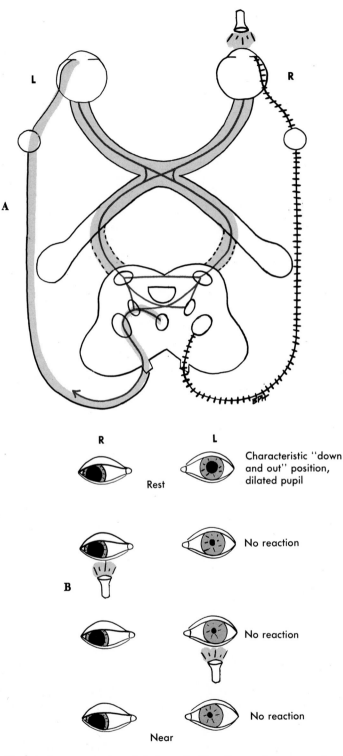

Fig. 4-15. Oculomotor nerve palsy. A lesion of either the oculomotor nucleus or the oculomotor nerve may produce third nerve palsy. There is an internal ophthalmoplegia combined with extraocular muscle disturbance and ptosis.

Oculomotor nerve palsy (Fig. 4-15). A lesion of either the oculomotor nucleus or of the oculomotor nerve may produce a variegated picture of oculomotor nerve palsy, in which the eye deviates "down and out" and the pupil is dilated and fixed. The differentiation of a nuclear from a nerve lesion is often difficult, and it becomes a problem for the neurologist to interpret the associated neurologic signs. The following generalities are diagnostic guidelines:

Oculomotor lesions
A. Nuclear lesions
   1. Rarely unilateral: both eyes usually have some type of disturbance
   2. Paralysis usually incomplete
   3. Pupil may not be involved
B. Nerve lesions
   1. Usually unilateral
   2. Paralysis usually complete except if the lesion is in orbit
   3. Pupil always involved to some extent

In considering oculomotor nerve lesions, the anatomy (Fig. 4-16) of its course offers four differing areas that can harbor discrete pathology: (1) en route to the cavernous sinus, (2) in the cavernous sinus, (3) in the superior orbital fissure, and (4) in the orbit.

The nerve leaves the midbrain in the basilar area and passes between the posterior cerebral and superior cerebellar arteries near the junction of the posterior communicating artery. A lesion in the basilar area will often produce bilateral signs because of the close proximity of the right and left nerves as they leave the floor of the midbrain. In this first area, the following lesions are most probable:

1. Tumors: gliomas and meningiomas
2. Aneurysms: posterior cerebral and posterior communicating arteries
3. Infections: basilar meningitis

The nerve then courses near the edge of the posterior clinoid process, where pathology usually produces unilateral signs, since the nerves are widely separated.

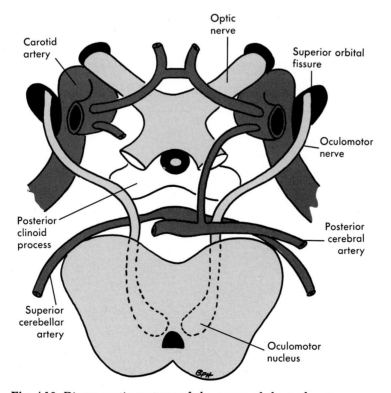

Fig. 4-16. Diagrammatic anatomy of the course of the oculomotor nerve.

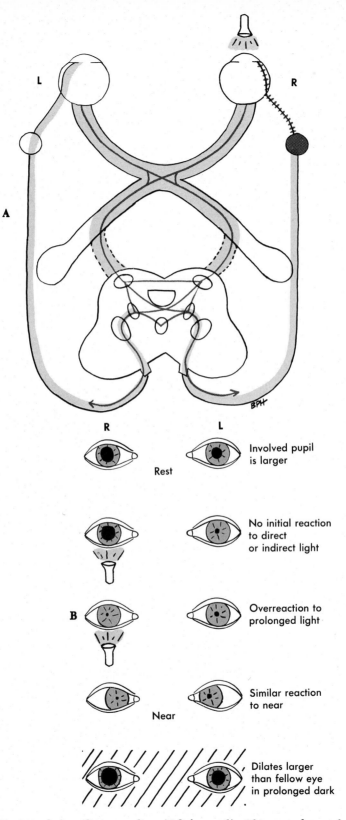

Fig. 4-17. Lesion of the ciliary ganglion (Adie's pupil). This may be confused with an Argyll Robertson pupil, but after prolonged stimulaton it is found to be a tonic rather than a fixed pupil. The methacholine (Mecholyl) test (see p. 67) will help with the diagnosis.

1. Tumors: meningiomas of sphenoid near posterior clinoids
2. Aneurysms: posterior communicating artery
3. Trauma: subdural or subarachnoid hemorrhage

The oculomotor nerve subsequently enters the cavernous sinus close to the trochlear, abducens, and trigeminal nerves and the carotid artery. Lesions within the cavernous sinus often produce oculomotor nerve palsy but with associated signs of damage to contiguous nerves and vessels.

1. Tumors: pituitary, meningiomas, metastatic, nasopharyngeal
2. Aneurysms: internal carotid artery
3. Infections: meningitis, cavernous sinus thrombosis
4. Others: carotid-cavernous fistula

The nerve continues to the superior orbital fissure and passes through to the orbit. In the orbit the oculomotor nerve divides into a superior division to the superior rectus and levator muscles and an inferior division to the medial rectus, inferior rectus, and inferior oblique, which in turn supplies the root to the ciliary ganglion. Pupillary signs in orbital disease are confusing because of the proximity of the anatomic structures. It is almost impossible to predict pupillary reaction from disease in the orbit because of the diffuse nature of the common pathology seen.

1. Tumors
2. Hemorrhages, trauma
3. Infections

All of the preceding lesions are destructive in nature and produce palsy of the nerve. However, there can be irritation of the oculomotor nerve characterized by sudden spastic miosis and lid retraction often followed by mydriasis and ptosis. This is seen early in the course of a massive insult such as meningitis, subdural or subarachnoid hemorrhage, and rapidly expanding aneurysms.

Ciliary ganglion (Fig. 4-17). Further along the efferent pupillary path is the ciliary ganglion. Disease of the ciliary ganglion can produce a myotonic or Adie's

pupil. Both structural and neuropharmacologic changes can cause Adie's pupil. The disease is usually unilateral and primarily affects young women. The typical myotonic pupil is larger than the fellow pupil. On initial stimulation the pupil does not react to direct or consensual light, but after prolonged illumination the pupil slowly constricts, then overreacts. There is a similar reaction to near. Dilation in the dark is also slow, but eventually it is of greater magnitude than the normal eye. The classic work of Scheie (1940) demonstrating the Adie's pupillary response to dilute (2.5%) methacholine (Mecholyl) has helped to differentiate Adie's pupil from the Argyll Robertson pupil with which it may be confused.

Argyll Robertson pupil	Myotonic pupil
Constricted	Dilated
Bilateral	Unilateral
No reaction with 2.5% Mecholyl	Constriction with topical 2.5% Mecholyl
Poor dilatation with atropine, cocaine	Prompt dilatation with atropine, cocaine

Sympathetic system

Horner's syndrome (sympathetic inhibition) (Fig. 4-18). The sympathetic system may be either stimulated or inhibited by a variety of lesions along its pathway. The classic picture of sympathetic inhibition is the syndrome of ptosis, miosis, and anhidrosis described by Horner in 1869. The pupil is reactive to light and accommodation, although the reactions are hard to observe because of the small pupil. A Horner's pupil usually will not dilate in the dark. Other significant signs in Horner's syndrome are seen in the following chart:

Horner's syndrome (ipsilateral sympathetic destruction)
1. Miosis (not pinpoint)
2. Usually unilateral
3. Normal reaction to near but difficult to observe
4. Narrow palpebral fissure
5. Ptosis
6. Enophthalmos (apparent, not real)
7. Anhidrosis and hypothermia of the same side of the face and neck
8. Brittle and dry hair

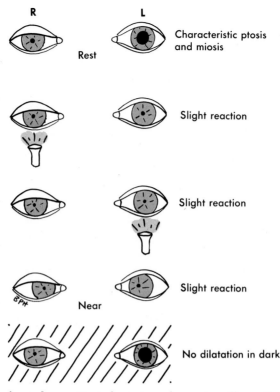

Fig. 4-18. Horner's syndrome. Typical ptosis and myosis will result from interruption of the sympathetic pathway to the eyeball. Usually the extraocular movements are intact.

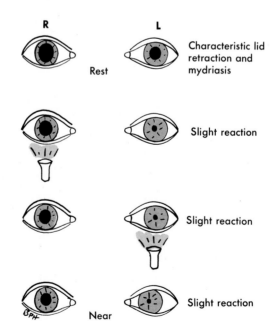

Fig. 4-19. Claude Bernard's syndrome. If the sympathetic path to the eye is stimulated, the physiologic opposite of Horner's syndrome will result. Claude Bernard's syndrome is usually short-lived since the stimulation often progresses to destruction and a Horner's syndrome.

9. Heterochromia iridis (especially in infants; lighter iris on affected side)
10. No dilatation in the dark

Horner's syndrome may be caused by many different lesions between the hypothalamus and the globe along the sympathetic pathway.

Etiology of Horner's syndrome

1. Pons: tumors, hemorrhages, infarcts, syringomyelia
2. Medulla: tumors, hemorrhages, syringobulbia
3. Cord: tumors, hemorrhages, trauma
4. Mediastinum: lung, esophageal and tracheal lesions, aneurysms
5. Neck: trauma (birth, postoperative), lymphadenopathy, aneurysms

The clinical picture produced by most of these lesions is similar, but associated neurologic findings may lead to the etiologic diagnosis. For example, Raeder's paratrigeminal syndrome presents a partial Horner's syndrome along with weakness of the jaw muscles and pain in the face and orbit of the same side. The lesion is often a tumor or aneurysm in the region of the trigeminal nerve and the carotid sympathetic plexus.

Claude Bernard's syndrome (sympathetic stimulation) (Fig. 4-19). A typical picture of sympathetic stimulation is produced by an irritative lesion along the sympathetic pathway. The symptom complex was investigated by Claude Bernard in 1869. The eye has a characteristic appearance of lid retraction and mydriasis, usually unilateral. The pupil reacts to light and near but not fully. The precise localization of the irritative lesion is often difficult, since there are no consistently helpful clinical tests. Associated signs of the syndrome often help in the diagnosis:

Claude Bernard's syndrome (sympathetic stimulation)

1. Usually unilateral
2. Mydriasis
3. Wide palperal fissure
4. Flushing of the same side of the face
5. Hyperhidrosis of the same side of the face
6. Appearance of exophthalmos (not measurable)

There are many possible etiologies of the condition, but few pathologic specimens have been available to demonstrate the causes.

Etiology of sympathetic irritation

1. Occasionally pontine and medullary tumors and hemorrhages
2. Usually apical lung lesions: infections, pneumothorax

Part two

Major disease areas

Chapter 5

The cornea and the sclera

PRELIMINARY INSPECTION

In every special area of examination, just as in the initial examination itself, a brief preliminary inspection must precede more critical and refined steps. The examiner should first note the lids for their texture, correct apposition to the globe, and position of the lacrimal puncta to furnish proper drainage of the precorneal tear film. Chronic infection in the lid borders should be noted for (1) production of irritation, (2) bacterial toxins damaging to the corneal epithelium, and (3) possible source of infection following any surgery. The amount and type of secretions on the lid borders or discharging down the cheek should be recorded. Just as important, note should be made of the *absence* of apparent tearing when the patient primarily complains of this. Clarity or injection of the conjunctiva in its bulbar, cul-de-sac, and palpebral divisions should be recorded for its relation to corneal health. Finally the brightness and clarity or gross vascularization and scarring of the cornea itself should be noted.

Thus the examiner should *not* first turn to the slit lamp without a preliminary flashlight inspection. Examination in direct daylight and the search for orderly reflection (catoptric image) of a windowpane from the corneal surface are too crude to merit any time except in underdeveloped areas of the world or in field conditions where ophthalmic equipment is not available.

Inspection in columnated or narrowed light such as from a penlight now replaces the older examination in "diffused illumination," just as the ever-present slit lamp itself now replaces the former inspection in "oblique illumination." The use of a spectacle-mounted loupe is helpful in preliminary inspection. The intermediate level of the old hand-held or portable slit lamps should be deferred to the full-scale table-based slit lamp, with the one recent exception of the new portable Kowa hand-held apparatus (Fig. 5-1),* which is valuable for mobile units or ophthalmic surveys under field conditions. Gross lesions are noted mentally from this light and loupe inspection.

SLIT LAMP EXAMINATION
Initial steps

The next step is the slit lamp examination. Of the valuable and ubiquitous instruments in ocular diagnosis, certainly the ophthalmoscope (1851) and the slit lamp (1911) are the most fundamental. Without exception, at least one modern model of each must be intimately familiar to every individual who examines patients (or sighted laboratory animals) for visual study or ocular evidence of structural and systemic disturbances.

Of all the laureates who have received the Nobel Prize in medicine and physiology since its inception in 1901, only three have been acknowledged for work directly in the visual field. The first of these was Allvar Gullstrand of Stockholm (1911) for his work in the dioptrics of the eye and his fundamental development of the slit lamp. Since 1911 there have been numerous re-

*Kowa Company, Ltd., Nagoya, Japan.

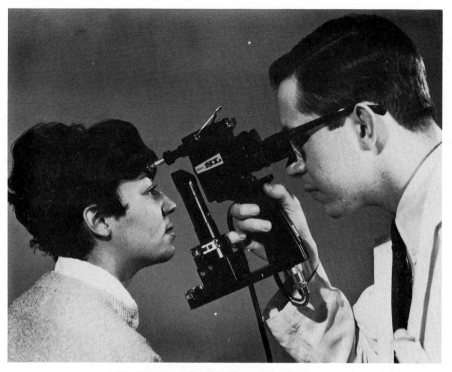

Fig. 5-1. Kowa hand-held portable slit lamp.

finements, enhancements in the illuminating system, and increased mechanical flexibility of the apparatus. Every modern model of the slit lamp, however, is based on the principles of the original Gullstrand instrument.

Before any slit lamp is brought into operation it is essential to ensure that several maintenance steps are observed. Mirrors and lenses must be kept free of dust with lens paper. The individual oculars of the biomicroscope should be focused for each eye of the observer with interpupillary distance adjusted. The proper bulb must be properly centered in its housing, and a spare bulb should always be kept with the instrument (plus a few others routinely kept in the office supply closet). Optimal efficiency is served if the slit lamp is brought to the patient in the principal examining chair without relocating him. Hydraulic, motor-driven, or counterbalanced systems are available for such mounting. When the convenience of a wall mount is used, it is essential (as with a projector chart) to be certain the wall is free of building vibrations.

Reassurance concerning sanitation is imparted by lifting off the topmost paper on the group of disposable chin pads just before the patient puts his head into position. If the patient must be moved to a nearby instrument table, the examiner should step behind the patient's stool to ensure its not sliding backward. He should also extend one hand in front of the foreheadrest so that the patient does not bump his eye while sitting down. The headrest is adjused to a convenient height for the patient, and the examiner accommodates himself to this position.

Some difficulty may be experienced in holding the lids open for corneal examination, particularly elevation of the upper lid for upper pole examination. The lid may be elevated with the thumb of the examiner's hand on the side of the eye under examination. A more delicate technique, however,

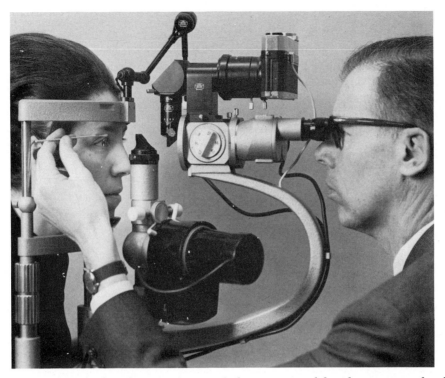

Fig. 5-2. Cotton-tipped applicator technique of elevating upper lid without pressure for slit lamp examination.

is the use of a sterile cotton-tipped applicator to lift the lid by gentle rolling of the applicator tip from the side (Fig. 5-2). This avoids undue pressure on the eye and also avoids contamination of or by the examiner's fingers.

Initial focusing should be done with an intermediate working magnification of about 16×. In the Haag-Streit instrument this is best done by keeping the high power oculars (16×) in place and the changeover lever controlling the objective at low (1×) power. When greater magnification is desired the objectives can be revolved within their holder to 1.6×, yielding a magnification of 25×. On the Zeiss instruments, the rotating drum can be advanced to 25× and rarely to 40× parfocal objectives, all of which are contained within a dust-free housing. Illumination should be kept below the maximum (5 or 6 volts rather than 7.6 volts on the Haag-Streit), which will prolong bulb life about fivefold and be better tolerated by the patient.

Illumination techniques

Examination is classically possible in seven slit lamp illuminating techniques:
1. Diffuse illumination
2. Direct (focal) illumination
3. Retroillumination or transillumination (direct or indirect)
4. Specular reflection
5. Indirect or proximal illumination
6. Scleral scatter
7. Oscillatory illumination

Diffuse illumination utilizes a wide illuminating slit slightly out of focus. It is a more stationary refinement of the preliminary penlight technique, making easily available the greater magnifying range of the microscope (Nikon zoom of 7× to 35×). This affords general localization of larger lesions on the cornea and orientation for more detailed techniques.

Direct or focal illumination is the most generally useful technique. It is achieved by critically focusing the narrowed beam onto the cornea from the right or left, depending on the examiner's habits and personal preference. The line of observation through the microscope can be adjusted from the infrequently desired complete coincidence (in most instruments) through an angular displacement up to 90 degrees.

The light, when sharply focused on the cornea, creates a brightly illuminated parallelepiped, with its anterior face corresponding to the precorneal tear film (closest to the side from which illumination is directed). The posterior face corresponds to the endothelial surface of the cornea and is in horizontal position nearer to the line of observation. Between these two curved faces are three normal lines of discontinuity anteriorly and two posteriorly.

The bulk of the depth between the surfaces is occupied by the stroma, which normally has a somewhat variable relucency. Under high magnification the stroma reveals a few delicately branching nerve fibers. A beautiful optic section of cornea is "cut" as the parallelepiped of illumination is narrowed and observed through an increased (45 to 90 degrees) angular displacement between the light and the line of observation. As the beam is narrowed the total intensity of illumination decreases, and therefore it may be necessary to increase lamp voltage during this step. Depth of lesions can be critically determined in such a narrow section. With higher magnification (18× to 25×) the three anterior lines of discontinuity are distinguished as (1) the precorneal tear film, (2) a darker or more optically transparent epithelial layer, and (3) the brighter or more relucent Bowman's membrane. Deep or posterior to the stroma can be seen the more relucent layer of Descemet and the less distinct endothelial line. This latter line of discontinuity is difficult to visualize in optic section without maximum magnification and illumination; it is more revealingly studied in specular reflection.

Retroillumination (less aptly called transillumination) is achieved by directing the light beam onto an opaque or reflecting surface (such as the iris, a lens opacity, or the posterior capsule) while focusing the microscope on the nearer tissue under study. The irregular reflection of light is particularly advantageous in bringing out corneal vacuoles, corneal bedewing, endothelial precipitates, or corneal blood vessels. When the light can be returned from a lens opacity or even the posterior capsule, this affords the best method of studying iris atrophy or loss of the pigment epithelium; such changes may be inapparent with diffuse or focal illumination. In the lens this may aid definition of small opacities and subcapsular vacuoles.

Color values are generally different in retroillumination than in direct illumination. Thus a minute blood vessel in the corneal stroma appears light gray in direct illumination but much darker when seen in retroillumination. The same is true of endothelial precipitates, asteroid bodies, and many opacities in the vitreous.

In further refinement of this technique, a lesion may be visualized by *direct* retroillumination (when it is precisely in the path of the reflected light) or by *indirect* retroillumination (when it is to one side of this path and therefore viewed against a darker background). This helps to differentiate opaque bodies by their obstructive properties from vacuoles or cystoid lesions that are refractive or dispersive. The former are centrally dark at all times, whereas the latter may appear light in their centers under direct retroillumination but change to bright crescentic edges under indirect retroillumination.

Specular reflection is the most critical of the various techniques and is the prime method for studying the endothelium. Specular reflection on the normally mirrorlike anterior corneal surface is a dazzling reflection and glare to direct ophthalmoscopy, particularly when the pupil is small. When focusing critically on the front corneal surface, this glare area (limited to a small portion of the parallelepiped) may be exploited in a narrow beam to reveal minute anterior corneal pits (concavities) or excrescences (convexities) far too small to be seen in diffuse light.

With the illuminating beam directed on this anterior specular reflection, the endothelial or posterior face of the parallelepiped must be suitably narrowed and medially displaced to avoid overlapping the anterior face. The focusing level of the microscope is then advanced the depth of the cornea to bring into clear view the somewhat darker and slightly golden endothelial surface just medial—or toward the observation line—from the line of illumination. The useful area illuminated in specular reflection is so circumscribed and critical that the reflected rays of light may center into only one of the two objective lenses of the corneal microscope. Therefore many observers, when utilizing specular reflection, prefer to close the nondominant eye, simplifying the focusing of the microscope and conducting this part of slit examination monocularly.

The normal mosaic-like pattern of the large endothelial cells is generally regular and slightly yellowish in tint. Hassall-Henle bodies are evident in the periphery of most adult corneas as nonreflecting areas or dehiscences in the mosaic. When these also involve the central area of the endothelium, this indicates the presence of the very common guttate corneal dystrophy. To examine various areas of the cornea within the circumscribed area of specular reflection, it is usually quickest and easiest to have the patient redirect the position of his eyes so that successive sites can be brought under focus.

Indirect (or lateral or proximal) illumination is obtained by focusing a fairly small beam adjacent to the feature under study and moving the line of observation to a wide angle from the line of light. Translucent deposits, foreign bodies, or similar small lesions stand out as darkened or shadowed areas in brighter surroundings. (This same technique is used with the ophthalmoscope to bring out subtle details in the fundus that would be "washed out" by the brilliancy of direct illumination.)

Scleral scatter utilizes the principle of indirect illumination by specifically focusing the light on the limbus and gaining a large amount of internal reflection and dispersion within the cornea. With properly incident light and a cornea of normal transparency, the entire limbal area seems to light up as a faint halo. Medium rather than high magnification is first used in the corneal microscope, and minute changes in normal corneal relucency or minute lesions are detected as they obstruct or diffract the otherwise uniform light pattern. Under scleral scatter corneal lesions generally appear larger than they are, and subsequent to their identification and localization by this technique they should be studied with higher power and direct illumination.

Oscillatory illumination with a small range of movement under moderate to higher magnification gives alternate direct and indirect illumination and creates changing shadows. This may reveal pinpoint defects in the cornea (also aqueous, lens, and retrolental space) that might otherwise be washed out by more static and diffuse illumination. This also conserves the photosensitivity of the examiner's foveal cones and facilitates his own ability to resolve minute details.

Measurement of thickness or depth (pachometry)

For sequential studies of corneal disease that may lead to thinning (keratoconus, congenital glaucoma, marginal ectasia, high myopia) or thickening (chronic inflammation, endothelial dystrophy, disciform disease, hyaline degeneration, phthisis bulbi), it is helpful to have an accurate record of thickness. At times, precise measurement of anterior chamber depth or lens thickness should be noted and accomplished by the same instrumentation used to measure corneal thickness. Early measurements of this type were derived to establish optic constants of the eye, but there is more practical need for anatomic measurements in relation to disease. Many techniques have been recorded, from refined tricks of inspectional estimation by Vogt,* to ocular micrometers, to complex photographic systems.

The simplest technique is that of direct or subjective slit lamp estimation of a thin optic section viewed at an angle of about 60 degrees. The slit beam length should exceed half the corneal diameter in order to afford comparison of central and peripheral thickness. Normally the central cornea appears slightly thinner than the peripheral cornea, and the maintenance of this relationship suggests an absence of pathology. Significant thickening involving the deep stroma almost invariably creates some wrinkling in Descemet's membrane as the inner curvature is flattened. Actually a lessened amount of Descemet's membrane and endothelium is needed to cover this surface.

A more quantitative method of estimating corneal thickness under the slit lamp is to place a corneal contact lens of known thickness on the eye. This constitutes a reference measurement in the slit beam, and corneal thickness is gauged accordingly.

Systems of corneal measurement are generally based on either the apparent optic depth or the real anatomic depth. Direct optic measurements using a microscope fitted with the Ulbrich calibrated drum (1914) suffer from disadvantages induced

---

*The Vogt technique of estimation (1930) is based on 20× magnification and halving the apparent width of the illuminated optic section because of angulation between the light beam and the line of observation. Thus with an assumed real corneal thickness of 0.6 mm. (Vogt actually erred on the high side with an assumed central corneal thickness of 0.8 mm.), the apparent width of the illuminated section would be 0.6 × 20 ÷ 2 or 6 mm. He would then mentally divide this apparent section into units of 1 mm., corresponding to actual distances of 0.1 mm., for localizing the distance of alterations in the cornea.

by movements of the patient's eyes, refractive distortion, and changes in the observer's accommodation. Anatomic measurements are calculated from optic measurements by formulas based on the average refractive power of the cornea and, in case of anterior chamber depth, the aqueous. High-frequency ultrasound with stand-off transducers offers a new type of reliability in real measurement.

Two recent instrumental refinements have been evolved by Professor W. Jaeger of Heidelberg, Germany (1952), from the astronomic technique of *doublement* utilized by von Helmholtz. These are practical, compact, and efficient slit lamp attachments manufactured by Haag-Streit. Either apparatus is mounted with a single screw atop the eyepiece in the position also used for a camera attachment on the Haag-Streit slit lamp. A single (right) ocular is used; this must be fitted with a 10×, split-image eyepiece. Two different depth-measuring attachments are manufactured. No. 1 measures up to 1.2 mm. for corneal thickness, and No. 2 measures up to 6 mm., as needed for anterior chamber depth.

The principle of measurement is based on doubling by two plano glass plates located edge to edge in front of the right objective and dividing the reflected light entering the microscope. The lower plate is fixed, but the upper plate can be rotated around a vertical axis by turning the scale segment of the device. A vertical diaphragm slit in an arm extending to the left of the measurement device reduces illumination to a thin knife of light and also ensures the predetermined angulation of 40 degrees between the line of observation through the right ocular and the slit lamp beam.

In use, the microscope and slit lamp are firmly coupled at a 40-degree angulation. The objective magnification lever is set to 1×. The slit must be projected perpendicularly to the surface of the cornea at the point of observation with the scale segment set in the zero position. The slit lamp is focused at the apparent center of the distance to be measured. Observations are made monocularly through the right ocular only. The scale segment is rotated to the left or up the scale, thus rotating the upper glass plate until the split images are positioned so that the measuring points coincide. This should be repeated a few times for consistency and then the value recorded.

For measuring the corneal thickness, the scale segment is moved until the anterior corneal or epithelial line in one image is brought into precise alignment with the posterior corneal or endothelial line in the other image. For measurement of anterior chamber depth, it is first necessary to establish the corneal thickness with attachment No. 1 and then, with attachment No. 2, to measure the anterior chamber depth from the reference point of the anterior cornea to the anterior surface of the iris or lens. Corneal thickness is subtracted to give the optic depth of the chamber.

Corrective tables (No. 1 and No. 2) must be used to derive linear measurement from the observed optic figures. Average normal corneal thickness is 1.1 mm. in the near limbal area and 0.6 mm. centrally.

VITAL STAINING OF THE CORNEA AND CONJUNCTIVA

Because the cornea and conjunctiva are both essentially transparent, minute breaks or losses of tissue are often difficult to identify even with moderate magnification. Surface staining becomes of great practical importance in diagnosing epithelial loss and impairments as with abrasions, foreign body injuries, ultraviolet damage, exposure drying, or tear deficiencies. Sodium fluorescein is by far the most practical and widely understood stain. It is used preferably in individual, sealed, dry, sterile paper strips rather than the solutions of years gone by, which were notorious for their growth of *Pseudomonas aeruginosa.*

Where there is a break, a scratch, an avulsion, or an area of devitalization in the corneal epithelium, the immediately underlying Bowman's membrane stains bright green, clearly demarking the extent of defect. Even if no breaks are being sought, the use of fluorescein to stain the precorneal tear film is an asset in thin optic sections to estimate uniformity and thickness of the epithelium, which appears as a dark or nonreluctent band between the green-tinged precorneal film line and the brightly relucent underlying Bowman's glass membrane.

In deep stromal ulceration it should be remembered that Descemet's membrane will not take fluorescein stain, though the stroma does absorb the dye. If excess stain remains in the conjunctival sac for several minutes, it may penetrate the intact epithelium and create a greenish flare in the aqueous. Very subtle staining is often seen better in short wavelength illumination, such as by inserting a cobalt glass filter (Wratten C) in front of the light source.

In injuries or chemical insults involving both the cornea and the conjunctiva, it must be remembered that fluorescein staining in areas of conjuctival epithelial loss will appear yellowish rather than green.

The next most valuable dye is probably a 1% aqueous solution of rose bengal, which keeps indefinitely. This has disadvantages of slightly greater irritability and a tendency of some distress to the patient for pinkish staining of the conjunctiva, lid borders, or even the lid skin that may persist for an hour or two. This dye is particularly valuable to demonstrate early areas of epithelial desiccation from tear deficiencies as in Sjögren's disease. A drop of topical anesthetic should be instilled first and then a small drop or glass rod application of the rose bengal made above the upper limbus. This promptly spreads throughout the lacrimal lake and should be flushed with sterile saline or irrigating solution. If allowed to pool in the inferior cul-de-sac, some punctate rose staining will occur even in normally moist eyes. Positive findings are indicated by fairly intense punctate staining throughout the corneal epithelium and bulbar conjunctiva.

Many other dyes of the aniline and

methylene blue families have been used largely as investigative tools or to aid in demonstration of corneal nerves. These may be quite irritating and are not of practical clinical importance.

CORNEAL SENSITIVITY

Sensitivity to pain, touch, or pressure in the superficial cornea is quite high and manyfold greater than in skin areas. This sensitivity is particularly reduced by lesions in the ophthalmic division of the trigeminal nerve and by the frequent invasion of herpes simplex virus. At least a gross qualitation of corneal sensitivity is therefore clinically important and can be achieved (Fig. 5-3) simply with a teased-out wisp of cotton a few millimeters longer than an ordinary cotton-tipped applicator. The patient should be instructed to look to the opposite side from the eye being tested. The examiner gently keeps the lids separated with the thumb and forefinger of one hand (to avoid undesirably contacting a lash) and then brings the cotton in from a lateral position, nearly parallel to the plane of the iris. This avoids the patient seeing the approach and making a visual avoidance response. When normal sensation is present, a lightly applied touch to either cornea should evoke (1) a blink reflex, (2) slight discomfort, and (3) increased lacrimation.

Quantitative tests of sensitivity were evolved in the past century by such devices as the graded von Frey hairs, but they have been superseded by the more stable and reproducible instruments based on durable nylon threads (Puglisi-Duranti, Boberg-Ans, Olah and Szarbo, Cochet and Bonnet). A simple and practical esthesiometer is that of Luneau and Coffignon,* based on a single nylon filament (Fig. 5-4). The instrument is held like a pencil with the examiner's index finger on the knurled wheel of a rack and pinion mechanism that adjusts the

*3, Rue d'Edinbourg, Paris 8, France.

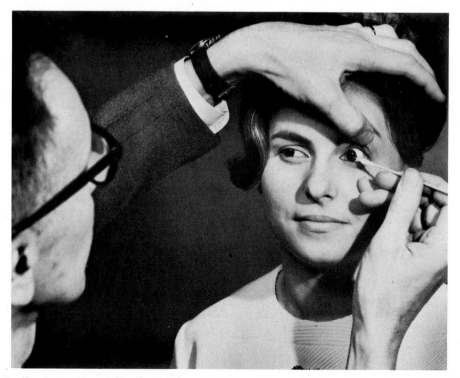

Fig. 5-3. Gross quantitation of corneal sensitivity to cotton wisp advanced laterally and beyond field of view.

exposed length of nylon. The longer the exposed filament, the less the pressure required to bend it. The tip of the filament is brought into perpendicular contact with the area of cornea to be tested, and initially a moderately long (40-mm.) extension of filament is used. The minimum amount of force is applied to cause a just visible bending of the filament. If no sensation is evoked, the filament is progressively shortened until the patient senses the contact. Sensitivity is then recorded as the length of filament. Immediately after use the filament should be completely drawn into the body of the instrument to protect it from accidental damage. Reading of filament length in millimeters (5 to 60) may, as in the reading of an indentation tonometer, be converted by nomograms to contact

values of milligrams per square millimeter.

Sensitivity of the cornea varies greatly in different areas and is highest in the thin optic center. Generally the sensitivity falls progressively from the center to the limbus, but it also is lower in areas of less frequent exposure. Thus the horizontal meridian tends to show greater sensitivity than the vertical, and the lower cornea is more sensitive than the upper, but these variations are only of small percentage difference.

CONTACT LENS DIFFERENTIATION OF VISION IMPAIRMENT BY OPACITIES VERSUS IRREGULARITIES

Visual impairments from corneal lesions are caused both by scars or opacities and

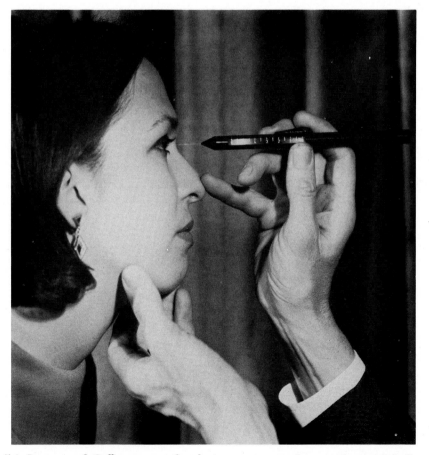

Fig. 5-4. Luneau and Coffignon corneal esthesiometer in actual use with extended filament directed perpendicularly into center of cornea.

by irregularities in the surface curvature. The latter is often underestimated in its amount of contribution to total visual reduction. In such cases vision should also be evaluated with a suitable diameter, plano strength, trial contact lens in place. For this type of trial refraction 1 drop of topical anesthetic should be used—assuming the patient is not in the habit of wearing contact lenses—and then the lens generously moistened with a wetting solution before insertion. Conventional refraction over such a lens in place may yield markedly improved vision, even in the presence of seemingly significant opacities.

CORNEAL CONFIGURATION

Any suspect abnormality found on preliminary inspection and slit lamp examination should be followed by progressively detailed studies. These generally advance through size estimates, curvature estimates, Placido techniques, and quantitative surface measurements.

Corneal dimensions

Viewed from the front, the cornea is slightly elliptic, with its horizontal diameter a little greater than its vertical. Estimates of corneal size render valuable clues to the overriding handicap of microphthalmos or the destructive bulbar enlargements of congenital glaucoma. These two disturbances in size are more frequent and of weightier prognostic importance than the relatively infrequent identification of microcornea or megalocornea, with or without megalophthalmia. The latter structural and optic deviations from normal have refractive and genetic implications but are safely diagnosed at leisure or with the aid of many subtleties of refractional and ultrasonic gear.

Clinical accuracy in corneal measurement cannot extend beyond 1.0 or 0.5 mm. because of (1) the difficulty in defining or identifying limbal limits, (2) irregularities of limbal scleralization, (3) impracticalities of bringing a ruler or caliper into close approximation or contact with the cornea, and

(4) restiveness on the part of pediatric patients, where such measurements are usually most important.

Just as the total eyeball increases much less (about threefold) than the entire body (about twentyfold) from birth to maturity, so the cornea shows very little size enlargement compared to the rest of the globe during this period. Most of the 1 or 2 mm. of postnatal corneal enlargement occurs during the second 6 months of life, and essentially all of it is achieved by the age of 2 years.

The horizontal corneal diameter is the most accessible and therefore the most frequently measured and specified. Normally this is 11 to 12 mm., whereas the vertical corneal diameter, like each of the diameters in the female, is slightly less. This is caused by greater scleral overlap at the vertical than at the horizontal corneal poles. Critical measurement of corneal diameter is not only restricted by vagaries of anatomic landmarks but is clinically far less important than measurement of intraocular pressure, which can be done with high accuracy and which identifies the sinister causative mechanism of corneal enlargement in early life. Small, hand-held, single-tube penscopes or eye gauge magnifiers* are available with built-in metric scales or graticules to facilitate diameter measurements. In use these superimpose the image of the cornea on the scale at the focal length of the lens and afford more repeatable, if not more accurate, measurements than does unaided visual inspection.

Horizontal diameter of 10 mm. or less may indicate simple microcornea or the more crippling hypoplasia of micropthalmia. A horizontal diameter of 12 mm. or more suggests the distending and destructive effects of congenital glaucoma, which affects the entire globe; the simpler megalocornea (macrocornea), which is clear, bilateral, nonprogressive, and almost exclu-

*Western Optical Co. (WO-1005A), Seattle, Washington 98109; Zeiss Jena (60-24-23) Keratometer, Jena, German Democratic Republic.

sively found in males; or else the rare and progressive thinning throughout the cornea designated as keratoglobus.

Topographic inspection is often assisted by (1) lateral examination aligning the observer's view in the plane of the iris to delineate better any abnormalities of curvature (the relatively frequent keratoconus or the progressively more rare megalocornea, keratoglobus, and cornea plana) or (2) inspection from above while the eyes are rotated downward. In this maneuver, the upper lids are retracted with the thumb and forefinger of one hand and the lower lid borders are brought to rest over the horizontal midline of the corneas. The use of the opaque lid border to outline the transparent cornea aids identification of gross disturbances in the anterior surface. Sharply forward or conic angulation as revealed by this technique is referred to as Munson's sign of keratoconus.

Corneal curvature
Normal values

The anterior corneal surface has a radius of curvature (7.6 to 7.8 mm.) slightly shorter than does the rest of the globe. This is particularly marked in the visually important optic portion, which is limited to approximately the central 4 mm. The transitional or peripheral zone is somewhat flatter (longer radius of curvature) though still more acutely curved than the sclera.

The posterior corneal curvature, on the other hand, is steeper, particularly in the central portion where the radius is about 1 mm. less than that of the overlying anterior corneal curve. Thus the high dioptric power (+44 to +46 diopters) of the cornea is actually a magnificently compensated base curve lens. The apposition of these dissimilar curves is associated with a normal central thickness of about 0.5 mm. and peripheral or limbal thickness slightly exceeding 1 mm.

Optic measurements of the anterior corneal surface are more important in the total refraction of an eye than are the measure-

ments of the posterior corneal curve. Both are now increasingly important in prescribing for contact lenses.

The anterior curvatures are easily measured and have received much attention since introduction of Placido's disc of concentric circles (1882) and the application of the old French astronomic measuring principle of doublement* by Louis Javal. This Parisian engineer turned physician devised the first practical keratometer (less aptly called "ophthalmometer") in 1881. Enduringly, the instrument has rightly borne his name and that of his distinguished ophthalmic student, Hjalmar Schiøtz of Norway.

Keratoscope or Placido's disc

Placido's disc can be made in many diameters and gives topographic mapping of the cornea over a wider area than is achieved by Javal-Schiøtz keratometer readings. Currently the most useful and popular model is the self-illuminating, power-handled Klein (1958) keratoscope (Fig. 5-5).[†] Minor irregularities in reflection of the illuminated rings near the corneal center or particularly distorting the horizontal axis suggest early keratoconus. In use, the observer looks through a small diameter plus lens (usually +6 diopters) in the center of the illuminated disc and approaches the patient's eye at the focal distance of this lens (about 3½ in.) until optimal clarity of the reflected image is obtained. The observer then notes the location or degree of distortion as he and the patient maintain fixation through the center of the instrument. To study peripheral areas of the cornea beyond visualization in this primary fixation, the patient is instructed to shift his fixation to a specified edge of the examining disc opposite the corneal area to be studied. This provides (1) a fixation point for the patient and (2) a

*Servington Savary, 1743; Pierre Bouger, 1748; John and Peter Dolland, 1754.
[†]Manufactured by Keeler Optical Co., London, England.

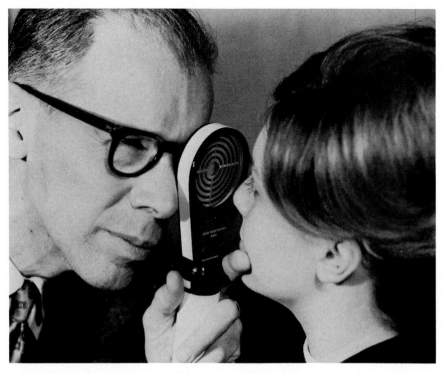

Fig. 5-5. Klein-Keeler keratoscope made on principle of Placido disc of concentric circles. This instrument is self-illuminated. Reflected images from the corneal surface are seen as the observer looks through the center condensing lens.

standard displacement distance that facilitates accurate comparison of corneal areas at later dates. Elegant and expensive photokeratoscopes* are also available for recording such topographic mapping, but they are not necessary for good clinical practice.

Keratometry

Keratometry is the instrumental measurement of corneal curvatures, which for clinical purposes is confined to the anterior surface. It is not ophthalmometry or optometry (though many instruments have been and are marketed under the names "ophthalmometer" or "optometer"), because it does not include measurement of the posterior corneal curvature, lenticular curvatures, and linear distances within the globe that are components of the total dioptric system of the eye. These are measured in summation by retinoscopy, total refraction, or allegedly with instruments such as the Hartinger Coincidence Refractionometer.

Unfortunately the term "keratometer" is sometimes applied to small instruments sold in the aim of more accurate measurement of corneal diameter (p. 82). They may also be used from a lateral position as a vertometer or distometer to measure linear distance between the corneal apex and the back surface of a trial spectacle lens.

Keratometry is based upon (1) the convex mirror characteristic of the cornea, which reduces the size of a reflected object in direct relation to its radius of curvature,* and (2) the astronomic technique of a double-image micrometer or "heliometer" for measuring short arcs (angular distances) in the celestial system. Both in the history of astronomy and in practical op-

---

*Corneoptor Corneagraph, Scientific Advances, Inc., Columbus, Ohio 43228.

*Thus if the radius of curvature is long (or the corneal surface flat), the image of the mire will appear larger. If the radius of curvature is relatively short (or the corneal surface steep), the image will be proportionately smaller.

tics, this measuring system is one of the most accurate ever devised. The illuminated objects used to obtain the double reflections have traditionally been called "mires" from the French astronomic term meaning "meridian marks." Basic components of the instrument are (1) a pair of illuminated mires that can be positioned at precise distances apart on a rotatable arc, (2) a doubling or Wollaston birefringent prism, (3) a compound telescope for observing the reduced images of the mires, and (4) a sturdy base to hold the components and provide rest points for the face of the patient. Literally dozens of modifications have been produced under a corresponding array of eponymic designations. Many of the modifications have concerned configuration of the mires. Demands of corneal contact lens fitting in the last decade have revived usefulness of the keratometer, which ordinarily is not a helpful portion of visual or refractive examination. Many table- or suspension-mounted production models are available.*

In use the eyecap of the observing telescope is first adjusted for the focus of the observer and the height of the chinrest adapted to the patient. Each eye is examined singly, the right eye first. The opposite eye is occluded. The patient and telescope are leveled so that the patient can fix on the reflection of his own eye (in some instruments a fixation light) in the objective lens axis. The examiner then aligns and focuses the optic axis of the instrument on the corneal center with the aid of cross hairs or concentric rings. Focusing of the mires is done by both rotation and adjustments in distance to bring their sharp image on the principal corneal meridian. The mires are then brought into apposition (on

the principal corneal axis or meridian) in accordance with the manufacturer's design of the contact points. The radius of curvature in millimeters may be read from the dial and the meridian or axis similarly noted from another dial. The entire component of mires and telescope is then rotated on its axis 90 degrees to read the second axis of the cornea. The adjustment in mire setting to achieve apposition on this axis gives the secondary radius of curvature. If the two mires are at identical positions on each radius, there is no anterior corneal astigmatism; if they are not equal, the difference between readings on the two axes measures the anterior corneal astigmatism.

All keratometers actually measure radii of anterior corneal curvature in millimeters. Many instruments, however, have imprinted on them conversion values (Tabo scales) suggesting approximate dioptric powers of these radii. This is based on a presupposed refractive index of 1.3375 in the human cornea, which may be either basically imprecise or inaccurate in terms of the eye under study.

There is some inherent inaccuracy in converting keratometric readings to dioptric values, and it is manifestly foolish to convert these figures to corrective cylinder strengths for spectacles. Unfortunately, a "Javal rule" and "Javal table" exist that seek to incorporate an average figure for posterior corneal astigmatism with the anterior corneal reading and then adjust this resultant for forward displacement of 14 mm., presumed to be the average distance from the back of a spectacle lens to the front of the cornea. This is of such limited accuracy that it should be abandoned. Another limitation of keratometry is that readings embrace limited linear distances of only 2.5 to slightly less than 4 mm., which is in proportion to radii of curvature measuring between 6.3 and 9.5 mm. A single pair of keratometric measurements therefore cannot encompass all the variously curved areas of corneal surface from central to limbal.

---

*Bausch and Lomb, Rochester, New York ("Keratometer"); Carl Zeiss, Oberkochen, Germany ("Ophthalmometer"); American Optical Company, Buffalo, New York ("Micromatic Ophthalmometer"); Zeiss Jena, German Democratic Republic ("Ophthalmometer"); and Haag-Streit, Berne, Switzerland ("Javal-Schiøtz Ophthalmometer"). The last two instruments use the three-step mires of the original French design.

Topogometers or toposcopes

Because the Javal-Schiøtz keratometers measure only in a restricted line of about 2.5 to 4 mm. and because the keratoscope of Placido gives a qualitative rather than quantitative reading, there is clinical need for geographically fuller measurements of anterior corneal topography. This is particularly indicated in prescribing contact lenses.

Topogometers are scaled and usually illuminated instruments* often attaching to a keratometer to extend accurate readings from the limited keratometric area throughout both central and peripheral portions of the cornea. With such aid it is possible to map the separate locations of the geometric, visual, and apical centers of the cornea. Of these three, the visual center (on the visual axis) can usually be measured satisfactorily without assistance of a topogometer. Around the apical center there can be identified a *limiting margin* or imaginary line that circumscribes the steepest curvature and beyond which is the progressively decreasing curvature of the *transitional zone*, leading to the flatter scleral curvature.

The Soper Topogometer (1963)† is particularly designed to clamp onto the large cylindrical end of the Bausch and Lomb keratometer just in front of its light housing. It consists essentially of a central fixation light assembly (with switch box and transformer that attach under the keratometer chinrest) and graduated vertical and horizontal decentration scales, each fitted with sliding indicator arms. In use, the sliding arms are initially positioned at zero on both the horizontal and vertical scales, and the patient's eye is directly aligned on the fixation light. This base situation is the same as when the eye is sighting directly on its image for visual center or visual axis readings without the topogometer.

Subsequently the patient continues to maintain alignment on the fixation light.

---

*Volk-Conoscope, Toposcope.
†Manufactured by the Topogometer Co., Houston, Texas 77027.

The corneal curvatures are systematically measured at decentrations of 0.5 to 1.0 mm. as the fixation light (and therefore the visual center) is moved by the sliding arms on the vertical and horizontal scales from the optic axis of the keratometer. After making readings at the visual center, the steepest corneal point or apex is sought and recorded both in millimeters from the visual center and in "K" (keratometric) readings. The horizontal and vertical meridians to each side of the visual center should be surveyed and the "K" readings recorded at significant decentrations, such as the limiting apical margin where flattening first appears. This should be noted by millimeters of decentration in the four principal meridians from the visual center. Measurement of the mean apical curve, plus important plotting of the apical diameter, and corneal diameter (by localization of the "keratometric limbus") greatly assist in fabricating both central and peripheral posterior curves of a contact lens.

TOPOGRAPHIC DIAGNOSIS

The anatomic position of defects and disease in the cornea often gives a specific clue to causative diagnosis. The immediate accessibility of the cornea makes this an easily apparent and recorded localization. The conspicuous, gross topographic considerations of the cornea are those of the frontal or presenting aspect, which is divisible into: (1) limbal, marginal, or peripheral area (superior, inferior, interpalpebral, medial, or temporal), (2) transitional or midzone, (3) central or pars optica, (4) interpalpebral (visible segments of the limbal, midzone, and central areas as exposed between the lid borders), and (5) total. Topographic classification should also be made, particularly with the aid of the slit lamp, in relation to the layer or depth of involvement: (1) epithelium or anterior layer, (2) Bowman's zone, (3) combined epithelium and subepithelium, (4) stroma (anterior, mid, or deep), (5) Descemet's zone, (6) endothelium (mesothelium), and (7) posterior surface (as keratic precipitates, epithelial down growths, or translucent strands).

Limbal, marginal, or peripheral area
Limbal areas generally

The limbal area is the initial site of Mooren's chronic serpigenous ulcer with its pain, relentless progression, characteristically undermined border, and predilection for the elderly. It is also the site of bilateral and symmetric marginal ectasia or gutter dystrophy, which tends to progress slowly and symmetrically to 360-degree involvement; irritative symptoms are minimal.

The common marginal or catarrhal ulcers generally are superficial, small, and usually separated from the limbus by a narrow area of less affected cornea. These may be related to infectious conjunctivitis or to allergic mechanisms. Fuchs' superficial marginal keratitis, which tends to be bilateral and appear after midlife, is more painful, serious, exacerbative, and complete in its encirclement of the corneal periphery. Either of these disease processes may coalesce into the visually destructive *ring ulcer* or a pyogenic deep stromal *ring abscess*.

The malignant changes of epitheliomas and intraepithelial epithelioma (Bowen's disease)—essentially unknown in the central cornea—almost invariably begin here.

Interpalpebral limbus (medial and lateral limbus)

The common white *limbus girdle of Vogt* occurs in the interpalpebral limbus. This delicate, lattice-like marking in Bowman's zone appears in the medial and temporal limbus, usually without symptoms and with no clear cornea between it and the limbus. It appears symmetrically and in increasing percentages of the population with advancing age. Rarely, it seems to be associated with early band dystrophic changes beginning in the interpalpebral corneal periphery and carrying an involutional prognosis. More often band keratopathy begins its untoward course in these

areas and extends horizontally across the cornea with pathognomonic, dark round holes at Bowman's level.

In parts of the world where onchocerciasis is endemic, the punctate keratitis associated with this *thread worm* usually begins its intermittently progressive course here.

Superior limbus

The superior limbus is practically the specific site for vascularization and pannus formation destroying Bowman's membrane in trachoma and leprosy. It is also the site for corneal manifestations of atopic processes such as vernal catarrh or neurodermatitis marked by Trantas points. By definition, it is also the site of superior limbic keratoconjunctivitis.

Vertical (superior and inferior) limbus

The age-related stromal deposits of arcus presenilis, arcus senilis (gerontoxon), or arcus lipoides first appear at the upper and lower near-limbal areas separated by a narrow rim of clear cornea (lucid interval of Vogt) from the limbus. Over many years, these arcuate deposits tend to extend in annular fashion, uniting medially and temporally to form a *circulus senilis*. There tends to be relationship to both familial incidence and hyperlipemia in various fractions. Lesions are generally symmetric in the two eyes.

Transitional or midzone

The transitional ring of the cornea can be identified by its curvature, which is flatter than that of the central or apical portions, but it generally is a subordinate or secondary area both in optic or disease consideration. It is commonly involved with dystrophies or other primarily central corneal disturbances that progress more widely. It is the site of copper accumulation in the deep cornea, which is known as the Kayser-Fleischer ring of Wilson's hepatolenticular degeneration. This is a familial and progressive disease of the cerebral cortex and basal ganglia developing in late childhood or the early decades of life with the striking and symmetric colored corneal rings that begin near the limbus and progress centrally over a distance of 2 to 4 mm.

Salzmann's nodular degeneration, which tends to be unilateral and following previous keratitis, predominantly involves this area through the anterior half of the cornea.

The very rare primary calcareous degeneration of Axenfeld spreads through a similar area of the cornea involving Bowman's zone and the anterior stroma, with similar distribution in both eyes.

Scalloped or map-like opacities associated with cryoglobulinemia involves the deep stroma in this area of the cornea.

Central area or pars optica

The central area of the normally avascular cornea is the furthest removed from the nutritive limbal vasculature and is a vulnerable site for many dystrophic changes and destructive invasion by bacteria and fungi (*Diplococcus pneumoniae, Pseudomonas aeruginosa,* diplobacillus of Petit, *Actinomyces, Candida albicans*). Anteriorly, this is the site of Cogan's microscopic cystic epithelial dystrophy, which has a predilection for healthy adult females. Neutrotropic keratopathies, evidenced by corneal anesthesia, generally begin in the central epithelium with clouding or vesiculation and commonly extend with superficial excavations throughout the cornea. The central area may also harbor the rare superficial reticular dystrophy of Koby, which causes painless and progressive loss of vision.

Mosaic degeneration or "crocodile shagreen" is almost exclusively limited to Bowman's membrane in its central part; it causes progressive visual loss that may be relieved by lamellar keratoplasty.

Somewhat more deeply in the corneal stroma, central lesions are represented by Groenouw's granular dystrophy (type I), lattice dystrophy, and hereditary crystalline dystrophy, which is very slowly progress-

ing and nonirritative. Rarer affections in this area are the central speckled dystrophies of François and Neeten.

In the deep stroma, the localized and nonsuppurative thickening of disciform keratitis follows an irritative course of nearly a year or longer. In the deepest layers of the cornea, dystrophies tend to be widespread rather than axial. Blood staining, however, resulting from hyphema and glaucoma is generally most dense in the central area and is uniformly preceded by some damage to the endothelium.

Interpalpebral area (visible segments of the limbal, midzone, and central areas)

The interpalpebral area of the cornea, again by definition, is the site of *exposure keratitis* of various types. It is particularly affected by actinic trauma (actinic keratitis) from welder's arcs or other sources of ultraviolet rays that are destructive to superficial cells. Chemical contaminants in the atmosphere similarly create identifying patterns of damage because the lids shield the upper and lower poles of the cornea. The usually unilateral, torpid, or sluggish lesions of Dimmer's nummular keratitis just under Bowman's membrane tend to be largely in the interpalpebral area and without conjunctivitis. Similarly, the more conspicuous changes of Sjögren's keratitis sicca affect the exposed interpalpebral area and the inferior corneal pole.

Meesmann's juvenile dystrophy, consisting of myriads of minute punctate opacities in the epithelium, appears in this area usually during the first 2 years of life. The vertical poles at the cornea are usually spared, and the painless, autosomal dominant process causes little visual loss until late life.

Total corneal involvement

Some of the incapacitating dystrophies and diseases that begin in the central portion spread widely throughout the cornea. Groenouw's macular dystrophy type II, seen less frequently than type I, is one of these beginning in the first decade of life, with clouding and surface irregularity in the central area. The process, however, rapidly spreads through all layers and the total area of the cornea, so that by the third or fourth decade there is major visual loss. The disease is an autosomal recessive trait marked by reduced corneal sensitivity and recurrent attacks of irritation and light sensitivity.

Fatty degeneration or corneal xanthomatoma, which occurs bilaterally in adult life, is often associated with increased serum cholesterol and ultimately affects all layers of the cornea.

The ring-like dystrophy of Reis and Bucklers principally distorts and destroys Bowman's membrane, with recurrently painful episodes beginning about the age of 5 and continuing through the second decade of life. Irregular mottling and opacification progress in subsequent decades with marked reduction in corneal sensitivity and in vision.

Lattice dystrophy of Biber, Haab, and Dimmer usually begins in childhood or early adult life with irregular linear opacities in the anterior stroma. The process may particularly involve the central area but spreads through the midzone and often through the periphery. Useful vision may be lost by the age of 40 in association with the increasingly dense opacities.

Keratoconus with its noninflammatory apical thinning usually affects the central area progressively from early adolescent life. It tends to spread through the midzone. Hemosiderin arcs in the epithelium frequently outline the base of the conical area and may form the incomplete Fleischer's ring, which appears as a dirty yellowish green color.

THE SCLERA AND ITS DISTURBANCES

"Do not shoot until you see the white of their eyes."
LEGEND OF THE BATTLE OF BUNKER HILL, JUNE 17, 1775

The sclera or the "white of the eye" derives its name from Galen's introduction of the Greek word meaning "hard." The sclera is a dense, largely inert, and almost acellular supporting coat of the globe. It is composed of elongated fibers that in turn constitute interlacing fiber bundles and lamellae. Their chemistry is predominantly collagenous, though some elastic fibers are found in the periphery of the fiber bundles. The role of the sclera is generally a passive one in local and systemic disease as well as in response to injury. Disorders of the sclera are comparatively rare, and primary diseases of the sclera are exceedingly rare. In common with the completely avascular lens and the normally avascular central cornea, but in sharp contradistinction to the vascular transition zone of the limbus, primary scleral neoplasms are essentially unknown.

Examination of the sclera must avoid easy confusion with disturbances of the overlying *bulbar conjunctiva,* the loosely fibrous and vascular *episclera,* and the fibroelastic condensation known as the *fascia bulbi* or *capsule of Tenon.* Within a few millimeters of the limbus, all of these anatomic layers tend to fuse with the sclera so that anatomic and pathologic differentiations are clinically less significant. Posteriorly, however, they may be separately involved in disease alterations, though inflammations often rapidly involve all the contiguous structures.

An important anterior landmark is the *external scleral sulcus,* which is just proximal to the limbus and which serves as a guide for anterior segment incisions. More important diagnostically is the corresponding *internal scleral sulcus,* whose posterior margin projects forward as the *scleral spur.* Gonioscopically this is seen as a whitish ring into which the anterior edge of the darker ciliary body normally inserts. The internal scleral sulcus is not specifically identified on gonioscopy because of the overlying trabecular meshwork.

The sclera varies widely in thickness at different areas within a normal eye, with changes of age, with physiologic differences among individuals, and with pathologic alterations. The thinnest and weakest area of the sclera is the posterior foramen, spanned only by delicate fibrils of the *lamina cribrosa* in order to permit exit of the optic nerve fasciculi. Here is where the increased intraocular pressure of glaucoma first causes pathologic distension. The sclera is also normally thin (about 0.3 mm.) in the areas proximal to insertion of the rectus muscles.

Beyond the age of 50 there is a widespread and increasing incidence of symmetric thinning and hyalinization just anterior to the horizonal rectus muscle insertions. These are asymptomatic and translucent *senile hyaline plaques* that permit the underlying darkness of the choroid to show through. The overlying bulbar conjunctiva is not involved and the plaques are only of cosmetic concern.

Another physiologic finding that occasionally misleads the unwary examiner is the presence of intrascleral nerve loops of Axenfeld (1902), which appear as two or three small dark spots beneath the bulbar conjunctiva 3 or 4 mm. from the limbus. These are branches of the long ciliary nerves that usually carry with them a few pigmented chromatophores from the suprachoroid or the cellular inner layer of the sclera, known as the lamina fusca sclerae. They are nearly always located superiorly and disclosed on elevation of the upper lid where they might be mistaken for foreign bodies. They occur rarely in other quadrants, and nearly always their true nature is confirmed by the presence of a single small blood vessel radiating from them.

Myopia in its progressive and higher degrees is commonly associated with scleral elongation and thinning that can be verified by ultrasound biometry. At times this may be visualized along the equator of the globe as increased transmission of the dark blue choroidal color through thinned sclera.

In logical extension of this alteration, the sclera may present serious pathologic stretching or ectasia diffusely or in localized portions. Outward movement of the

underlying choroid and ciliary body into such areas creates the ominously dark *staphylomas* of adult life, which may cause retinal detachment or even perforation of the globe. Such staphylomas when present anteriorly or as intercalary lesions (between the iris and ciliary body) are more viciously progressive than are similar defects at the equator.

Inflammatory disturbances of the sclera generally represent collagen systemic diseases of obscure origin and should be provisionally described by their morphology as: diffuse or brawny scleritis, deep scleritis, nodular scleritis, anterior scleritis, annular scleritis, sclerokeratitis, necrotizing scleritis, posterior scleritis, scleromalacia perforans, and so on. More superficially there may be nodular episcleritis or episcleritis fugax. More posteriorly there may be sclerotenonitis or tenonitis with its painful effects on attempted rotation of the globe. Rarely there may be true pyogenic or bacterial scleritis from extension of similar enophthalmitis or exogenous agents ranging from the common *Staphylococcus* and *Streptococcus* to the granuloma-producing organisms of tuberculosis, syphilis, or leprosy.

In the presence of suspect pyogenic infections, attempts should be made at identification of organisms by smears and cultures.

Masses appearing as granulomas in the sclera or on the scleral surface may at times be extensions of intraocular malignancies such as malignant melanoma of the choroid, which is the most common intraocular malignancy. This usually represents advanced and neglected disease with preceding visual loss and growth through the small scleral emissary channels that normally transmit nerves and vessels. The basic diagnosis is clearly suggested by ophthalmoscopic discovery of a large single or multilocular dark tumor mass within the eye. Ultrasound will show a solid pattern of irregular echoes throughout such a mass.

Pigmentation or color changes in the sclera present accentuated values because of its normally alabaster white coloration. The inertness of the sclera precludes it from early participation in most diseases accompanied by biologic staining. Jaundice is commonly associated with yellow coloration over the white of the eyes resulting from bile pigment deposits. Careful examination with the slit lamp reveals that such color changes, like those of argyria or silver staining, are overwhelmingly confined to the bulbar conjunctiva and are merely rendered more conspicuous by the white scleral background. This is confirmed by noting that the maximum amount of discoloration is located peripherally or in the fornix areas rather than in the near limbal region.

Blue sclerotics represent a congenital and hereditary abnormality of the sclera and other connective tissue. The sclera has increased translucency and may at times be thinned, causing the blue color of the choroid to show through uniformly. This is not a pigmentary abnormality. The anomaly is associated in a high percentage of patients with multiple fractures, deafness, and joint dislocations.

Ochronosis (congenital alkaptonuria) is indicated by bilateral and generally symmetric patchy deposits of yellow greenish pigment in the interpalpebral sclera and episclera. Associated darkening and discoloration in the cartilage of the pinnas and the nose is seen in the third or fourth decade of life (though it may appear either earlier or later) and tends to be progressive. This usually causes no visual difficulty.

Chapter 6

Ocular motility

Ocular motility examining techniques encompass study of both the sensory (afferent) components and the motor (efferent) components. Therefore ocular motility is actually a subdivision within the neuroophthalmic examination. This embraces afferent pathways along cranial nerves II (visual and pupillary) and V (corneal, conjunctival, and lid sensitivity). Efferent pathways are along cranial nerves III (oculomotor), IV (trochlear), VI (abducens), and VII (facial). Examining routines and techniques are identified by legions of literature and enormous eponymology, reflecting inherent inadequacies in the peripheral approach (muscles, tendons, and fascia) to what is far more frequently a central problem (vision, binocularity, fusion, and motor control). This attack via the end-organ has perforce characterized strabismology from the birth of modern ophthalmic study up to the findings of recent decades from investigations into electromyography, electroencephalography, better sensory diagnostics, and developmental neurology of lower primates.

Many diagnostic tests duplicate or overlap in their spheres of usefulness. In general, the simplest and most physiologic maneuver should be selected to minimize introduction of abnormal or instrumental conditions. Thus the Bagolini striated glass is preferable to the multiple Maddox rod because it maintains more usual or physiologic conditions for vision.

PRELIMINARY GENERAL INSPECTION

Preliminary general inspection in the area of ocular motility presupposes the examiner's full understanding of ocular and orbital anatomy and should note (1) activity pattern of the patient (hyperkinetic pattern in children, head-nodding in infants, aimless movements of the mongoloid patient), (2) normal versus abnormal head and cervical spine positions (usual freedom of cervical motion, contracture of a sternomastoid muscle, ankylosis or deformity of the spine), (3) gross positioning of the eyes (apparently normal versus internal deviation, external deviation, and so on), (4) presence of chronic ocular movements (pendular nystagmus in severe congenital impairments of vision, jerk nystagmus in central and vestibular lesions, vertical nystagmus in subtentorial lesions, random movements of blindisms), (5) position of the lids (protective ptosis in acquired diplopia, levator impairment associated with localized muscular dystrophy involving the superior rectus, lid lag in hyperophthalmic Graves' disease).

PRELIMINARY OCULAR INSPECTION

Preliminary ocular inspection in the primary position of gaze (direct or straight ahead) establishes the following points.

Usual positioning of the face and head. Position of the head should be checked for normal attitude versus chin-lifting in ele-

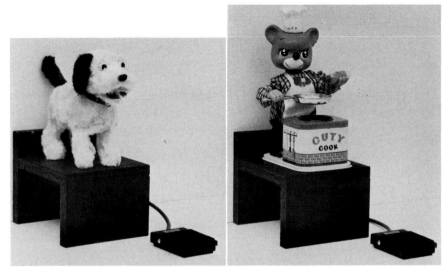

Fig. 6-1. Electrically activated and illuminated remote fixation devices to attract attention of child. Foot control illuminates eyes and activates components of each toy. (Made by Jenkel-Davidson Optical Co., San Francisco, California 94119.)

vator paralyses, face-turning in abducens palsy, and head tilt in oblique impairment.

Anatomic characteristics of the orbits influencing strabismic appearance (pseudostrabismus). The factors influencing pseudostrabismus include facial or orbital asymmetry, hypertelorism simulating exotropia, epicanthus simulating esotropia, small interpupillary distance also simulating esotropia, traumatic deformities, disturbances of tumors or possible tumors, enophthalmos following orbital floor fractures, and vertical asymmetry simulating vertical imbalance.

Angle kappa. Much of preliminary ocular inspection is based on observation of the corneal light reflex, the reflection of the examiner's inspection light held in front of the patient. The corneal light reflex (reflection) generally appears on the shiny cornea of the normal eye in its visual or fixation axis. For practical clinical purposes the visual or fixation axis is the principle visual line that extends from the object of regard, through the corneal light reflex, to the fixating portion of the retina (normally the fovea). The examiner must estimate the angle formed between the visual axis and the apparent pupillary center or pupillary axis. This is usually designated as *angle kappa*. Rarely are the visual and pupillary axes the same, at which time angle kappa is zero.

When the corneal reflex is slightly nasal to the pupillary center or pupillary axis, the angle kappa is positive.* A positive angle kappa of 3 to 5 degrees may be physiologic in emmetropia, whereas higher degrees of angle kappa are seen in hyperopia. Light

---

*Of the series of angles in strabismometry, angle kappa (between the visual axis and central pupillary line) is the most important (Landolt, 1878). This is a familiar and practical approximation of what in more precise terms is the angle between the optic and fixation axis (angle gamma) at the center of rotation, but the optic axis is essentially impossible to locate clinically. Academic minutiae in definition of the optic axis (the theoretic line through the centers of curvature of all refracting surfaces), the visual axis (line from fixation point through nodal points to the fovea), and the fixation axis (line from the fixation point to the center of rotation) have led to theoretic and insignificant clutter of the literature with designations such as angle alpha (angle at the anterior nodal point between optic and visual axes) or the less familiar angle lambda of Glenn Fry (a clinical expression for angle kappa).

reflex temporal to the pupillary axis, which may be seen in myopia, is called negative angle kappa.

Positive angle kappa tends to simulate slight divergence or exodeviation, while negative angle kappa may simulate slight convergence or esodeviation.

Angle kappa, for practical clinical purposes, is adequately measured by the examiner's estimation. More precise measurements may be made, if desired, objectively in degrees on an arc perimeter or subjectively in a major amblyoscope using slides with horizontally aligned targets at 1-degree intervals. Usual practical needs of measurement are served by the examiner's direct visual estimation of the distance between the apparent pupillary center and the corneal light reflex seen in monocular fixation. Normally the right and left angles kappa are essentially equal unless there is marked anisometropia. Thus if loss of fixation ability precludes measurement of angle kappa in one eye, it may be estimated from measurement in the isometropic opposite eye.

Estimation of fixation. Gross estimation of the fixation pattern of each eye to a stimulus such as a small light bulb or for young children a small animated toy or squeaker (Fig. 6-1), is made with both eyes open.

Fixation may be:
1. Normal, centric or foveolar, and binocular
2. Normal but influenced by significantly positive (simulating exodeviation) or negative (simulating esodeviation) angle kappa
3. Unilateral
4. Eccentric (caused by strabismic amblyopia, macular lesion, displaced or ectopic macula)
5. Alternating
6. Absent or nonfixing, as in a blind eye

In the cooperative adult and older child showing the second through the fourth types of fixation as estimated by the corneal light reflex, it is often helpful to clarify these patterns by Visuscopic or Projecto-scopic measurements of fixation targets projected on the fundus (pp. 101-102).

Evaluation of deviation. Gross evaluation of deviation of the eyes from parallelism is observed objectively by the position of the corneal light reflex.

Cover test for each eye to detect heterotropia

The simple qualitative cover test is a refinement in observations of the corneal light reflex and should be the examiner's first, and almost automatic, maneuver following preliminary inspection. With a fixation light in one hand and facing the patient frontally for careful observation of the corneal light reflexes, the examiner brings an opaque cover, held in his other hand, over one eye. The test presupposes fixation ability in each eye. If the *uncovered* eye makes a movement of redress or realignment to the fixation light, this eye has been deviating (in a direction opposite to its movement of realignment) and is now taking up fixation. If a deviating eye is covered, there will be no movement of the fixing eye. Therefore the test must be applied to each eye in turn while the fellow eye is under observation. An accommodative target or stimulus must be used in near range testing.

If there is no movement of either eye while *uncovered,* there is good binocular balance (relative orthophoria) or anomalous retinal correspondence of the harmonious type.

The test is more critical and diagnostic in near than distance range, but it is preferably recorded also with the aid of a fixation light at least 20 ft. away, because some deviations appear only at distance. Though the test is useful at every age, small deviations of a few prism diopters or so may not be detected and will require further diagnostic refinements of the subjective type, which are generally not possible until the age of 4 or 5 years.

This cover test may also be executed in each of the other eight cardinal positions of gaze to elicit deviations not apparent in the primary position. It may be used to separate *primary deviation* (that of a squinting eye while behind the cover or while it is not fixing) from *secondary deviation* (that of a nonsquinting eye while behind the cover or while the paretic eye is forced to fix).

Cover-uncover test to detect heterophorias

The cover-uncover test is an immediate extension of the cover test, predicated upon fixation ability in each eye. However, attention is given here to the covered eye *as* the cover is removed, rather than to the uncovered eye. In this test the cover serves to disrupt fusion and thereby a heterophoria or latent tendency to squint may be revealed by deviation of the eye under cover.

Each eye is tested separately. Careful observation is directed to the eye as its cover is removed. If the eye under cover has not deviated, relative orthophoria is present; if the eye moves in recovery of fixation, heterophoria is present. For example, if the eye moves outward to fixate as the cover is removed, an esophoria is present; if the left eye moves downward to fixate, then a left hyperphoria is present. Again, though applicable at all ages, this rather primitive dissociation procedure may miss small heterophorias, particularly in the vertical direction, but these can be elicited in patients older than 5 or 6 by subjective tests such as the Maddox rod test (p. 106).

Estimate of rotations

"Just what to look for almost defies description and there is no substitute for experience."

RICHARD SCOBEE, 1947

Techniques

Just as soon as the estimates of fixation and gross evaluation of deviation have been made, the examiner assesses the rotational ability of the eyes. Required equipment consists only of a fixation light, an occluder (often most easily the examiner's hand), and a near or accommodation target carrying print or small figure details.

Quantitation of rotation is usually done by one of three techniques: (1) visual approximation based on the Hirschberg estimate of corneal light reflex displacement, (2) measurement of the fixation field based again on position of the corneal light reflex but with more precise localization on an arc perimeter, or (3) prism cover neutralization test. The first method is obviously most simple, appealing, and rapid. It fails to quantitate minute degrees of deviation, but such specificity in a variable and fatigable neuromuscular feat is of doubtful validity. The arc perimeter adds more critical evaluation in units of approximately 5 degrees and may also be used to standardize the selected distance from the primary position for reproducible positions in which to measure. This is far more time consuming than the Hirschberg estimate and requires a quiet and attentive child.

The orthoptically traditional and venerated neutralization of deviation in the cardinal positions with prism and cover yields specific numbers in terms of a few prism diopters. Such measures usually have their significance eroded by (1) vagaries in patient attention and effort, (2) influence of fatigue or medical factors, (3) mechanical difficulty in keeping the back surface of the prism perpendicular to the visual axis, (4) alterations in prism strength by tilting, (5) manual problems of properly holding horizontal and vertical prisms when both are needed, and (6) compounding errors in each of these items as the need for prism strength exceeds 20 or 25 diopters. The comic term "FFP" test (fist full of prisms) was born with reason.

Diagnostic positions

In addition to preliminary ocular inspection in the primary or straight-ahead position of gaze, the other eight *principal* or *diagnostic* positions of gaze must be utilized. This evaluates each of the twelve extraocular muscles in the six specific directions of their maximum action (right, left, up and right, down and right, up and left, down and left) and in the two functionally important positions of straight up and straight down.

Versions

Versions are conjugate or yoke movements of the two eyes executing gaze directions in response to normally equal innervation (Hering's law, 1879). These are commonly evaluated first as the patient fixes with his nondeviating or preferred eye, if one is preferred. The patient is asked to follow, or with small children hopefully to be attracted to, a small inspection or fixation light. This enables the examiner to gauge the position of the eyes by maintaining a close watch on the corneal light reflexes, rapidly alternating his own observation from the patient's right to left cornea. The primary position of gaze is straight ahead with remote fixation.

Versions are commonly designated (1) dextroversion (right gaze), (2) levoversion (left gaze), (3) supraversion (straight-up gaze), and (4) infraversion (straight-down gaze). These move the eyes into "secondary" positions. A "unitized" name is not available for the equally important oblique rotations of gaze: (5) up and right, (6) down and right, (7) up and left, and (8) down and left. These move the eyes into "tertiary" positions. It is necessary to examine in each of these positions. If the corneal light reflex on either eye appears to slip forward of the visual axis in the direction toward which rotations are being tested, then that eye is not rotating fully with its fixating fellow eye.

After testing with the preferred or nondeviating eye fixing (to quantitate the *primary* deviation), an attempt should be made to repeat these same eight rotations with the nonpreferred or deviating eye fixing (to quantitate the *secondary* deviation). To achieve this, it may be necessary to cover the preferred eye briefly or even intermittently. In comitant, nonparalytic, or older and compensated paretic heterotropia, the primary and secondary deviations will be essentially the same. In paretic heterotropia, secondary deviation (of the

nonsquinting eye) will exceed primary deviation. Where only small and uncertain inequalities exist between amounts of primary and secondary deviation, intermittent cover helps to bring out these measurements.

Cycloversion. The two types of cycloversions (dextrocycloversion and levocycloversion) are named by the rotation of the upper corneal poles. Torsional concomitant squints or cyclotropias are exceedingly rare, usually difficult to quantitate, and may escape detection unless special studies are made on a major amblyoscope.

On the basis of supranuclear lesions there may be gaze impairments related to the type of version stimulus. Thus versions in response to *command* may be impaired by a lesion in the descending pathway from the midfrontal convolutions. Versions in response to *attraction* may be impaired by lesions in less well-defined pathways from the occipital lobes. Versions in response to *following* apparently represent the lowest level of internuclear coordination and may persist in the absence of both command and following versions.

A and V patterns. Particular attention should be given to variations in amount of horizontal heterotropia on execution of versions straight upward (supraversion) and straight downward (infraversion). For standardization in evaluation of these two important diagnostic positions of gaze, it is desirable to make the upward measurement about 25 degrees above the primary position and to make the downward measurement about 35 degrees below the primary position. Normally there is a slight tendency for increased convergence in infraversions and a slightly greater tendency to increased divergence in supraversion. Measurement of A and V patterns at distant fixation eliminates accommodative components that may confound diagnostic findings at near. To do this, the examiner tilts the patient's face upward or downward to obtain, respectively, depression or elevation of gaze while maintaining fixation on a small light source at least 20 ft.

away. Near testing of an esodeviating patient in these positions should be with an accommodative target to bring out maximum overconvergence. Similarly, to elicit the maximum cosmetic deviation when testing an exodeviating patient, a nonaccommodative target or light should be used.

The A or V pattern may be present with or without horizontal deviation in the primary position. Strong V esotropia in downward gaze may be accompanied by habitual chin-tucking, particularly in the reading position, to avoid the convergent area. Significance probably should not be attached to variations with horizontal position in supraversion and infraversion unless a difference of at least 15 or 20 prism diopters is found with V esodeviation or V exodeviation. Similarly there should be a difference of at least 10 prism diopters in establishing A esodeviation or A exodeviation.

The A or V pattern, with or without horizontal deviation in the primary position, must be identified because of symptoms it may produce, compensatory chin-tucking or chin elevation that may be used by the patient, and difference in surgical correction that may be required. A and V patterns will commonly be found in association with disturbances of the oblique muscles, which will require correction in their own right. Thus the inferior oblique muscles, which act as abductors in upward gaze, tend to decrease esotropia or to increase exotropia in supraversion if these muscles are overacting (or if the superior oblique muscles are underacting). When specific abnormalities are not present in the oblique muscles, it may be necessary to correct these patterns by supraplacement or infraplacement of the horizontal recti, according to the precise diagnosis established. In general these patterns will be found to be symmetric and therefore require symmetric surgery. Supraplacement or infraplacement of the horizontal muscles in recession correction will be in the direction where most correction is desired. Thus in a V esotropia without oblique muscle defects, it is usually indicated to combine the recession surgery with infraplacement.

Observation should be made for antimongoloid slant (outer canthi downward) of the interpalpebral fissures, because this is frequently associated with V pattern.

Vergence

Vergences are disjunctive or disjugate movements in which the two eyes move in opposite directions. Clinically the most significant, the most demanding, and the most easily measured are the horizontal vergences: divergence and convergence. These relate to two major and frequent motility problems, divergence excess and convergence insufficiency. The first, a common disturbance in children, should be evaluated by directing the patient to remote fixation by looking out a window at a landmark several miles away. This effect is enhanced by the brightness of a sunny day and is significantly masked by examination in a dimly lighted room at a test distance of 20 ft. or under. Measurement is best accomplished by noting the position of the corneal light reflexes.

Convergence should be measured at the reading distance of about 13 in. by determining the near point of convergence (NPC). It is essential to use a finely detailed target commanding the patient's focusing effort in the near range. The patient must wear his distance spectacle correction. Convergence is usually increased by (1) tonic factors, (2) accommodative efforts, (3) the proximal stimulus (nearness to an object), and, in some people, (4) voluntary effort.

The NPC is influenced by the interpupillary distance, requiring less convergence effort when this distance is small and more when it is large. Theoretically, therefore, the NPC should be measured from a convergence base line that connects the centers of rotation of each eye. For practical purposes this base line is equal in length to the interpupillary distance when the eyes are in the primary position, but it is located about 13 mm. posterior to the corneal apices. Measurements made from the nasal bridge should therefore have added to them an amount to compensate for the height of the bridge anterior to the corneas, plus the additional 13 mm. In clinical testing, a small accommodative target is advanced toward the patient along a ruler edge (Prince, Duane, Gulden, Foster) extending from the bridge of the nose. The examiner watches both eyes of the patient for the first evidence of one breaking from convergence (moving laterally); this represents the NPC. An intelligent patient may also be instructed to report the moment the target appears to double; this will confirm the measurement.

Generally, each eye adducts similarly in response to convergence stimuli. The NPC should be expressed in millimeters and is significant primarily when interpreted in the light of age, refractive errors, and horizontal imbalance. As a rule of thumb, the NPC is normally less than the near point of accommodation for the single emmetropic (or corrected) eye and about equal to the interpupillary distance.

Analysis of vergences should also note and record the infrequent vertical divergence when present. These are right sursumvergence (right eye higher), sometimes called positive vertical divergence, and right deorsumvergence (right eye lower), sometimes called negative vertical divergence. Near versus distance fixation generally has no effect on vertical vergences. In conjunction with change from distance to near, or from primary position down to the reading position, there may at times be significant cyclovergences. If the upper corneal poles rotate nasally, this is incyclovergence (conclination or adtorsion), and if the upper corneal poles rotate laterally, this is excyclovergence (disclination or abtorsion). Infrequently, this is important in the presence of a high cylindric refractive correction, which must be prescribed at different axes in separate pairs of glasses for distance and near use. Cyclovergences and cyclotropias can be best measured with the major amblyoscope but can also be quantitated with the Maddox double-rod procedure (red and white Maddox rods placed before each eye while looking at a bright light source).

Prism vergence, or ability to maintain single binocular vision against increasing

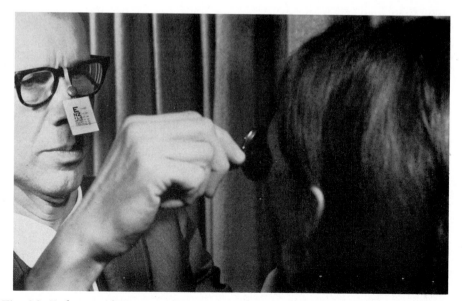

Fig. 6-2. Technique of measuring horizontal prism vergences with near fixation targets suspended on bridge of examiner's spectacles. Risley rotary prism is held horizontally to measure base-in or base-out prism power.

prismatic obstacles (base-out for convergence, base-in for divergence), is another quantitative measuring technique. However, it is largely an abnormal or instrumental hurdle and may relate more to comfort factors in sustained near work than to precise diagnostics in motor aspects of fusion (Fig. 6-2).

Ductions (active and passive)

Ductions are monocular rotations evaluated in each of the six directions of maximal action corresponding to the six extraocular muscles. The fellow eye must be occluded to minimize any inhibitional palsy from that eye. Ductions are generally less diagnostic than versions because each muscle has approximately 100 times more strength than is needed to move the globe (Lancaster, 1941). Thus, a significant number of muscle bundles may be knocked out, and ductions still appear fairly normal. Measurement may be made by estimation from the corneal reflex or by perimeter arc determination of the fixation field. Such fixation fields are of significance primarily in comparison with those of a fellow eye.

Active ductions on command or following provide limited information and need not be done routinely, but passive or forced ductions with forceps under topical or general anesthesia are of highly specific value in differentiating an innervational paralysis from a mechanical obstacle to rotation (such as an adherent superior oblique tendon sheath or incarceration of an inferior oblique in an orbital floor fracture).

In planning surgical procedures for reoperations, the analysis of rotational limitations on forced duction is often crucial to successful correction. Similarly, as the planned surgery is executed at the table, reevaluation of forced ductions will indicate the effectiveness of the procedure or the necessity of additional steps. If the surgeon cannot rotate the globe in forced ductions following a corrective intervention, certainly the patient will be unable to do so.

To test forced ductions in most adults, a topical anesthetic must be instilled several times. The patient is instructed to look in the direction to which the eye under examination is to be moved. A toothed forceps is used to engage the conjunctiva and episclera near the limbus, and effort is made to rotate the globe by direct mechanical action. Generally children will not tolerate this procedure. Many adults will complain of discomfort, and usually a small conjunctival hemorrhage remains for a few days at the site of forceps application.

Forced ductions are more easily and reliably performed under general anesthesia, which excludes voluntary eye movements and eliminates pain. Under these conditions firm fixation can be made with the forceps into the tendinous insertion of one of the rectus muscles. Alternatively, pressure can be exerted with the broad portion of a squint hook into the conjunctival cul-de-sac in line with the direction of action of the muscle under examination. This also tends to produce a series of small conjunctival hemorrhages in the area of pressure application.

Recording rotations

Methods or schema of recording rotations are almost as numerous as the population of strabismologists. A simple diagram should be part of every record and should indicate increased or decreased functions in the nine diagnostic positions. Specifically, quantitative notations in degrees or prism diopters should be emphasized in the primary, the straight-up, and the straight-down positions. The older record systems that omitted straight-up and straight-down positions were oblivious to the A, V, and X components that enter so many cases of heterotrophia. Therefore they should not be used.

Quantitative measurement of the degree of deviation

Fundamentally, reliance in establishing diagnoses should be based on objective procedures in preference to tests requiring subjective responses or participation. Although precision is an inherent element of all scientific measurements, practicality and true understanding dictate the level of exactness to be sought. Thus the width of a prism is not measured in inches nor the power of spectacle lenses in tenths of a diopter. Similarly, at surgery, the insertional line of an extraocular muscle cannot be measured in tenths of a millimeter from the limbus. Because of hour-to-hour and day-to-day variability in most strabismus, and because of the influence of attention, concentration, and relaxation, it is misleading to measure most deviations in units of less than 5 degrees and a waste of time and effort to measure in units of less than 5 prism diopters. Valid exceptions, however, exist in Visuscopic measurements of eccentricity of fixation, or prism measurements of small deviations in the primary position.

The *Hirschberg estimation* (1875) of the angle of deviation, based on the position of the corneal light reflection from an inspection (fixation) light held at the near or reading distance (33 mm.), is a sheet anchor measure used particularly in young children or uncooperative patients. This requires attention and fixation ability in at least one eye. Estimates are based on simplified geometry of the cornea, equating each millimeter on its surface with slightly more than 7 degrees or 15 prism diopters. Thus displacement of the corneal light reflex to a position just beyond the limbus equals about 45 degrees (90 prism diopters) of deviation; displacement of the light reflex midway between the corneal center and limbus equals about 20 degrees (40

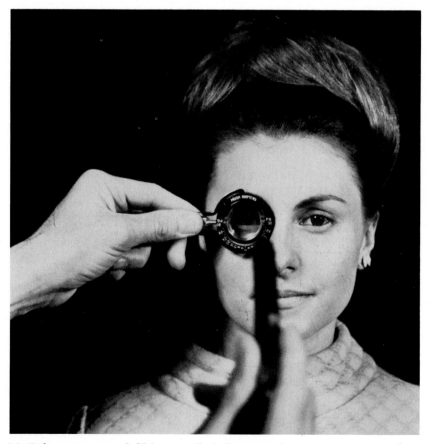

Fig. 6-3. Risley rotary prism held horizontally before patient's eye in position to induce 0 to 30 degrees of horizontal prism.

prism diopters) of deviation. Though not precise and prone to miss deviations under 7 degrees (1 mm.), this may be the best or only method usable in infants, toddlers, or hyperactive children. In deriving Hirschberg figures, it is necessary to correct for a large angle kappa or for a small "physiologic" positive angle kappa that simulates a small exodeviation or obscures a small esodeviation.

The *Krimsky measurement* (prism reflex test, 1943) derives the prism power needed before the fixing eye (apex in the direction of duction) to induce yoke movement of the opposite eye, which moves its corneal light reflex from an eccentric to a centric location. This requires attention and ability of the patient to fixate with his preferred eye, but it is advantageously independent of any fixational capacity of the other or deviating eye. Findings are slightly more precise than with the Hirschberg method, but they require the back surface of the prism to be kept perpendicular to the line of fixation. Results are progressively less precise as high amounts of prism are required. Measurements for distance are imprecise because the examiner's face, which should be directly in front of the patient, must be moved to one side.

The *Duane alternate prism and cover test* or parallax test (1889) combines the fusional interruption achieved by rapidly moving an opaque cover from one eye to the other while placing before one eye a prism with the apex in the direction of deviation. Beginning always in the primary position, increasing amounts of prism are placed before the deviating eye until all movements of redress or realignment are neutralized or compensated for by the prism. Mechanical difficulty in testing is reduced in deviations under 30 prism diopters by use of a Risley or Hughes rotary prism; this is held in one hand so that the thumb and forefinger operate the knurled knob, varying the prism strength from zero to 30$^\triangle$ (Fig. 6-3). Though awkwardly requiring more drawer or storage space, a prism set (1$^\triangle$ to 40$^\triangle$) or a Berens plastic prism bar* (vertical, 1 to 25; horizontal, 1 to 40) can be used for the same purpose. Small sets (5$^\triangle$, 10$^\triangle$, 20$^\triangle$) or small bars (vertical, ½ to 10; horizontal, 1 to 20), though less expensive and easier to store, often are inadequate when most needed. This test may also be extended to each of the other eight cardinal positions of gaze and may be carried out with prisms, first over the deviating eye (preferred eye fixing) and then over the nondeviating eye, to separate primary and secondary deviation.

DETAILED MOTILITY EXAMINATION

The preceding tests are generally objective in nature and require little on the part of the patient other than obtaining his fixation. In addition to the standard steps of examination (history, vision, refraction, fundus examination), this may be all that can be obtained from a young and restless patient. It may be an adequate working amount of information in many simple, initial, or uncomplicated patients with heterotropia. Depending, however, on the age and level of cooperation of the patient, vagaries or uncertain aspects of particular functions in the case, and personal preference of the examiner, a further series of progressively detailed examinations may follow.

Objective quantitative diagnostic measurements

These objective diagnostic measurements include primarily the identification and measurement of monocular fixation patterns and angular strabismometry.

Monocular fixation patterns

In the cooperative adult and older child, the estimates of fixation behavior based on position of the corneal light reflex often need to be refined by the ophthalmoscopic projection and localization of a macular target graticule (such as a "Linksz Star")

---

*Manufactured by R. O. Gulden, Philadelphia, Pennsylvania 19117.

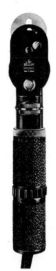

Fig. 6-4. Visuscope by Oculus Products combines features of direct ophthalmoscope with star test in concentric circles at 20-second separation to measure fixation patterns. Interchangeable retinoscope and transilluminator heads are available (6 volts; 6 watts).

on the posterior pole. This is indicated principally when vision is reduced or fixation is unstable. Testing is done with a modification of the direct ophthalmoscope such as the Oculus Visuscope or the Keeler Projectoscope, or most elegantly with the recording assistance of multiple fundus photographs (Fig. 6-4).

This is a monocular test and the opposite eye should be occluded. The patient is instructed to look directly at the projected star, asterisk, small ½-degree ring, or other device being used. The examiner notes, or photographs, the position of this target in relation to the foveola on the basis of several repeated fixations. The following are the patterns of monocular fixation that may be noted and differentiated.

1. Normal centric or foveolar fixation. The target is held steadily on the foveal center. Three or four types of minute, involuntary, and physiologic ocular oscillations or tremors may be identified and recorded while a patient is holding normal and steady fixation. These should be ignored in the identification of pathology, and differenti-

ated from nonphysiologic micronystagmus that may account for reduced acuity even in the absence of strabismus.

2. Eccentric fixation. Eccentric fixation may be parafoveal, perifoveal, or peripheral. (a) In parafoveal fixation the fixation target is off the fovea centralis but maintained within the vessel-free concavity (or clivus) of the central area. (b) In perifoveal (or paramacular) fixation the fixation target is at the far edge of or beyond the clival slope into the small vessel area. Fixation becomes progressively less steady as the target is imaged farther from the foveola. (c) In peripheral fixation the fixation target is beyond the fiber layer of Henle and beyond the luteal pigmented portions of the central area. Unsteadiness or inconsistency of fixation may extend through an area 2 disc diameters or more in size. Patients with persistent fixed esotropia of 25 to 30 prism diopters at distance and at near and using the optic nerve head scotoma or blind spot mechanism (Swan) to avoid diplopia in binocular vision do not fix the Visuscopic target on their blind spot but rather may have good monocular acuity and centric fixation.

3. Paradoxic fixation. In this condition the fixation target is in the opposite direction from the fovea to that which would be anticipated on the basis of ocular deviation. Thus an esotropic patient may fix the target temporally rather than nasally, as would be expected. This is more apt to be found after surgical corrections, after overcorrections, in spontaneous (consecutive) change of a deviation as from esotropia to exotropia, or some times without apparent cause.

Accommodative convergence/accommodation ratio (AC/A ratio)

Patients with horizontal, nonparalytic deviations should always be studied both at near and at distance fixation targets when wearing their full, distance refractive correction. In children this necessitates refraction after complete atropinization and then a suitable interval for the effects of atropine to wear off. Several factors may influence differences in degree of deviation for near and for distance. One significant though variable factor is the ratio of accomodative convergence to accommodation (AC/A ratio) in the particular patient. Convergence responses are closely linked with accommodative efforts, as illustrated by the uncorrected hyperopic individual who must exert extra diopters of accommodative effort to focus for near and far; he will generate extra convergence impulses and may show excessive *accommodative convergence* in relation to his particular AC/A ratio.

Normally the amount of accommodative convergence to accommodation varies between 3 and 5. Thus 3 to 5 prism diopters of accommodative convergence occurs with each diopter of accommodation. High ratios tend to be associated with convergence excess or accommodative esotropia as well as myopia without strabismus. Low AC/A ratios tend to be associated with convergence insufficiency as well as hyperopia without strabismus. The AC/A ratio, however, does not depend on refractive errors, heterophoria, or heterotropia and may remain constant in an individual even through presbyopia.

Interpupillary distance also affects the manifestations of AC/A ratios, because a high interpupillary distance demands greater AC/A ratios to achieve bifoveal fixation in the near range. Conversely, narrow-set eyes need less accommodative convergence per diopter of accommodation.

In use the AC/A ratio is first assessed by measuring the deviation at distance and near with the alternate cover test. If the results are essentially the same at near and distance, the AC/A ratio for that patient is normal. Differences should be established numerically with prism neutralization of movement during the alternate cover test. Measurement at ⅓ meter calls for 3 diopters of accommodation as compared to measurements at infinity or its simulation at 6 meters. Thus, to determine the AC/A ratio, the difference in prism diopters of deviation as measured at 6 meters and at ⅓ meter is divided by 3.

The basic ratio is not altered by orthoptic exercises, prisms, spectacle correction, or bifocals. Lenses as well as miotic drugs, however, may have profound effects on the apparent position of the eyes when properly prescribed for abnormal AC/A ratios. Similarly, surgical changes in the extraocular muscles will significantly alter the findings on clinical measurement of the AC/A ratio.

Angular strabismometry

Angular strabismometry, begun by the Parisians Landolt (1875) and Javal (1896), has gone through countless perimetric techniques and short-lived tangent scales, tapes, anglometers, linear gauges, transparent rules, measuring bridges, pupillometers, deviometers, tropophorometers, minor amblyoscopes, and so forth. All of these have been clearly superseded by the more adap-

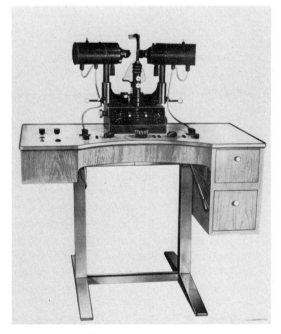

Fig. 6-5. Synoptophore, standard model, with integrated table, is shown from operator's side. (Manufactured by Oculus Products, Dutenhofen, Federal Republic of Germany.)

table and flexible major haploscopes or amblyoscopes, which afford measurement of both objective and subjective angles of deviation as well as considerable analysis of the sensory components in strabismus. Such instruments may also be used to a lesser degree for orthoptic training as an adjunct to other, more major methods in treatment. These instruments include the Orthoscope and the table-top Synoptophore with a plug-in but separate electric control by Instrumedic, Ltd.,[*] and the completely integrated table and Synoptophore by Oculus Products.[†] Other generally similar table-top models are the standard No. 11 Synoptiscope and the 5000 Synoptiscope (1970) by Cuprax and the Troposcope by American Optical Company (Fig. 6-5).

Instruments establishing fixation points by meridians and linear distance from the primary position are valuable in obtaining reproducible measurements on subsequent examination. The Owens deviometer has been helpful for this, and more recently the Soll strabismalite manufactured by Jenkel-Davidson serves a similar purpose (Fig. 6-6). The table-stand Lavat Deviometer,[‡] utilizing double luminous points on a fully rotational axis, affords standardized measurements that may be recorded on pads of diagrammatic sheets furnished with the instrument.

Dissociation tests

> "Finally, the confusion is rendered greater by the underlying fact that we do not know what we are measuring but are certain that we are measuring different things with different tests."
> STEWART DUKE-ELDER, 1949

The individual with good vision in each eye (20/40 or better), asymptomatic binocularity, and cosmetically acceptable appearance does not usually come for an ocular motility examination. Many factors such as visual fixation, the high cerebral function of fusion, and the unacceptability

[*]London W1H, OHS, England. Instrumedic, Ltd. is the successor to both Clement Clarke and Theodore Hamblin.
[†]Federal Republic of Germany.
[‡]Luneau and Coffignon, Paris 8, France.

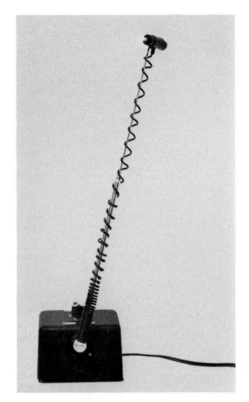

Fig. 6-6. Soll Strabismalite may be set in nine diagnostic radii to establish reproducible measurement sites. (Made by the Jenkel-Davidson Optical Co.)

of diplopia are strong curbs against strabismus or ocular deviation. However, the patient complaining of ocular use discomfort, variable diplopia, poor vision in one eye, or intermittently manifest squint requires not only careful evaluation of the optic components of refraction (which may be abnormal) and the preceding preliminary inspections (which may appear normal) but also examination of the eyes while interrupting fusion or dissociating the images of the two eyes in various ways. With such testing, latent (heterophoric), intermittent, or subtle impairments in binocularity are uncovered, in some fashion quantitated, and then interpreted as to significance.

The major amblyoscope or haploscope is traditionally the ally of the twentieth century orthoptist in deriving rather minute numerical values in measurement of both objective and subjective angles of squint.

All such measurements, however, like the photograph of one ultrasonic echo, represent only one brief moment in the course of a process that may be highly variable. Amblyoscopic figures also inevitably are distorted by the influences of such extraneous factors as instrumental convergence and the near or proximal reflex.

Classifications of objective and subjective angle measurements include test findings without and later with dissociative measures to interrupt fusion. Many methods may be employed to produce dissociation. Each yields a level or type of dissociation that is difficult or impossible to quantitate numerically but that should be designated by the name of the test method and assigned somewhat of a rank order or degree of magnitude designation. Thus the Bagolini lenses produce one of the most subtle and physiologic forms of dissociation. The stroboscopic flash-afterimage tester produces one of the most coarse and least physiologic dissociations, and its use is becoming less popular.

In general, dissociation is commonly produced by (1) complete exclusion of the field of one eye from the other, as by an opaque cover, in the cover-uncover test, (2) use of color differences between the two eyes, as in the Lancaster red-green projection test, (3) distorting one image, as with the Maddox rod test, (4) displacing one image, as with a prism of a few diopters before one eye aligned at right angles to the major direction of deviation, or (5) adding subtle markers over the usual visual fields as with Bagolini striated glass. Less commonly it is produced by polarized illumination of the test objects and Polaroid lenses at opposite angles before each eye, or dissimilar bright stimuli generating afterimages, as with the electronic flash afterimage tester. The orthoptist turns most frequently to different, partial or fusional test targets presented to each eye through the separate arms of a major amblyoscope.

One of the most precisely quantitative expressions of dissociation is the angular measurement of stereoscopic acuity or "stereoacuity." This may normally be developed to a very high degree (a few seconds of arc), but it is closely dependent upon visual acuity and is unrewarding to test in the presence of poor vision.

Both causative mechanics and corrective procedures necessitate measurement of deviation at near and far. Near fixation distance has generally been standardized at 13 in. or 33 cm. Distance measurements should be at a stated distance of 20 ft. or 6 meters and, for all questions of divergence excess, should be repeated while the patient is "looking out the window" or fixing on an object at least a few hundred yards away.

Differentiation may further be made between *true divergence excess* and *simulated divergence excess*. This is done after initial measurement of the exodeviation for near and for distance by occluding the dominant eye with an opaque Elastoplast patch for at least an hour. The patch is then removed and measurements of the exodeviation repeated at near and distance. Remember, however, that permission of even brief binocularity on removing the patch may reinstate strong convergence mechanisms; therefore, a cover or occluder paddle should be placed over the nonpatched eye before removing the patch.

Testing then proceeds with a routine of the alternate cover technique using an estimation of corneal light reflex position or measurement in prism diopters. If there is no increase in near exotropia on removal of the patch, this suggests a *true* divergence excess. However, if the manifest exotropia at near is increased after patching, this is a *simulated* divergence excess. Along with the weighing of other factors such as amblyopia or orbital asymmetry, the simulated divergence excess will more likely require unilateral surgery (medial rectus muscle resection and lateral rectus muscle recession), whereas the true divergence excess constitutes a more specific indication for recession of both lateral rectus muscles (von Noorden, 1969).

Maddox rod test

The multiple Maddox rod test (1890) still stands as the most widely familiar dissociation procedure and has been used as an official measurement in the U. S. armed services for many decades. It is applicable only in the measurement of heterophorias (not heterotropias) and is more accurate and valuable in vertical than in horizontal phorias. A relatively bright light (usually brighter than afforded by a projection acuity device) and a darkened room are necessary to achieve visualization of the line, which appears at about half intensity compared to the brighter dot seen by the eye not behind the rod.

Use is facilitated by a phoropter or major refractor that includes swing-away Maddox rods and Risley rotary prisms before the apertures for each eye. Testing should be for distance and for near. First the patient's distance refractive prescription is set in the phoropter and then the Maddox rod presented before one eye. To enhance contrast, a red Maddox rod is usually used with a white light. With both eyes open, the patient is instructed to fix on a small bright light 20 ft. away and to describe the position of the red line he sees through the Maddox rod in relation to the light. For vertical testing the bars are set vertically and the patient sees a horizontal line (at right angles to the bars of the Maddox rod). If the line appears to run through the light, there is no vertical heterophoria. If the line does not run through the light, then the Risley prism is placed over the aperture with the rod and its zero line set horizontally. Vertical prism power is introduced base-up or base-down, as needed, to move the line into coincidence with the light. The examiner may have to interrupt the image of the fixation light by briefly placing his thumb before this eye in order for the patient to attain visualization of the relatively less-bright line.

If the test is elected to estimate horizontal phorias, the rod is rotated so that its components are horizontal and the resulting line, as visualized, appears vertically. Fu-

sional impulses, however, will affect horizontal, quantitative measurements.

Similar Maddox principles can be tried to diagnose and measure cyclodeviations by positioning a red Maddox rod vertically before one eye and a white Maddox rod, also vertically, before the other eye. For this procedure, the phoropter (or trial frame) must be aligned precisely so that both rods are in accurate vertical alignment. Again with both eyes open, the patient fixes on a bright light 20 ft. away. If there is no vertical imbalance and no cyclodeviation, the patient sees only one horizontal pinkish line—a blending of the red line from one eye and the white line from the other eye. This may be verified by placing a 3- or 4-diopter prism base-down before either eye. Two separate horizontal lines (one red and one white) will then appear to the patient. These will be horizontal and parallel if there is no cyclodeviation. If one eye tends to intort or extort, however, the line before it will appear rotated in the opposite direction to the torsional disturbance of the globe. The Maddox rod (not a prism) is then rotated by the examiner or the intelligent patient until the two lines appear parallel. The amount of cyclodeviation is read in degrees from the trial or phoropter frame. This test, however, does not differentiate between cyclophorias and cyclotropias.

Maddox rod testing may also be repeated in the near or reading range. For this measurement the phoropter is less suitable than the trial frame because it does not permit the usual downward deviation of the eyes common in near use. The refractive correction and any needed near point add should also be in place before near readings are made. Cycloplegics are, of course, contraindicated in these near measurements.

Bagolini striated glass test

A more physiologic test, presenting less instrumental disturbance in the test situation, is the examination with Bagolini lenses (1960). These are plano lenses sized for in-

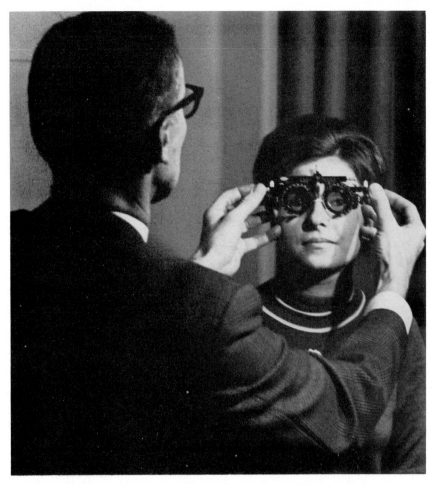

Fig. 6-7. Bagolini striated lenses being placed in position with conventional trial frame.

sertion in the cells of a trial frame and containing almost imperceptible striations that do not obscure visualization of the environment. They may be likened to glass that has been lightly but unidirectionally streaked with slightly oily fingers. Point light sources visualized through these lenses appear as luminous stripes at right angles to the lines of striation. This is the same directional relationship as with the Maddox rod. Simplicity of the procedure makes reporting easy even for children, and the patient's eyes are observable throughout the test.

In use, the room light should be slightly subdued and the fixation light should not have other light sources nearby. By convention, the Bagolini lens before the right eye has its striations oriented at the 45-degree axis, and the lens before the left eye is oriented at the 135-degree axis (Fig. 6-7).

The patient is asked to report the position of the lines he sees. A perfectly intersecting X indicates no suppression and either no deviation or deviation with harmonious, anomalous retinal correspondence (ARC). An interruption in one line suggests foveal suppression or a macular lesion. Absence of either line suggests suppression throughout the area of conscious regard, and possibly peripheral suppression.

When a perfectly intersecting X is reported, the cover test is used on top of the Bagolini lenses to differentiate normal retinal correspondence (NRC) from harmonious, anomalous retinal correspondence (ARC). If the cover test shows no shift of the uncovered eye and if fixation is central, then NRC is present. If the cover test shows shift of the uncovered eye, then harmonious ARC is present. Unharmonious retinal correspondence cannot be diagnosed by this method.

Afterimage test

Perhaps the least sensitive or least subtle and most unphysiologic dissociation procedure is the afterimage test (Hering, 1868; Bielschwosky, 1938) to a bright light filament.* The test is unrestricted by modest limitation of acuity or opacities in the media but requires fixation ability in each eye and cooperation to describe, or preferably draw, the appearance of linear afterimages. The electronic flash, hand-held tester gives instantaneous stimulus exposure, though old, filament instruments are still available in many places in lieu of the electronic flash.

In use, the nonpreferred eye is first covered. The patient then fixes with the better eye on an opaque central marker in a horizontal light source for an electronic flash, or filament exposure of about 20 seconds. The cover is then transferred to the better eye, the light is rotated to a vertical position, and fixation and stimulus are held as before. The light is extinguished, the occluder removed, and the patient instructed to draw the position of the afterimages as they appear against a blank wall. The gap in each linear afterimage corresponds to the visual direction of each fovea, *if* central fixation is present. A perfect cross indicates normal retinal correspondence or deeply entrenched eccentric fixation with harmonious ARC.

When central (foveal) fixation is still retained in each eye in spite of heterotropia, the relative position of the afterimages will be displaced (outward in exotropia, inward in esotropia) because ARC is present and the two foveas no longer have a common

*Electronic flash, After Image Tester, manufactured by Nytronics, Inc., Kutztown, Pennsylvania.

visual direction. In the intermediate stage, designated as *eccentric viewing* (rather than the more deeply entrenched level known as *eccentric fixation*), the two foveas retain their common visual direction. Though the patient may use an extrafoveal area in casual viewing, the relative position of afterimages is displaced (NRC is present).

In full *eccentric fixation,* the visual direction and motor orientation are firmly associated with an extrafoveal retinal area, even though the patient has the sensation of looking directly at an object. In this situation, afterimages intersect precisely because of the ARC.

Subjective dissociation tests based on color

The subjective dissociation tests based on color as introduced by Javal in 1880 include: (1) the red glass diplopia test and tangent scale measurements, (2) the Lancaster red-green projection test (1939), (3) the Hess screen test (1908-1916), and (4) the Tschermak congruence test (1899-1903).

The use of medium-density color filters (such as red, green-blue, and Snellen glasses) to achieve visual dissociation of the two eyes while using the same geometric stimulus has a record of usefulness in sensory evaluation from the latter nineteenth century.

1. The red glass test is the simplest of these procedures and is first used for subjective (diplopia) measurement of heterotropia (in which case a light- to medium-density red is used to minimize uncovering or eliciting heterophoria) with normal retinal correspondence. In use, the patient holds the red glass before his better eye while fixing on a pocketlight (Fig. 6-8) or similar light source at the intersection of the vertical and horizontal arms of a Maddox tangent scale (1890), which is marked in degrees of angular deviation for a predetermined test distance of 1 or 5 meters. With normal retinal correspondence, both foveas have a common visual direction. Therefore

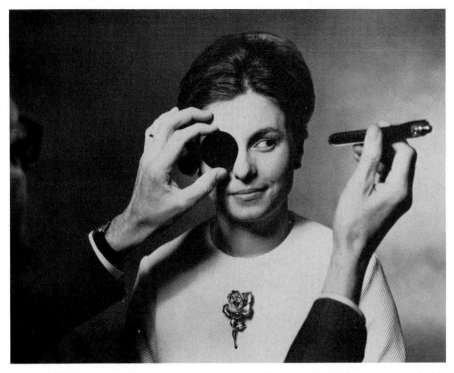

Fig. 6-8. Red glass tests with filter held before patient's right eye while fixating on flashlight in left lateral position of gaze.

the linear separation of the red and white images, either in space or on the tangent scale, indicates the angular deviation. The observation of a single "pink" image indicates no deviation and no diplopia. The test may be done in all principal positions of gaze to elicit incomitant deviations. A linear target light also enables identification of torsional (oblique) deviations.

The red glass test may also be used to estimate suppression and retinal correspondence. Here a medium- to high-density red is needed and the tangent scale is omitted. Just as for the subjective measurement of heterotropia, the red glass helps the patient identify the images from each by changing the value of one. If the red image falls on a scotomatous area, then suppression, anomalous retinal correspondence, or a local pathologic lesion may be present. To differentiate between suppression and ARC in such cases, a 3- or 4-diopter prism is placed vertically before the red filter. The red image is then vertically separated (subjectively appearing toward the apex

of the prism) from the white fixation light. In heterotropia with NRC it is displaced opposite the direction of the squint. In heterotropia with ARC, the red image is aligned with the fixation light. Suppression, however, can be more reliably determined on the major amblyoscope and correspondence is better determined with the Visuscope.

2. The Lancaster red-green projection test is the simplest, least affected by subjective elements, most productive of diagnostic information, and easiest to interpret of all tests in this group. It may be used against any dull, dark, and homogeneous wall or with a marked tangent screen supplied for a predetermined testing distance, usually 1 meter. In use (Fig. 6-9) the patient wears the red-green glasses and usually begins with red over the right eye. A red and a green torch projecting linear images are used (Foster penlight torches containing streak retinoscope bulbs beneath a focusing sleeve; larger Welch-Allyn torches with transformer-supplied light sources; or the

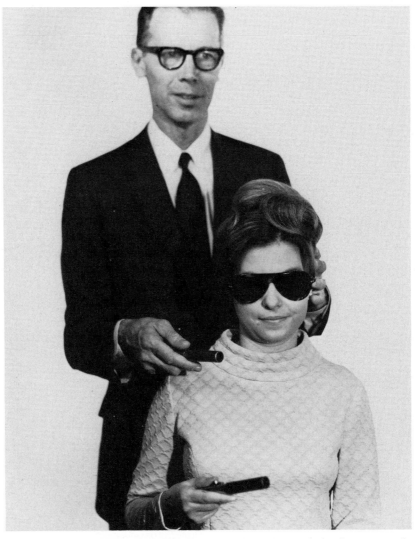

Fig. 6-9. Lancaster red-green projection tests showing patient wearing red-green goggles and responding to fixation with eye behind colored glass corresponding to examiner's colored torch. Patient's head is steadied by examiner's left hand to avoid movement during testing. Images of each torch are projected on screen in front of patient.

Strabismometer,* which uses the identical red-green principle by projecting a circle from one flashlight and, fitting the central hole in the circle, a solid disc of complementary color from the other).

Room lights are dimmed. The examiner, standing behind the patient, projects a red line on the wall or screen. The patient sees this red line (through his red lens) only

*Allied Ophthalmic Products Co., Morton Grove, Illinois.

with his right eye and therefore fixes with his right eye. With the green projection torch in his hand, the patient then superimposes the green slit, as seen with his left eye only, over the position he relates to the red line. Torsion and displacement of the slit directly indicate the corresponding position of the eyes (when NRC is present). When the normal eye is fixing, the primary deviation is demonstrated; when the red-green lenses are reversed, the secondary deviation is demonstrated. Deviation in each cardinal position is quickly and easily quantitated. Even small children enjoy the "game" and provide data that cannot be elicited with the more subjective red-green procedures. If neither the inexpensive Foster torches nor the expensive Welch-Allyn Lancaster or Allied sets are available, the examiner may quickly make suitable torches from a pair of flashlight pointers (or two old streak retinoscopes) by covering them with appropriate red and green cellophane.

3. The Hess screen (1908-1916) is an accurate, wall-mounted tangent screen made of black or gray felt with red stitching, scaled for use at ½ meter. Alignment of suspended green threads or use of a Law or similar green pointer provides the two color components. In use, the red-green Snellen (diplopia) glasses are worn and may be reversed for measurements of primary and secondary deviation. Torsional components can be identified, particularly if the linear green threads are used instead of a nonlinear pointer. The test is somewhat cumbersome and is fixed to the distance for which the screen is designed.

4. The congruence test of Tschermak, even after 65 years, is used very little, and less in the United States than in Europe. It requires a retroilluminated box with extending opaque vertical shields for each eye. It cannot be adapted to projection devices. It presents an illuminated white cross to both eyes, a vertical red extension above to the left eye, and a vertical green extension below to the right eye. Rather than requiring red-green glasses, the projecting opaque shields secure the colored line extensions to the respective eyes. Though accurate, this test requires considerable explanation and subjective reporting not needed in other tests.

Small base-out prism test for verification in small angle esodeviation

Patients who may have small central scotomas (under 2 degrees) or who show uncertain abduction of a questionably esodeviating eye when the fellow eye is oc-

cluded may be better diagnosed and better understood by small-degree image displacement testing. Uncertainties particularly arise in small-angle esotropia and microstrabismus or following surgical correction of a larger deviation. This technique necessitates a very small fixation light that will fall within a minute central scotoma. It may be employed for near or distance so long as the patient can follow the fixational instructions of the examiner.

A weak base-out prism—conventionally 2 to 4 diopters—is successively placed before the right and left eyes to displace the image of the fixation light temporally, but within an area of suspect central scotoma. An orthophoric individual shows an immediate binocular movement or version away from the side of the prism, followed by a slower fusional movement or duction of the fellow eye in the reverse or return direction to correct for the image displacement.

If, when placing the base-out prism before the right eye, both eyes move in levoversion, there is no foveal suppression in the right eye. If a subsequent slow fusional duction of the left eye occurs, there is no foveal suppression of this eye.

If, when the prism is placed before one eye, both eyes show a version to the opposite side, but the fellow eye makes no secondary fusional duction, then the fellow eye has a central scotoma. This is confirmed on changing the prism to this eye and noting that neither eye moves (the prism has merely displaced the image within the scotoma).

The test will thus confirm the presence of small degrees of esotropia and small central scotomas. It is not applicable in large deviations, absence of fixation ability, or established eccentric fixation.

Stereoscopic acuity or stereoacuity

Identification and quantitation of "fusion" is often confused because it entails two distinct though overlapping components: (1) the motor component or motor power, which may be quantitated over its widely variable range by prism vergence amplitude testing with rotary prisms, and (2) the sensory component of bifixation, which may be quantitated through gross tests such as the Worth four-dot test (1903) to minute measurements of stereoacuity.

Stereoacuity is simply the least fractional change in depth that can be detected binocularly. This is the most precise clinical measure of sensory fusion. It is inversely proportional to the square of the distance an object is away from the eye and directly proportional to the interpupillary distance. (Thus range finders are built to increase interpupillary distance by several feet.) Because of the marked effect of distance, there is a *near range* where stereopsis is accurate and critical, a *medium range* where stereopsis is poor, and a *far range* beyond 500 or 600 meters where there actually is no stereopsis. Horizontal, rather than vertical, disparities appear responsible for stereoacuity, but it is also asymptotically related to illumination levels and increases with exposure time by a factor of 4 from exposures of .004 seconds to 1 second. Beyond this time period there is no further enhancement by additional exposure.

Instruments used in measure of sensory fusion and stereoacuity,* in order of increasing precision, are:

1. Worth four-dot test for distance and the Hardy (1937) near modification for gross testing of extramacular fusion
2. Targets for either macular or extramacular fusion and stereopsis in a major amblyoscope
3. Polaroid vectograms (Wirt-Titmus, 1947), which are double-printed with

------

*The Howard-Dohlman aligning box for testing at 6 meters with two pegs separated by about 10 minutes of arc (64 mm.) is extremely crude and affords neither quantitative measurements for a strabismic patient in the near range nor correlation with performance in far ranges. It has been abandoned by civilian and military transport examiners for inapplicability. The Verhoeff battery-powered, hand-held Stereopter affords a qualitative judgment of near stereopsis but does not give quantitations (Fig. 6-10).

polarizing axes at right angles to each other (These are inspected through polarizing filters worn over each of the patient's eyes and oriented at right angles to each other.)

The Worth four-dot (paramacular) test presents one red, two green, and one white disc, usually subtending a visual angle of 1 to 1.5 degrees at 20 ft. The patient wears a matching red filter before one eye and green filter before the other. Thus the green lights are seen only through the green filter and the red light through the red filter. The normal patient will see the white light through both filters and may report it as a blend of changing red and green because of retinal color rivalry. The normal individual with normal vision in each eye may also report the white to appear predominantly red, regardless of which eye is wearing the red filter. This is because psychophysically most individuals perceive the color red as dominant to that of green. The patient with moderate to severe amblyopia in one eye will usually report seeing no lights with that eye and the appropriate two or three lights with his better eye. The heterophoric or mildly heterotropic patient will often report seeing five lights, two red and three green, appearing in crossed positions with exotropia and uncrossed positions with esotropia. The Hardy flashlight modification (Fig. 6-11) of this test has similar value for identification of bifixation and elementary paramacular fusion in the near range. The test should always be repeated with the red-green glasses reversed for confirmation. This test subtends too broad an angle to detect suppression limited to the fovea.

The major amblyoscope (haploscope) has the advantage of being able to present countless variations of target designs and sizes. Foveal targets should subtend 1 or 2 degrees at the most, and paramacular targets should subtend no more than 5 to 7 degrees. Targets for peripheral function generally should be larger than 7 to 10 degrees. In order to grade very fine degrees of stereopsis, however, horizontal disparity

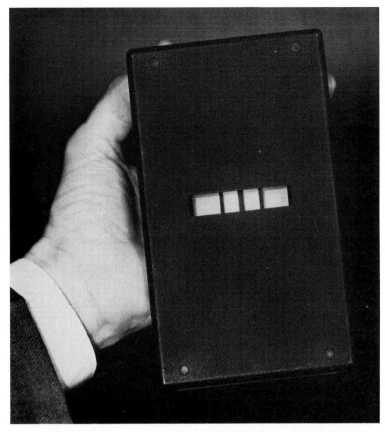

Fig. 6-10. Verhoeff stereopter showing three vertical rods in front of translucent white glass (as viewed by patient).

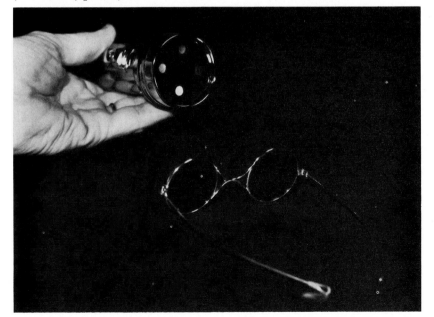

Fig. 6-11. Worth four-dot test modified by Hardy for near range, paramacular fusion. Patient wears red-green Snellen spectacles as shown.

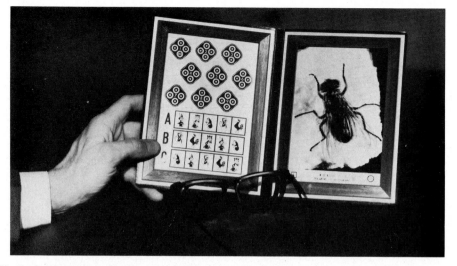

Fig. 6-12. Wirt-Titmus double-printed Polaroid vectograph for quantitating stereoacuity through Polaroid spectacles.

of targets in small fractions of a millimeter must be achieved. Irregularities in slide bindings and necessary clearance to lift target slides in and out of an amblyoscope exceed these differences, and therefore finer grading of stereoacuity must be done with the Wirt type of printed vectograms.

The familiar Polaroid stereoscopic fly test* is a simple and direct measure of third-degree fusion but is relatively gross and can be perceived in true stereopsis by an individual with up to 3,000 seconds (50 minutes) of arc disparity. Thus a patient with as much as 10 or 15 prism diopters of manifest exotropia in the near range may be able to visualize the Polaroid fly satisfactorily. The series of quantitative stereoacuity targets double-printed as Polaroid vectographs by S. E. Wirt are available (Fig. 6-12) in a booklet or folder (Titmus) convenient for both child or adult patients. Polaroid spectacles are worn with the polarizing axes of the two lenses oriented 90 degrees from each other to correspond with each of the printings of the vectograph. This permits gradation of stereoacuity in a series of nine steps down to 40 seconds of arc. (The initial Wirt series went to 14 seconds of arc.)

*Titmus Optical Co., Petersburg, Virginia.

Project-O-Chart vectograph slides are also manufactured by the American Optical Company with eccentric circles to measure stereoacuity to 60 seconds of arc but at far range test distance. In use, a nondepolarizing screen is necessary, and the patient wears Polaroid glasses. More critical vectographs measuring down to 15 or 20 seconds of arc can be produced, and the limits of stereoacuity with good central acuity may be measured down to a few seconds of arc under laboratory conditions.

One of the recent and rewarding diagnostic developments in strabismology has been identification of the involved mechanisms in patients with mild amblyopia whose eyes appear to be straight or who do not show a fixation movement of the uncovered eye when either eye is subjected to the cover test for heterotropia. A movement of realignment may or may not be apparent on the cover-uncover test for heterophoria. Clinically, such patients usually have mild to modest anisometropia (exceeding 1.5 diopters), an antecedent history of manifest esotropia that may have been approached surgically in early childhood, and peripheral fusion with amplitude if amblyoscopic examination is done. This is sometimes designated as small-angle strabismus or microstrabismus (Helveston and von Noorden, 1968). Measurement of foveal stereoacuity reveals distinct limitations but better performance than in heterotropic patients with macular suppression and worse than in those with bifixational heterophoria or orthophoria.

Thus it is diagnostically helpful in patients with straight or nearly straight eyes and with uncertain amblyopia to measure stereoacuity. High-grade stereoacuity is found only in the presence of bifixation and enhances the outlook for functional improvement. Contrariwise, very poor stereoacuity limits the prognosis for full functional restoration, particularly when the history of strabismus is from early infancy or birth.

Special tests and procedures

The examinations discussed in the preceding pages yield a satisfactory diagnosis and plan for treatment in the large majority of motility problems. The perceptive examiner culls from these procedures those most productive of diagnostic data and least fatiguing to patient and to self. Thus he should prefer the Lancaster red-green projection test to the more cumbersome Hess screen test or the old congruence test of Tschermak. He should try to avoid the gross afterimage testing of Hering-Bielschowsky. In practicality of testing he also tries to avoid the "fist full of prisms" tests, favoring rather the best analysis of corneal light reflexes by simpler means.

Yet there remain many other tests of value that the individualist will espouse and that, at times, an individual patient will require.

The Bielschowsky head-tilt test (1935) and its three-step elaboration by Parks (1958) are specifically valuable in differential diagnosis of vertical, or preferably designated "cyclovertical," impairments. The Bielschowsky maneuvers are particularly diagnostic in isolating the offending muscle requiring surgery, whether impairment is recent (without secondary contracture of the homolateral antagonist or the contralateral yoke muscle or disturbances in the antagonist of the yoke) or long standing (with such secondary changes or with loss of the distinction between primary and secondary deviation). Parks' three-step procedure may be inapplicable following long-standing secondary changes or surgical interventions.

Bielschowsky head-tilt test

The Bielschowsky test is applicable only in cyclovertical paresis, where good sensory fusion or distaste for diplopia stimulate a compensatory head tilt. This is more conspicuous in oblique than in vertical rectus muscle impairment. Therefore quantitative responses noted while testing will be more marked in oblique than in vertical rectus impairment. When a superior oblique muscle is underacting, its normal incyclotorsional tone is reduced, the eye consequently is extorted by the less opposed action of the homolateral inferior oblique muscle, and the patient takes up head-tilting to the opposite side to restore verticality to the 6 to 12 o'clock axis of the involved globe. Forcibly tilting the head to the side of the palsied superior oblique (reversing the spontaneous tilt) in the Bielschowsky test increases the excyclotorsion; this calls on the homolateral superior rectus, which has a minor incyclotorsional component in its action, to make a compensatory contracture. A greater component of action in the superior rectus, however, is elevation. Therefore the involved eye shoots upward (positive Bielschowsky test).

If the superior rectus—rather than the superior oblique—is at fault, spontaneous or compensatory head-tilting (to the opposite side) is distinctly less conspicuous. There is theoretic depression of the involved eye resulting from unopposed action of its superior oblique. On forcible tilting of the head to the involved side, the eye does not elevate and may even show some depression. This identifies the superior rectus as the impaired muscle.

The test is also applicable in the presence of impairment of the inferior oblique and the inferior rectus muscles, which have, respectively, major and minor components of extorsion. Paresis of either of these muscles tends to permit some intorsion of the globe and to stimulate compensatory tilting of the head to the *same* side. The amount and clarity of these cyclovertical findings is less with the inferior than with the superior pair of muscles and least with the inferior rectus. Forcibly tilting the head to the opposite (uninvolved) side increases the incyclotorsion of the affected eye, and thus if the inferior oblique is at fault, the compensatory contraction of the homolateral inferior rectus leads to a diagnostic downward displacement of the eye.

The complete objectivity of the findings in the Bielschowsky test makes it particularly valuable to use at any age and with almost any degree of interest on the part of the patient.

Three-step test of Parks

The Parks' test is done to identify nonoperative and nontraumatic cyclovertical palsies. The tests are best done with distant fixation and good light with which to observe movement of the eyes.

Step I   Identify whether the right or the left eye is higher by direct inspection or by use of the cover-uncover test if necessary. This eliminates four of the eight muscles that can be suspect in vertical palsy. Thus if the patient has *right* hypertropia, only one of the following four muscles can be paretic: right superior oblique, right inferior rectus, left superior rectus, or left inferior oblique.

Step II   Determine whether the vertical deviation increases in dextroversion or in levoversion. This eliminates two of the remaining four suspected muscles. Thus if the right hypertropia increases in dextroversion, only one of two muscles (those now in the field of maximum action) can be paretic: the right inferior rectus or the left inferior oblique.

Step III   Determine whether the vertical deviation increases on tilting the head toward the right or the left shoulder. This may be apparent in direct inspection (particularly when a superior oblique muscle is paretic) or may require alternate cover to elicit the difference. Thus if the right hypertropia increases on tilting the head to right, the paretic muscle is the left inferior oblique, and the left eye has been rotated downward by compensatory contraction of the left inferior rectus, as explained under the Bielschowsky test.

CONCLUSION

Some component of ocular motility evaluation is an integral part of every complete eye examination. This is initiated by the leads communicated from the patient in his chief complaint. It is more specifically oriented by the ocular and central nervous system history. The examiner then progresses step-by-step from preliminary inspection through the minimum number of separate tests needed to establish either normal ocular motility or the presence of abnormality. In the presence of disorder, a reasonably quantitative anatomic and functional diagnosis must be made. The examiner who dares to pass up a small amount of acquired esodeviation in a child with a passing assurance of improvement with age will make some catastrophic errors. The otherwise silent brain tumor first evidenced by partial paralysis of one lateral rectus muscle must always be considered in either the history or the finding of convergent strabismus.

In the presence of diagnostic uncertainties, highly variable findings, or inconsistent results from different tests, the examiner may often attain valuable clarification on the basis of a reexamination or two. At times, specific instructions to a mother or a mate as to what to watch for may greatly aid an otherwise vague history.

There is no substitute for the penetrating history augmented by careful and searching observation of the patient. In the restless child or infant those steps that should be limited to preliminary inspection of the older individual may constitute the entire field of information obtainable. In spite of this, the examiner still must achieve satisfactory data to rule out malignant possibilities and to institute appropriately constructive programs.

Chapter 7

Glaucoma

INTRODUCTION
Definition

Glaucoma is a complex of many causative disease mechanisms having a common pathologic factor of increased intraocular pressure. The disease may be acute or chronic, primary or secondary, painful or painless and may cause temporary or permanent impairment of visual fields, night vision, and visual acuity. It is one of the most frequent causes of visual loss in our older population and one that produces far too much needless impairment. Suspicion of glaucoma should be part of the perpetual set of the examiner, and diagnostic steps with this in mind should be part of *every* eye examination. Glaucoma is not only a photophobic enlargement of the globe in infants, and an excruciatingly painful crisis in angle-closure episodes, but it also is a frequent, unsuspected concomitant of maturity or an occasional subtle devil in the progressively myopic patient.

Minimum diagnostic examinations

1. In every initial examination of the globe, an estimate must be made of chamber depth centrally and angle depth peripherally. This is first done as part of the inspection in focal light by directing a flashlight beam along the plane of the iris from the temporal side. If the chamber is shallowed by the iris bowing forward, only the temporal half of the iris will be illuminated and the nasal half will be shadowed. This warns of a narrow angle anatomy and calls for careful contact lens gonioscopy. Conversely, a broadly illuminated iris gives some reassuring index of safe chamber depth for pupillary dilatation with little danger of angle-closure glaucoma.

Between estimation of depth by illuminating the iris surface and by careful gonioscopy, reliable measurement of depth may be secured with the slit lamp beam. This is easily and directly done in the center of the chamber. For more critical estimation of angle depth, a vertical beam should be focused nearly perpendicular to the corneal surface and positioned as close as possible to the limbus at one of its horizontal sites. The beam must be as narrow as possible and viewed from an angle of approximately 60 degrees. The optic section of the cornea thus illuminated is used as a unit for estimating angle depth on the basis of peripheral chamber depth at the entrance to the angle (Herick, Shaffer, and Schwartz, 1969).

If the distance between the illuminated endothelial curve of the cornea and the anterior surface of the iris is equal to or greater than the depth of the corneal section seen in this slit beam, gonioscopy will always show a wide open or grade 4 angle. If the distance is only half the width of the slit beam, the angle is incapable of closure and may be estimated as grade 3. When the width is equal to one-fourth of the corneal section, this is probably a grade 2 angle and merits careful gonioscopy. If the width is less than one-fourth the slit beam, the angle is functionally a grade 1, and gonioscopy will usually confirm an extremely narrow angle.

117

This is an excellent premydriatic test to avoid medically induced angle-closure glaucoma. Such a simple step incorporated in routine slit lamp examination of the anterior segment will also eliminate the danger of overestimating angle depth in the presence of a plateau-type iris, where the chamber is deep centrally and most of the iris plane may be illuminated in the simple test of a flashlight beam directed from the temporal aspect. With such a plateau iris, there is danger of angle closure even though chamber depth centrally appears superficially reassuring.

2. Every ocular examination—even if only for a slight increase in a schoolchild's myopic correction or similar increase in a presbyopic patient's reading aid—must include an intraocular inspection for glaucoma. The prime target is the optic nerve head under ophthalmoscopic inspection. Here the basic anatomy of the nerve head and the strength of diastolic pressure constitute a twofold defense against nerve fiber atrophy induced by increased intraocular pressure. The ruddy and small nerve head with a small or no physiologic cup, as in the hyperopic eye, is most difficult to damage by glaucoma. The large disc with large cup and less capillarity, as particularly seen in the myopic eye, is more vulnerable to small increases in pressure. Systemic blood pressure, particularly at the sustained diastolic level, is important in maintaining adequate circulation to the axon fibers. Thus a drop in blood pressure, especially if diastolic, has a similar effect to that of increased intraocular pressure in creating ischemia or nutritional compromise, which damages the optic nerve fibers. Knowledge of blood pressure is of both diagnostic and follow-up importance in glaucoma. By the same token, the family physician or internist caring for a hypertensive patient who also has chronic or open-angle glaucoma should not abruptly reduce the patient's blood pressure.

In any pair of eyes, suggestion of glaucomatous change or susceptibility is evidenced by (1) inequality in the size of the right and left optic cups (the larger is more likely to prove glaucomatous now or in years ahead), (2) broad saucerization of the cup approaching the disc border, even in the presence of apparently good capillarity, (3) nasal positioning of the major vessels on the nerve head, and (4) angulation or knuckling of the vessels as they go over the nerve head rim into the cup.

The examiner will helpfully force himself to be more analytic about the size of the cup in the optic nerve head if he notes and records a specific cup/disc ratio expressed in decimal notation from 0.1 to 1.0. This is best accomplished on the basis of an imaginary horizontal line extending across the maximum width of the disc. If, on such a horizontal line, the cup appears to be half the total width of the disc, it should be recorded as 0.5. If the cup has almost completely involved the width of the disc, it would be recorded as 0.9. This gives a comparative value for subsequent examinations. Usually it is easy to localize the nasal edge of the cup, but difficulty is experienced in establishing the temporal limit of the cup when there is a gently sloping or saucerized configuration. Under such circumstances, the examiner should attempt to estimate a point at which the slope has come up to what would be the level of the unaltered rim or else estimate an arbitrary point near the disc border. A more adverse prognosis is suggested when the temporal extension of the cup is directed below the imaginary horizontal line. This may be associated with nasal field defects found on tangent screen examination.

3. Any of these suspect findings should be followed by corneal tonometry, preferably of the applanation type. Remember, however, that normal applanation tonometry (10 to 22 mm. Hg) may be found in the presence of disc changes, or vice versa. In either event the patient should be continued under observation at least twice a year as a glaucoma suspect.

4. The fourth step in the minimum diagnostic series is central visual field examina-

tion on a tangent screen at a distance of at least 1 meter, with a white target of 2-mm. diameter. Frequently the location of suspect alterations in the optic nerve head points to areas of probable field impairment. Careful tangent screen examination should be made for reductions in the superior nasal outer isopter, a Rönne nasal step, or Bjerrum arcuate defect. If a laterally inverted nerve head is present, these defects are more likely to be found in the temporal than in the usual nasal field.

Beyond these minimum steps of (1) chamber depth estimation, (2) optic nerve head inspection, (3) tonometry, and (4) tangent screen study of the central fields, there are many other sophisticated and specific examinations that must be included in many glaucoma work-ups or the consultation examination. Knowledgeability, alertness, suspicion, and experience by the examiner, however, are frequently more valuable than many routinely performed tests of variable interpretation.

MEASUREMENTS OF INTRAOCULAR PRESSURE

A series of progressively critical techniques is available for diagnostic measurements of intraocular pressure. These are:

1. Digital palpation (tactile tension)
2. Indentation tonometry
3. Applanation tonometry
   a. Optic
   b. Electronic
4. Tonography
5. Provocative testing
6. Diurnal curves
7. Ballistic tonometry (viscoelastometry)

Digital palpation or tactile estimation of ocular tension

Tactile estimation of ocular tension is a qualitative method with which every physician should be familiar. It cannot begin to approach the accuracy of instrumental tonometry, but it is a substitute for quantitative methods when corneal scars, irregularities, or infections preclude instruments. This technique requires experienced palpa-

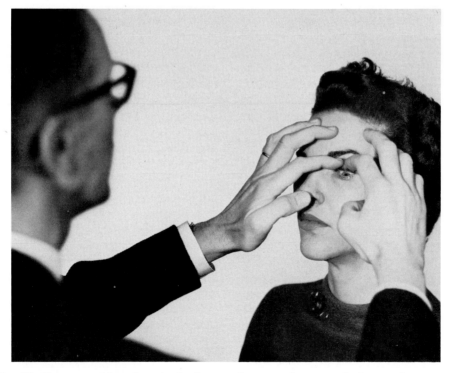

Fig. 7-1. Correct position of patient's downward gaze and examiner's fingers above tarsal plate for digital tonometry.

tion plus instrumental confirmation on many eyes before even such coarse gradations as increased +1, +2, +3 or decreased −1, −2, −3 can be made. In emergency situations or under field conditions it can be vitally helpful. Proper diagnosis of the unconscious diabetic patient who may be in either insulin shock or diabetic coma can be pivotally assisted by palpation of the soft globe consequent to the hyperglycemia of diabetic coma.

For digital tonometry (Fig. 7-1), the patient must look down with both eyes open. In some patients the protective tendency to close the lids, causing the globes to roll upward in Bell's phenomenon, will be reduced by having the patient fixate on his own hand held at waist level.

The third and fourth fingers of the examiner's hands are rested on the patient's brow to sustain the weight of his hands. This gives maximum freedom to the pulp tips of the index fingers, which then palpate the globe *above* the tarsal plate and *above* the limbus. An estimation of fluctuation of the globe is made by alternate and light indention (not ballottement) with one finger while gently steadying the globe with the other. Tactile sensation is impaired if palpation is done through the tarsal plate. A misleading sense of undue firmness is introduced by palpating against the cornea rather than the sclera. The reverse is true of instrumental tonometry, where the normal cornea should be used for sensitivity, consistency, and maximum accuracy of reading.

Indentation tonometry

Instrument. Though many instruments and many modifications create an international history of bioengineering from 1863 (von Graefe, Donders, Gradle, McLean, and so on), by far the best standardized and critically evaluated indentation instrument is that of Schiøtz, introduced in 1905. It has undergone modest refinements of design: multiple weights (1924); convex plunger x-model (1926); Harrington scale mangification (1941); Sklar mirror scale to re-

duce parallax in reading, and epicycloid lever (concave upward) to reduce friction (1948); Friedenwald refined nomograms for converting scale readings to millimeters of mercury (1955); Allen (Gulden, Pilling) modification to hold the plunger in elevation prior to contact with the eye (1964). The Schiøtz tonometer can be purchased from many sources for $40 to $90, including the necessary verification and certification.*

Technique. For indentation tonometry, the patient should be recumbent, comfortable, and without any constrictions of clothing at the neck that may impede venous return from the jugular system and artificially increase intraocular pressure. Men often need to loosen their neckties and collars. A drop of topical anesthetic such as proparacaine hydrochloride (0.5% Ophthaine, or 0.5% Ophthetic) or benoxinate hydrochloride (0.4% Dorsacaine) is instilled. These short-acting agents neither burn nor soften the epithelium as does cocaine, which is contraindicated. While the reaction from this drop is quieting down, the Schiøtz instrument may be quickly checked for zero reading on the steel test block furnished with the instrument. Plunger freedom should be quickly checked with the fingertip and then the contact area of the instrument should be dry wiped on an unused tissue. The patient may be instructed to fixate a mark on the ceiling directly overhead—if there is adequate sight in a fellow eye—or to fixate a fingertip on his hand extended at arm's length above his face. The hand fixation technique is essential in a one-eyed patient or in the presence of heterotropia where a compensatory version is needed to bring the cornea under examination into a proper horizontal plane.

The thumb and forefinger of one hand hold the lids away from the eye and against

---

*University Hospital of Cleveland, Department of Ophthalmology, Cleveland, Ohio 44106; Electronic Testing Laboratories, University of Tubingen, Tubingen, Democratic Republic of Germany; Physikalisch-Technische, Bundesanstalt Institut, Berlin, Federal Republic of Germany; Ross Foundation, Edinburgh, Scotland.

the orbital rim, carefully avoiding any pressure that may be transmitted to the globe. With the thumb and forefinger of the other hand, the vertically held tonometer is brought to rest on the center of the cornea. Touching the lashes can stimulate both blink and Bell's responses and so must be avoided. Freedom of plunger in the sleeve is evidenced by rhythmic transmission of the cardiac impulse in the indicator needle. To reduce inaccuracies at low- or high-scale readings, an appropriate weight (the normal 5.5 or the accessory 7.5, 10, or 15 gm.) should be used to obtain, if possible, scale readings of 4 to 10 units. The right eye is traditionally read first and then the left (Fig. 7-2). The patient should be routinely cautioned not to hold his breath and, if he appears tense, should be

asked to breathe through his mouth. A brief complimentary word as the chair back is returned to vertical or as the clinician checks the conversion table imparts to the patient a feeling of cooperative accomplishment and makes the procedure easier the next time.

Results are most appropriately expressed as a fraction, with the test weight being the denominator and the scale reading the numerator. Many physicians and patients, however, have a more comfortable feeling in a pressure notation expressed as millimeters of mercury. Generally it is preferable to tell the patient his pressure as it is recorded. The intelligent individual appreciates this participation in the studies, and it is a help to him if he needs eye care in some foreign port at a later date.

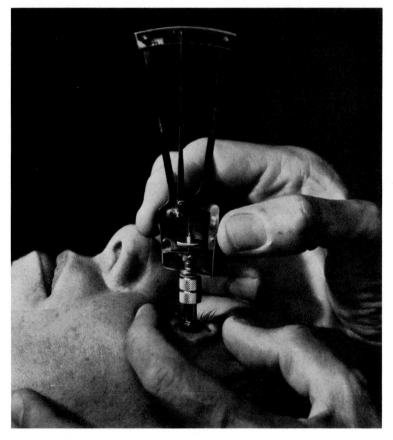

Fig. 7-2. Correct positioning of Schiøtz indentation tonometer vertically and directly centered on cornea of supine patient. Lids are gently retracted against bony orbital rim above and below, avoiding all pressure against globe.

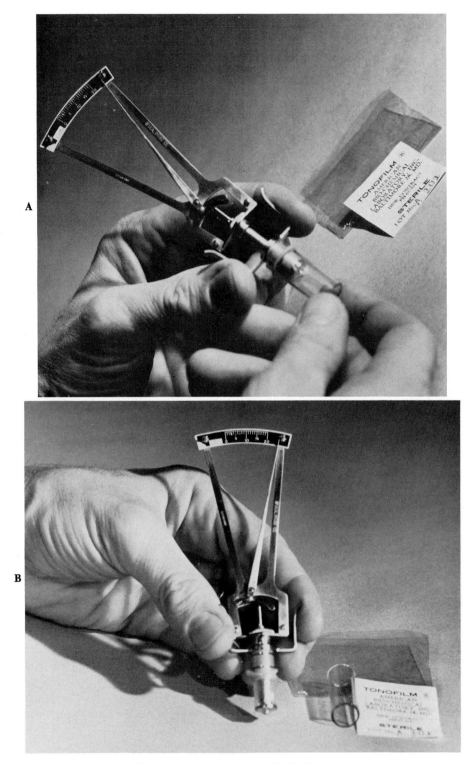

Fig. 7-3. A, Sterile tonofilm within clear plastic cylinder being inserted over footplate of Schiøtz tonometer. **B,** Tonofilm in place over footplate of tonometer. Clear plastic cylinder has been withdrawn and discarded to right.

Instrument sterilization. There is no way to achieve total and safe sterilization of a tonometer in clinical use other than to shield its operating footplate and plunger within sterile Tonofilm* so that no direct contact is made with the cornea or lids (Fig. 7-3). Such a film, affixed before each use and discarded immediately thereafter, is also an almost complete safeguard against corneal abrasion and an indispensable protection in mass screening programs. Cold sterilizing (Berens) solutions, if concentrated enough to be bactericidal and viracidal, present a caustic threat of residual chemical between the plunger and cylinder. Alcohol presents the same threat plus ineffectiveness against certain viruses. Flaming or other heat devices (Bell, Sklar) have been employed with occasional inadvertent coagulation calamities. Ultraviolet (Stirne, Rosner) does not penetrate the recess between plunger and cylinder nor any waxy secretion that might remain on the tonometer. In practice, workable safety against transmission of infection is achieved by never using the instrument on a suspect or frankly infected eye, wiping the instrument clean and dry after each use, and firmly wiping the dried instrument before each use.

Contraindications to tonometry and tonography. The following conditions, which contraindicate instrumental tonometry, relate to either possibilities of infection or conditions that render the procedure inaccurate.

1. Ocular infection or discharge: suspect, frank, or resolving
2. Recent ocular injury, perforation, corneal abrasion, or chemical burn
3. Herpes on the face or lids
4. Corneal edema, which both predisposes to epithelial displacement and makes reading inaccurate
5. Marked nystagmus
6. Corneal distortion, thickening, stromal loss, or major scarring

7. Significant apprehension, blepharospasm, or strong Bell's phenomenon as an avoidance response
8. Constant and uncontrollable coughing
9. Endemic outbreaking of ocular infection such as shipyard keratoconjunctivitis (adenovirus type 8)

In each of the preceding, a carefully performed digital estimation of ocular tension is of qualitative value and should be recorded. The examiner, of course, must wash his hands after touching any infected eye.

Applanation tonometry

The introduction of applanation principles by Weber in 1867, and more enduringly by Maklakoff in 1885, followed the primitive indentation instruments of the earlier 1860's. Maklakoff's carefully weighted applanation rods with no moving parts had simplicity in their favor, but they were subject to considerable variation in findings dependent upon lightness or crudeness of the examiner's hand and vagaries of stains and papers with which disc-like imprints (called "tonograms") were recorded from the cornea. Though modified by Filatov and Kalfa, they have been subject to much challenge of accuracy. Recently Posner and Inglima have revived interest in these weights of 5, 7.5, 10, and 15 gm. (available in a "Tonomat" kit*) for home evaluation of ocular tension. Families capable of understanding topical anesthetic procedures and use of such instruments, however, may derive more exact comparative data, particularly on the same patient, by purchasing a Schiøtz tonometer for instructed, home use.

Optic measurement. The niceties and advantages of minimizing instrumental deformity or indentation, however, have been fostered by the applanation principle and long championed by Frederick Verhoeff, using the simple Souter (American Optical Co.) tonometer of 1916. Dr. Verhoeff would apply this variable force applanator against

---

*American Bio-Chemical Laboratory, Inc., 1173 N. Rolling Road, Baltimore, Maryland 21228.

---

*Ocular Products, Inc., Seattle, Washington 98101.

the anesthetized cornea of a seated patient while watching for the first distortion of a windowpane reflection on the cornea. From these Maklakoff and Souter principles, Hans Goldmann in 1954 presented unquestionably the most significant and accurate advance in tonometry of modern times.

The Goldmann applanation tonometer* can be mounted on nearly any slit lamp, though most easily of course, on the Haag-Streit 360 or 900, where it may be used as an auxiliary attachment (Model T 900) and stored in an accessory box when not in use or as a permanent attachment (Model R 900) pivoted on top of the microscope objectives. The R 900 tonometer must be lifted off its pivot support if the photographic attachment or depth measuring device, which attach to the same pivot, are to be used. With a small bracket or metal mounting plate the tonometer can be attached to the Thorpe (Bausch & Lomb) and the Campbell (American Optical Co.) of the United States or the Carl Zeiss and the Zeiss Jena of Germany. Gams of Lyons, France, and a few other manufacturers now produce competitive models.

Currently the Goldmann is the most accurate tonometer available and presents large theoretic and practical advantages. Weight applied to the eye and the resultant area of flattening or distortion are much less than with Schiøtz indentation. Actually the area of flattening with the Goldmann flat plastic face is essentially the size of the Schiøtz plunger (disregarding the footplate), and the volume of intraocular contents displaced is about one-thirtieth of that caused by Schiøtz indentation. The distension characteristics or ocular rigidity of the globe are essentially of no concern in the minute disturbances effected by applanation. Similarly, intraocular pressure during tonometry is so nearly identical to the pressure (P_o) before the tonometer was applied that the instrument can be used on a cooperative patient at almost any time after intraocular surgery.

---

*Manufactured by Haag-Streit, Berne, Switzerland.

In actual testing, both patient and examiner are comfortably seated at a slit lamp. Topical anesthesia is induced as for Schiøtz measurement, avoiding tetracaine and cocaine, which cause some softening and staining of the epithelium. A thin film of fluorescein is obtained by touching the tip of a dry sterile fluorescein paper (Ful-Glo, Fluor-I-Strip) to the outer canthal conjunctiva of each eye. A theoretic equilibrium of 0.25% in tears should be achieved as evidenced by bright and solid yellow-green fluorescence. The small fixation light may be positioned closely in front of the eye not being tested to keep both eyes directed steadily forward.

The cobalt blue light filter is brought into the light beam and the slit diaphragm opened fully. The light arm is angulated to focus on the applanation prism in the region of the encircling black line near its tip, and at an angle of about 60 degrees to the line of observation. The voltage is turned to maximum and the low-power microscopic system is focused through the plastic prism so that its front face is clearly seen through the one (right or left) eyepiece as chosen. The pressure knob of the tonometer is turned to 1 gm. (10 mm. Hg), bringing the prism arm to its forward stop so that when corneal contact is made the prism will be exerting only light pressure. Room light is lowered.

The patient's eye and the applanation prism are watched from the side (or with the eye not sighting through the microscope) as the instrument is brought forward by the "joy stick" control until gentle contact is made between the prism face and the corneal center. This is evidenced by an immediate bluish glow throughout the limbus. With the single eye aligned through the microscope, the examiner then sees two blue semicircles (actually encircling the flattened area of cornea), each bordered by an arc of green light and pulsing synchronously with the cardiac rate. Small vertical or horizontal adjustments may be needed to center the pattern.

If there is distortion of high anterior corneal astigmatism (about 4 diopters or more), the scale reading on the applanation prism should be rotated so that the minus cylinder axis coincides with the red mark. The semicircles should be of equal size and their width about one-tenth the diameter of the flattened surface contained within either one. If the semicircles are grossly widened, excessive tears are present or the prism was probably wet before contact and therefore must be withdrawn, dried, and reapplied. If the semicircles are grossly narrowed, the tear film has dried excessively, the prism must then be withdrawn and the patient instructed to blink several times before recontacting the cornea. If the semicircles are so broad as to extend beyond the illuminated field, there is excessive flattening and the slit lamp must be drawn back.

Readings in the presence of this ever-changing pattern should be taken at approximately the midpoint between systole and diastole, when the inner (concave) boundaries of each semicircle just meet in contact, or as they rhythmically glide past each other through excursions of equal distance. Adjustment to the reading point or end point of properly located and sized semicircles is finalized by rotating the pressure knob back and forth. With applanation pressure exceeding intraocular pressure, the semicircles overlap excessively. With applanation pressure lower than intraocular pressure the semicircles are too small to intersect.

At the actual end point there is a flattened disc area 3.06 mm. in diameter within the 7-mm. diameter of the prism face. Here the attractive power of the tears toward the prism is balanced by counterpressure of the elasticity or springiness of the cornea, and at this point the grams of force applied through the prism (indicated on the pressure knob) are directly convertible when multiplied by ten into millimeters of mercury, expressing intraocular pressure. With this instrument the average ocular tension of a seated patient is 14 to 17 mm. Hg.

After use, the tonometer should be carefully wiped dry and rotated to either side (or folded upward on the Bausch & Lomb model) if the slit lamp will then be used for other purposes. The pressure adjustment should also be verified every few weeks with the test weight or metal balance bar provided. This is attached to the main pivot above the pressure knob. With the test bar at its zero (center) position, the prism should move on rotating the pressure knob either plus or minus 0.1 gm. With the test bar decentered backward to its first black line (two position), the prism should move when the pressure knob is advanced to 2 gm. With the test bar decentered backward to its last black line (six position), the prism should move when the pressure knob is advanced to 6 gm.

A hand-held model* of this equipment has been devised (1966) by J. Draeger particularly for use in the operating room under general anesthesia or in field survey conditions. Its greatest utility seems to be for children who cannot be examined in usual clinical settings but who require general anesthesia. The instrument is rugged, simple in construction, and completely free of any relation to vertical or horizontal positioning of either the patient or the instrument.

Electronic measurement. The electronic applanation tonometer of Holcomb (1970), a new corneal applanation tonometer, has been developed in prototype (1967-1969) at the Wilmer Eye Institute. It is electronic rather than optic in its measuring principles. The applanating face of this instrument is a small, mirror-smooth, semiconductor strain gauge. The patient holds a neutral electrode in his homolateral hand as the tonometer probe is touched to the cornea (Fig. 7-4) under unaided visual control of the examiner. Current flows in direct proportion to area of contact between the instrument face and the cornea. In relaxed and cooperative patients this may be done without topical anesthetic drops, but

---

*Hand-Applanation Tonometer, manufactured by J. D. Moller Optische Werke, Federal Republic of Germany.

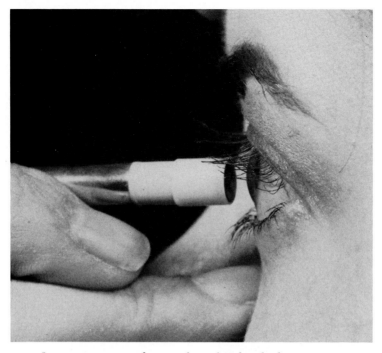

Fig. 7-4. Mirror-flat, strain gauge applanation face of Holcomb electronic tonometer tip being applied with patient in seated position. (Distributed by Codman and Shurtleff, Inc., Randolph, Massachusetts.)

most commonly the drops are needed. In response to the quantity of current flow, the indicator needle of the hand-sized display unit reads directly in millimeters of mercury and holds the maximum reading until the needle is manually reset. Two alternate ranges are provided to indicate intraocular pressure from 0 to 50 or by the flip of a switch from 0 to 100 mm. Hg.

Holcomb values correlate with those of the Goldmann applanation tonometer at a level of .94 to .95. Errors can be induced by blinking, eye movement, dirt on the probe, incomplete contact between probe and cornea, or significant variations in thickness of the tear film. The values obtained in a series of five readings should be averaged after discarding any inconsistently high or low reading. The entire instrument is self-contained and may be operated from small penlight batteries. It offers an intriguing advantage in miniaturization, portability, and freedom from the need of either a table-model or a portable slit lamp.

Tonography

Massage or pressure against the eyes has been recognized as reducing ocular tension since the work of Donders and of Pagenstecher in the 1870's. Similarly, Schiøtz and Priestly Smith in the early years of this century noted that holding a tonometer on the globe or repeatedly measuring ocular tension would lower these values, apparently by expressing some of the intraocular fluids. Quantitation of this "rate of ocular drainage" in terms of duration of application of the tonometer was begun by Gelder (1911) and Schoenberg (1912). This was improved somewhat by Kronfeld and his colleagues (1934) using a 2-minute application period. In the late 1940's two diagnostic aids, the electronic tonometer by Mueller and the practical understanding of gonioscopy evolved by Troncoso, laid the groundwork for modern, recorded tonography against a constant weight applied to the globe. In 1950 Moses and Bruno, as well as Morton Grant, presented mathematic foundations and prototype instruments for recording the "rate of outflow" over a standardized 4-minute period.

Tonography is an extension in time of Schiøtz indentation tonometry and therefore incorporates the problems of indentation tonometry such as (1) ocular rigidity, (2) problems of clogging versus corneal attraction in the space between the plunger and footplate cylinder, (3) variations introduced by atypical or irregular corneal curvatures, and (4) defects of instrument manufacture or maintenance. In addition, the electronic tonometer and its recording equipment are subject to line voltage variations, influence of nearby metal masses or electric fields from other sources, drifts in electronic circuitry, and variations in function before complete warm-up. More than a thousand models of strip recorders are available for adaptation to electronic tonometers, though generally the narrow types are superseding the wide because of economy achieved at the expense of vertically compressing the tracing and making the reading of smaller variations difficult. Newer instruments contain well-matched recorders and often have built-in line voltage stabilizers,

In addition to continuous refinements by Mueller (nuvistor circuitry, 1963), other quality instruments are available: Crescent Instruments'* transistorized circuits (1960), Berkeley Tonometer Company's† low center of gravity plunger head (1965), Schwarzer Corporation's‡ table-model and console stands, and Takata Instrument Company's§ small tonometer with built-in narrow strip recorder.

In use, the patient must recline on a suitably padded cot, stretcher, or tilt-back lounge chair, which must be relaxing and comfortable. A fairly large, and preferably luminous, ceiling fixation device should be centered above the patient's eyes. Drews

---

*Crescent Engineering and Research Co., El Monte, California 91731.
†Berkeley, California 94710.
‡Germany and 46 Salmi Road, Framingham, Massachusetts 01701.
§Japan.

recommends a decorator's handsome, four-bulb, frosted glass ceiling fixture about 12 to 24 in. square with an opaque knob in its center. The technician should be supplied with a comfortable stool with a backrest and should have some structure or available edge of the cot where she can steady her forearms. A foot switch for the recorder is highly desirable to reduce distracting movements around the patient. All disturbances of buzzers, telephones, intercoms, and incidental traffic must be excluded from the area during tonography. The recorder and tonometer dial must be positioned to be seen by the technician with no more than eye movement, because head movements are distracting to the patient.

The tonometer calibration should be checked before each run and before the patient is brought into the room, in accordance with the manufacturer's instructions. Gentle and reassuring explanation should be given as the patient is positioned. The patient's face must be parallel to the ceiling and must be maintained in this position without blinking or ocular movement for the 4 minutes of the test. Both local and vocal anesthesia should be administered as for Schiøtz tonometry. Tear evaporation from the open, fixing eye may create an unpleasant problem of drying and visual obscuration, which may be reduced if the patient shifts gaze, but only within the fixation target. Grant prefers to reduce tear evaporation by fixing a thin sheet of clear plastic Saran Wrap over this eye.

After achieving good patient understanding and relaxation, the tonometer must be lowered very slowly and gently onto the anesthetized right cornea, avoiding any mechanical bang or impact touch. The heel of the technician's hand should rest on the patient's forehead. Conversation cannot be allowed during the tracing, though the technician may have to remind or reassure the patient softly during the procedure. At the conclusion of tracing, the tonometer is gently lifted away, cleaned, and dried. A little movement, a compliment to the patient, and a few more drops of anesthetic in the left eye will prepare for the second tracing. The technician should not comment on the quality or the implication of the tracing, both of which the physician must interpret to the patient. As a single laboratory test, this is only one component in the study of the disease.

The finished tonogram must bear (1) calibration marks, (2) patient's name, (3) date, (4) hour, (5) eye, (6) weight used, and (7) technician's name. The tracing itself is a complex of superimposed variables including the falling slope of intraocular pressure induced by the tonometer, the clearly visible cardiac pulse, the Traube-Hering slow undulations in systemic blood pressure, and the respiratory pattern. To plot the reading, a smooth line is drawn through the center of the tracing, averaging out the extraneous variations. Gross artifacts should be excluded, as should abrupt changes in slope at either the beginning or the end of the tracing. The averaging line is almost always a gentle curve and practically never a straight line. Once this has been constructed, or merely located visually, the scale readings (R) at the beginning and end of the 4-minute run can be read. In relation to the weight used, it is then possible to calculate the initial or opening intraocular pressure (P_o), which is assumed to have been present before the tonometer was applied, by use of the Friedenwald nomogram* based on the 1955 Friedenwald tonometer table. This should be essentially the same as applanation tension recorded before tonography. The difference between initial and final scale readings is then calculated and this figure ($\triangle R$) located in the row across the top of the table for the appropriate weight employed. The number in the column below this ($\triangle R$) difference, which lies in the row across from the initial scale reading (R), is the facility of outflow (C).

For the clinician these two values, P_o and

C, are the most important facts to be derived from tonography. Corrections for the influence of ocular rigidity on P_o and C are not clinically significant. Similarly, other numerical values derived by manipulation of P_o and C have statistical interest and value but do not merit the mathematic labors of derivation for individual patient care.

C values above 0.18 are generally normal, those between 0.13 to 0.18 are borderline, and those below 0.13 are abnormally low.

A crude or fixed pressure form of tonography is the bilateral Bulbar Compressor Test* of Berens and Tolman (1959). Applanation tension is measured in each eye and then a pressure of 50 gm. is applied simultaneously to each eye through the concave base of two spring-loaded compressors placed 7 mm. proximal to each limbus and below the lateral rectus borders. The examiner maintains these compressors in radial position for 2 minutes, then removes them and immediately repeats the applanation readings. Simultaneous testing theoretically avoids the possibility of pressure on one eye unduly affecting the other. Results should be expressed as the change in ocular tension. Normal values are not well documented, but generally normal eyes may be expected to show a greater drop than those with glaucoma or reduced facility of aqueous outflow.

Provocative tests

Provoke: (from Latin) to irritate; to offend

"Don't challenge and thus gamble with the vitality of the patient by quickly subjecting him to more tests and treatments than he can tolerate with reasonable safety."
DAVID SEEGAL, 1964

Provocative tests—such as the Marlow prolonged occlusion technique for heterophoria, intravenous curare in suspected myasthenia gravis, digital compression of the carotid artery to evoke amaurosis fugax, or the mydriatic examination in narrow-angle glaucoma—are generally secondary

---

*The Tonography Table of Moses and Becker based on the eye of average ocular rigidity and normal radius (7.8 mm.) of anterior corneal curvature may also be used to derive P_o and C.

---

*Matalene Surgical Instruments Co., New York, New York 10017.

procedures and should be avoided if possible. Each of these examples has been followed at times by near catastrophic results. Resort to such methods to establish a diagnosis generally suggests inadequate development of the state of the art or the state of the examiner. More widespread use of modern applanation tonometry, gonioscopy, and tonography have lessened the need for provocative testing in individual patients, though such procedures may have both predictive and statistical value.

The possibly intermittent character of open-angle glaucoma (elevated P_o or depressed C values) in its early stages may at times yield negative provocative procedures as well as standard tests. In such patients, the longitudinal studies and follow-up observations of the regularly attending ophthalmologist may be of greater value than the one-time or "cross sectional" view of the consultant, even though the latter has the virtues of *freshness* and possibly unencumbering *set* from previous experience with the particular patient.

Provocative tests are subdivided in correspondence with the major types of glaucoma into those applicable to open-angle glaucoma and those applicable to narrow-angle glaucoma. Anatomically narrow iridocorneal angles, however, can be present incidentally in an eye with the underlying fault of open-angle glaucoma, and thereby both major forms of the disease may be present at the same time.

When anatomically narrow angles cause glaucoma (in the absence of open-angle defect) it is by the mechanism of angle closure or forward displacement of the peripheral iris blocking access of aqueous flow into the trabecular drainage meshwork. This may be independent of or secondary to a pupillary block, wherein the iris sphincter adheres to the anterior lens surface physiologically (such as with increased convexity of the lens surface and rigidity of the iris), pharmacologically (such as with tight sphincter contraction by strong miotic medications), or anatomically (such as following inflammatory adhesions of iritis). The symptoms of pain, blurred vision, and tearing, as well as the signs of deep conjunctival injection and increased ocular tension, initially tend to be intermittent and frequently mild until a major angle closure occurs with subsequently intense pain, nausea, and vomiting. Gonioscopic inspection with a contact prism identifies the anatomic proximity of the iris to the corneal endothelium and should define the likelihood of acute glaucoma being induced. In some patients, either during or between angle-closure episodes, the acute iridocorneal angulation of 10 degrees or less is so apparent (closed, Shaffer grade 0; extreme narrow angle, Shaffer grade 1) as to leave no doubt in the examiner's mind concerning the induction mechanisms. In other patients, the reverse end of the scale (wide open angle, Shaffer grade 4) is so obvious that closure is impossible. Between these extremes lie the moderately narrowed configurations with angles of approximately 20 to 40 degrees (Shaffer grades 2 and 3) where the examiner might wish to quantitate better the closure potential. Basically two provocative tests are suitable under these conditions.

The *dark room test* is the most conservative provocative procedure. Initial applanation measurements are made with or without tonograms, as desired, and then the patient is placed in a totally dark room. Both eyes are covered lightly with patches or a bandage. The test cannot be done on one eye at a time, as is done in mydriatic tests. After 60 minutes, the dressings are removed and very prompt applanation readings are made again, but with the added precaution that lighting is kept very dim and directed away from the patient. An increase of pressure exceeding 5 mm. Hg should be considered positive. Generally the degree of dilation by this technique is less than with topical drugs, and it is progressively less in advancing years as iris rigidity increases and physiologic miosis develops.

Mydriatic testing generally produces larger pupils, more positive results than does dark room testing, and greater likelihood of induced glaucoma necessitating surgical relief. Because of this danger, only one eye should be tested at any examination. Long-acting drugs such as atropine, difficultly reversible drugs such as 10% Neo-Synephrine, or rapid and potent drugs such as 1% cyclopentolate (Cyclogyl) should be avoided. Shorter acting and weaker mydriatics such as 3% eucatropine hydrochloride (Euphthalmine), 0.5% tropicamide (Mydriacyl), or 1% hydroxyamphetamine (Paredrine) are preferable. The pupil should be brought to a midposition of dilation (diameter of 5 to 7 mm.) thus avoiding the tendency for the iris to fall back on the receding lens surface as occurs in extreme dilation. Ambient light is not important, but the pupillary diameter should always be recorded before and after the dilation period. Results may be considered positive when ocular tension increases by more than 8 mm. Hg, when there is distinct flattening of the tonogram, and when gonioscopy shows the angle to be closed. Following this test it is necessary to instill a weak miotic such as 0.5% or 1% pilocarpine and have the patient remain in the office long enough to see that the dilation has been reversed. This may require 30 to 45 minutes. Strong miotics are contraindicated because of their ability to cause pupillary block and subsequent angle-closure glaucoma.

In the presence of distinctly wide or open angles, or where a concomitant open-angle defect is suspected in the presence of anatomically narrowed angles, two provocative procedures are again available.

The water provocative or hemodilution test, as all of these procedures, requires tonometry and preferably tonography before the test. Manifestly, if the tonography is abnormal there can be no additional information obtained by hemodilution, and the test is not indicated. The patient should be off all medication that may affect pressure and should be restricted from all food and liquid for at least 4 hours before the test. The test is often thus best scheduled for an early morning office appointment.

Fourteen milliliters per kilogram of body weight, or approximately a quart, of water is then drunk as rapidly as comfortable. Practically all beverages are hypertonic to water; therefore, they will have a lesser effect and should not be used. Repeat tonometry is done 15 and 30 minutes after ingestion of the water or until the pressure starts to fall. A rise of at least 8 mm. Hg in ocular tension should be interpreted as positive. The effects are bilateral. Of the provocative procedures, this is the least apt to be followed by complications. To obtain mathematical indices such as P_0/C after water drinking, it is, of course, necessary to do repeat tonography.

Steroid testing may not only evoke positive pressure increments in a given patient, but such reponse in apparently nonglaucomatous members of a family may yield statistics on predisposition and the three known phenotypic patterns for inheritance of steroid responsiveness. This seems to be a recessive trait. Though various topical corticosteroids have been employed, most testing has been done with 0.1% betamethasone and 0.1% dexamethasone, 1 drop in each eye three or four times a day. Tensions are checked weekly and drops may be continued until a significant increase is noted or for a maximum of 6 weeks. Modifications of this routine for more frequent instillations on a short-term basis may prove to yield similar responses. Steroids administered systemically generally do not have this capacity to elevate intraocular pressure. Though topical steroids are also known to "provoke" subclinical or latent herpes simplex, this has appeared to be of little clinical significance thus far. There is a further potential for topical steroids to cause lens opacities, which the physician must always weigh in the extended use of these drugs.

Diurnal variations

Glaucomatous elevation of pressure may be intermittent but may also vary with the time of day and the cycle of ocular rest or reduced mobility during sleep in comparison to the massaging action of waking hours. Diurnal fluctuations are more marked in eyes with impaired outflow facility than those with normal facility and therefore seem related more to alterations in secretory than in drainage capacity. Careful measurement by the same instrument and same examiner every 2 or 3 hours around the clock may reveal significant diurnal rises that would be missed during routine office hours only. The patient is commonly hospitalized for such studies, but he is reassured and less disturbed if this can be done in a self-care or convalescent unit. In some medical centers, a type of "Medical Inn" of motel design serves well for such studies.

Normal diurnal fluctuations are usually within 2 to 4 mm. Hg, but in open-angle (chronic simple) glaucoma they may reach 15 to 20 mm. Hg. Commonly the greatest rise in pressure is in the early morning hours of 4 to 7 A.M., but there may be reverse cycles with highest pressure in the late afternoon. Differences between the two eyes particularly raise suspicion of the eye with the greater increase.

Ballistic tonometry or viscoelastometry

Since the late 1950's several refinements of measurement (vibration tonometry: Hargens, Keiper, Sarin, 1965; viscoelastometry: Hargens, Keiper, G. Spaeth, 1962) have been designed to extremely minute disturbances of the globe and self-recorded information (signatures drawn automatically on an oscilloscope with X and Y axes representing strain and stress) of deformation and reformation or viscous and elastic moduli. Permanent records are obtained on Polaroid camera film. Such equipment yields a new dimension in study of both tissue characteristics and pressure factors within the globe, but it is expensive and cumbersome as yet. These new concepts, however, have far more potential that did earlier attempts in the modification of indentation techniques (fixed indentation: Maurice, 1958; microplunger movements: Mackey-Marg, 1960) or use of the less sensi-

tive—and less consistent—scleral portions of the globe (Wolfe, 1948). At present, however, such equipment in practical or production models is not available.

GONIOSCOPY

Gonioscopy (Greek *gonia*, angle, and Greek *skopein*, to examine) is a contact lens technique of visualizing the anterior chamber recess or filtration angle, which is hidden to direct inspection by the overhanging opaque scleral limbus and obscured to view from the opposite limbus by internal corneal reflections and often by forward bulging of the peripheral-most or "last roll" of the iris.

Gonioscopic visualization of the iridocorneal or filtration angles has led to probably the most fundamental advance of this generation in understanding and diagnosing causative mechanisms in glaucoma. This has also produced far more rational and effective therapy. Basically this is the identification of the anatomically narrow angle mechanism and its precipitating role in both acute and progressive angle closure. Gonioscopy thus affords direct and immediate differentiation of such pathology from chronic simple or open-angle glaucoma. Unfortunately the presence of narrowed angles or the catastrophe of angle closure does not exclude coexistence of open-angle mechanisms or "mixed glaucoma." On the other hand, a wide open and accessible angle does rule out likelihood of angle closure episodes. It is therefore important to examine gonioscopically all glaucoma patients and those with suspect episodes of pain, blurring, or congestion. Progressive thickening of the lens throughout life also has a narrowing effect, both on the anterior chamber and on the angle itself. A progressive or "creeping" angle closure may occur; this calls for repeated gonioscopy in open-angle glaucoma patients at intervals of a year or so.

Gonioscopy is also essential in the location of small, radiolucent foreign bodies whose concealment in an angle recess may cause localized corneal edema. Similarly, it is vital in the study of peripheral iris or angle recess tumors to determine their invasion into the angle and the possibility of excision by methods less than removal of the eye.

Modern practical gonioscopy has been made possible by the contact lens designs and procedure introduced by Troncoso for "direct" visualization of the angle (1925). Technical evolutions were spearheaded by Salzmann (1914-1915) and by Koeppe (1919-1920), primarily in the area of circular or 360-degree (direct) goniolenses for use with the recumbent patient. Koeppe also developed early contact lenses for use at the slit lamp with the patient seated, and Goldmann in the mid-1930's presented the first of his mirrored or "indirect" contact lenses for slit lamp use. These became the prototypes for more recent refinements such as the Goldmann three-mirror lens, which is now one of the most widely used models. In the mid-1930's, Barkan also began a series of handled and truncated lenses to facilitate surgical introduction of a knife for goniotomy under visual control.

Lens designs

Goniolenses are divided into those for examination with the slit lamp or gonioscope, and those for surgical use with the operating loupe, microscope, or other mechanically mounted gonioscope (Troncoso, Heine, Haag-Streit, Barkan floor stand).

Gonioscopy is one of the most fundamental or pivotal examinations in both diagnosis and control of glaucoma. It should be part of every initial work-up and repeated in controlled patients about once each year.

Techniques of use are modified according to the design of the retention mechanism for the lens:

1. Smooth, nonflanged base for retention with fingers and capillarity. The Zeiss four-mirror lens, the Barkan surgical lenses, the Thorpe four-mirror lens, and the Haag-Streit Goldmann three-mirror lens are of this type.

2. Flanged or scleral haptic base for retention between the lids. Early models of the Goldmann three-mirror lens (and the earlier single-mirror version), the Koeppe, the Troncoso, the Franklin, the Sarwar, the Richardson, and the four-sided Allen-Thorpe are of this type and therefore contribute to their own self-retention. A silicone rubber or similar plastic surface to the flange reduces the likelihood of corneal abrasions.

3. Vacuum retention lenses. These lenses (Lo-Vac) of J. G. F. Worst are small, light lenses of original design (direct goniolens with tilted flat anterior surface allowing nearly a 180-degree view of the angle; six-mirror indirect goniolens; double-focus lens for gonioscopy with direct or indirect ophthalmoscope) or modifications of classical designs (Barkan and Koeppe), each fitted with connections for plastic tubing through which a small amount of vacuum is generated after the lens is placed on the cornea.

4. Hand-held lenses. This includes the Cardona goniofocalizing lenses, some of the Barkan lenses, the Unger holding fork for the Zeiss four-mirror lens, and the Swan.

Various diameters are available in several lens designs for use in children or those with small eyes: Koeppe 17, 19, and 21 mm. outside-flange diameter; Cardona small, medium, and large; Goldmann three-mirror, small and large; Worst spherical goniotomy lens, small and large.

In use, the adult must have a topical anesthetic such as Ophthaine or Ophthetic instilled. Infants and small children require light general anesthetic under proper preparation and with appropriate resuscitation safeguards immediately available. A small amount of 2% to 6% methylcellulose solution is placed in the concavity of the corneal surface of the lens both to complete the lens-corneal contact and to reduce possible edge trauma. When the sitting position is used for slit lamp gonioscopy, the

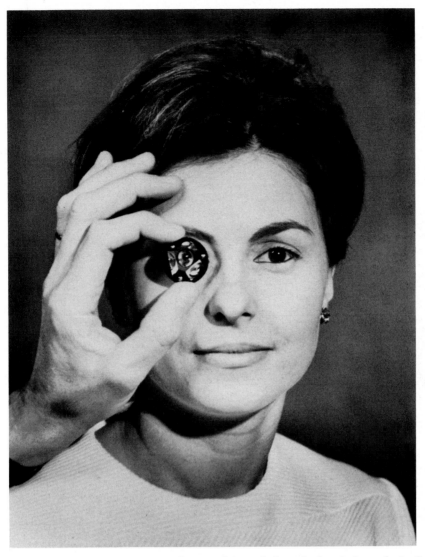

Fig. 7-5. Goldmann three-mirror contact lens in place with the aid of topical anesthetic. Small semicircular mirror shown in upper position is angulated for inspection of the filtration angle.

patient is first positioned on the chinrest and the slit lamp turned on. With the lens held between the thumb and forefinger of one hand, the thumb of the opposite hand is used to draw down the lower lid while the patient looks upward. The lower edge of the goniolens is then inserted against the center of the lower lid border, and the hand is moved to draw the upper lid away from the globe. At this time, the goniolens is rotated upward, bringing its concave surface against the patient's cornea. At the same time, the upper lid is released to drop against the upper surface of the lens. The patient is initially asked to maintain the primary position of gaze and not to squeeze his lids (Fig. 7-5).

Illumination and technique

Light is no problem with indirect lenses used at the slip lamp, but for direct lenses used with a supine patient it is necessary to have a small focal light source such as the Barkan illuminator (Fig. 7-6) or the illuminators built into the Troncoso, Heine, and Haag-Streit binocular gonioscopes. For

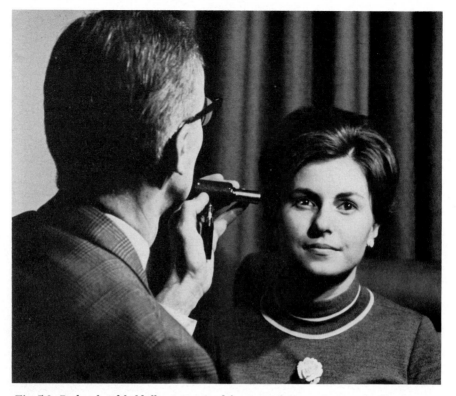

Fig. 7-6. Barkan hand-held illuminator used for external inspection or gonioillumination.

slit lamp gonioscopy, the light and line of observation are brought to coincidence first on the reflecting surface positioned at the upper pole in order to study the lower angle. It is generally necessary to tilt the lens at various points of examination in order to visualize the angle fully. Initial contact should be quite light against the eye, to avoid unknowingly manipulating open an angle that has been physiologically closed. The entire circumference of the angle is then inspected by rotating the goniolens and the illuminating and observation systems or with multiple mirrors by moving the light and line of observation to successive mirrors.

Indirect slit lamp gonioscopy of the upper angle is at times slightly more difficult than the lower, and focusing into the medial and lateral areas is the most difficult because it affords the least latitude in aligning the light and observational axes. Sclerotic scatter (p. 77) may be used in the horizontal recesses if it seems impossible to obtain illumination and visualization in good coordination. The Leydecker (1969) goniolens directs light into the angle by incorporated fiber optics and has the added benefit of not requiring contact fluid between the lens and the cornea. This is an advantage at surgery as well as at examination in that one additional step is deleted from the technique.

Diffuse or broad-beam illumination should first be used in identification of the landmarks of the angle and major pathologic alterations. The beam should then be narrowed to a fine slit in order to demonstrate in optic section the precise curvature of the iris surface into the angle.

Landmarks

The landmarks should be sought serially from anterior (corneal) to posterior (iridic). They include:

Schwalbe's line. Schwalbe's line (anterior

border ring) or termination of Descemet's membrane appears as a whitish line, often projecting slightly into the anterior chamber.

Trabecular meshwork. The trabecular meshwork extends from its anterior limits at Schwalbe's line to the blending of its posterior (uveal) portion with the anterior iris surface.

Schlemm's canal. Found beneath the junction of the middle and posterior thirds of the trabecular meshwork, Schlemm's canal sometimes appears as a faint gray line or a blood-filled line deep to the trabeculum.

Scleral spur. The scleral spur is the most anterior projection of the sclera and often appears through the trabeculum as a gray-white line of varying width at the outer end of the angle recess.

Ciliary body band. The ciliary body band is a stripe created by the anterior portion of the ciliary body when it is within gonioscopic view. It usually appears to extend from the root of the iris to the scleral spur, but in some eyes it is completely veiled by the overlying posterior trabecular meshwork. In darkly pigmented individuals the band appears to be dark gray, and in light individuals it may be unpigmented. In angle recession, the ciliary muscle is torn from the scleral spur, and therefore exposed scleral whiteness may be seen in this area. The narrower the angle, or the farther forward the iris is attached, the narrower or less visible will be the ciliary body band.

Iris processes (pectinate fibers). The iris processes bridge the angle recess from the anterior iris surface to the trabeculum, usually in the scleral spur area. Some processes, however, may run as far forward as Schwalbe's line. The processes are pigmented and more conspicuous with brown irides; with blue irides they appear light gray and are difficult to identify.

Trabecular pigment band. The trabecular pigment band often appears in the proximal meshwork just anterior to the scleral spur. This results from uveal pig-

ment being carried through the trabeculum with the aqueous flow. It is seen more commonly (1) in the inferior trabeculum, (2) in darkly pigmented eyes, (3) in advancing years, (4) in the presence of a Krukenberg spindle, (5) in the diabetic patient, (6) in eyes with anterior melanomas, (7) following uveitis, and (8) in pigmentary glaucoma. The width and intensity of this pigment band is graded from 1 through 4, and in the most advanced grade it fills about half or more of the trabecular width.

Adhesions (synechiae). Adhesions occur between the iris surface and trabeculum or farther anteriorly. They may vary widely in appearance from small and tent-like types from localized injury, through columnar or broad adhesions of previous narrow-angle glaucoma attacks, to essentially circumferential apposition, or extensive strands and broad processes arching forward from the anterior iris surface to Schwalbe's line, as in the congenital anomaly of Axenfeld (1920).

Blood vessels. Vascular patterns vary widely in the angle. The normal radial iris vessels appear as irregularly corkscrew structures in the peripheral iris, particularly if pigmentation is light. Anomalous knuckles or hairpin loops of normal vessels may emerge through the iris or ciliary body. Pathologic or new vessels tend to be on the surface of the iris or trabeculum at indiscriminate angulations and with some fibrous proliferation about them.

Grading of iridocorneal angle

Accurate observation should be made of the openness or depth of the anterior chamber angle or iridocorneal angle. This is graded from 0 through 4. Unfortunately, contradictory systems exist for numerical designation of the width of the angle. The classification on the following page, sometimes known as the Shaffer System,* is in

---

*Adopted by the United States Public Health Service Committee on Glaucoma and by the Symposium on Primary Glaucoma of the American Academy of Ophthalmology and Otolaryngology.

Shaffer System

Numerical grade	Terminology	Description
0	Closed	Anterior iris surface is in contact with peripheral corneal endothelium and trabeculum, or it is sufficiently displaced forward so as to preclude visualization of any anatomic details of the trabecular area. The lens is well anterior to the ciliary body ring. The central, endothelial iris surface is snug against a major area of the anterior capsule.
1	Extremely narrow	The iridocorneal angle is reduced to approximately 10 degrees, or "slit-like" appearance. It will close with slight iris edema or additional bombé, such as from physiologic pupillary block. Closure is probably inevitable in time. The lens is anterior to the ciliary body ring and a large area of endothelial iris surface is in contact with the anterior capsule.
2	Moderately narrow angle	The iridocorneal angle is approximately 20 degrees. The iris surface appears to be modestly convex but anterior trabecular details can usually be visualized without excessive tilting and manipulation of the goniolens, though these maneuvers may be necessary to inspect the narrowed posterior depths of the angle. The lens is slightly anterior to the ciliary body ring, and there is moderately broad contact between the endothelial iris surface centrally and the anterior capsule. Closure is certainly possible, and the earlier in life such angles are seen, the greater the likelihood of angle closure in later life. Such angles are more commonly found in later years of life and with hyperopia.
3	Open angle	The iridocorneal angle is approximately 30 degrees and there is only a little convexity of the iris surface. Anterior trabecular details are easily apparent, and posterior trabecular details can be seen with only modest tilting or angulation of the goniolens. The lens is approximately on a level with the ciliary body ring. Closure is most unlikely or impossible. This angle configuration is more likely in myopia than in hyperopia.
4	Wide open angle	The iridocorneal angle is approximately 45 degrees. All details of the trabecular area and recess are visualized with ease. The iris extends from its attachment at the inner anterior border of the ciliary body and generally appears flat. The lens is on a level with or slightly posterior to the ciliary body ring, and there is minimal contact between the endothelial iris surface centrally and the anterior lens capsule. Physiologic pupillary block and angle closure are both essentially impossible. This type of angle is commonly seen in youth, myopia, and aphakia.

wide use and logically considers the zero angle to be the closed angle.

In quantitating the width of the iridocorneal angle and to avoid distortion of trabecular details by oblique inspection, the observer's line of view should be as nearly parallel as possible to the surface of the iris. In narrow-angled eyes (grades 1 and 2), however, the necessarily oblique view precludes critical evaluation of structures beneath the trabeculum and gives a foreshortened illusion of the extent of the meshwork.

Recording angle characteristics

Just as inflammatory adhesions may be limited to specific areas of the angle, so may the anatomic characteristics differ in various portions. At times the entire 360 degrees will be fully open grade 3 or 4, and in the presence of certain catastrophies the angle may be 0 throughout. The ophthalmologist should note configuration of the angle by quadrants or positions of clock hours. More detail may be displayed graphically and in fewer words by use of a sche-

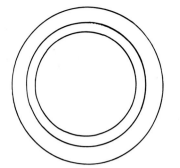

Fig. 7-7. Scheme for diagramming details of the anterior chamber angle. Outer circle represents Schwalbe's line with trabecular meshwork extending to the middle circle, which represents the scleral spur. The angle recess is represented by the space extending to the inner circle, which indicates the iris root or iris insertion. The position and height of synechiae are recorded by drawing in radial lines to their anterior limit. The grade of angle width, 0 through 4, is noted by placing the appropriate number in each quadrant or clock position adjacent to the outer circle.

matic set of three concentric circles in which the outermost represents Schwalbe's line, the middle represents the scleral spur, and the innermost represents the angle recess (Fig. 7-7).

Chapter 8

The uvea and its disturbances (inflammatory diseases of the choroid and retina)

Differentiating the red eye of intraocular inflammation from the generally less serious external infections of conjunctivitis and the major problem of congestive, acute, or subacute glaucoma presents an immediate and pressing problem. Probably the most pivotal sign is the pupil: this usually is normal in external infections, tends to be smaller and somewhat irregular in uveitis, or larger and somewhat vertically ovalized in acute or angle-closure glaucoma. Thus a normal-size and reactive pupil tends to rule out acute or severe intraocular disturbances in the presence of a red eye. Secretions also furnish some guide: external infections produce tenacious or purulent secretions with matting or adherence of the lids on awakening; both uveitis and glaucoma produce excessive secretions, but these are clear, watery tears. Pain is generally mild in posterior uveitis and conjunctivitis, moderate in anterior uveitis, and severe in acute glaucoma. Severe uveitis in childhood, however, may be deceptively devoid of discomfort.

Diagnosis in any illness is best made on the basis of specific cause. Often, however, in uveitis no specific cause, either local or general, is identified even after extensive search. In studying disease manifestations and in considering prognosis, it is important to make at least a morphologic description and classification of the ocular process. The following interim classification provides valuable working data:

Classification of uveitis

A. Anatomic area of inflammation
  1. Anterior uveitis or iritis: swelling and inflammatory signs confined primarily to the iris and circumcorneal area
  2. Iridocyclitis: inflammatory disturbances involving both the iris and ciliary body (This is more frequent than iritis alone, generally produces uncomfortable disturbances of accommodation, and causes ocular hypotonia because of impaired aqueous secretion.)
  3. Posterior uveitis (chorioretinitis): appears in many forms and should be specified as to whether the retina or the choroid is primarily inflamed (Disturbances in the retina commonly produce marked cellular debris in the vitreous.)
    a. Macular or posterior polar involvement: an almost exclusive localization
    b. The pars plana (pars planitis): may be principal site of involvement
    c. Peripheral or disseminated involvement: primary localization of pathology
B. Stage of activity
  1. Acute: sudden onset of findings in a previously clear and quiet eye
  2. Subacute: modest or mild onset without sudden, disabling symptoms
  3. Chronic: persistent inflammation, though subject to variations in severity
  4. Recurrent: intermittent inflammation with complete clearing and quieting between episodes

C. Degree of severity
  1. Mild: slight discomfort, little lid edema, minimal disturbance of vision, and almost no disturbance of pupillary reaction
  2. Moderate: discomfort requiring medication and particularly troublesome at night, mild lid edema, significantly depressed vision, small and irregular pupil (if involvement is anterior)
  3. Severe: pain not completely controlled by simple or oral medications, marked lid edema, poor vision, pupil small and caught by inflammatory adhesions to the lens capsule (if involvement is anterior)
D. Type of inflammation (this may vary from time to time)
  1. Nongranulomatous: usually diffuse edema without lumpy infiltration of uvea; small gray or slightly pigmented inflammatory deposits on corneal endothelium
  2. Granulomatous: chronic inflammatory signs with localized thickening of the uveal tissue; fatty or lardaceous deposits on the corneal endothelium

Such notations produce an orderly ocular base on which to seek associated systemic disturbances and to obtain special tests. Previously many clinicians felt that a diagnosis of uveitis was automatically an indication for a "uveitis survey" or "uveitis work-up." This has often been time consuming, uncomfortable for the patient, and fruitlessly expensive. Instead of widely scattered and frenetic activities, from general physical examinations through exotic serologic tests for leptospirosis (which can cause uveitis), the examiner should (1) recheck his questions concerning previous medical history for any inflammatory disease associated with uveal inflammation (such as histoplasmosis, tuberculosis, toxoplasmosis, sarcoidosis, rheumatoid arthritis in children, or syphilis), (2) inquire into any active focal infection that may be troubling the patient (periapical dental inflammation, sinusitis, prostatitis, or tonsillitis), and (3) order such x-rays or laboratory tests as may be related to the type of uveitis or suspect areas of medical disturbance. Thus an active granulomatous process particularly involving the retina at the posterior pole suggests skin sensitivity tests and agglutination tests for toxoplasmosis.

The appearance of so-called candle wax drippings about vessels in the posterior pole particularly indicates study of the long bones and serum albumin–globulin ratio for sarcoidosis. Chronic dental sepsis in the presence of acute serous anterior uveitis suggests dental x-rays for periapical abscesses.

Skin tests for sensitivity to tuberculoprotein, histoplasmin, or toxoplasmin are significant to indicate a previous exposure to the organisms of these diseases. On the other hand, skin testing for sensitivity to *Streptococcus* is a remote and almost desperate last-ditch search for an unlikely cause after more logical efforts have failed.

In examining the eye with uveitis, the slit lamp is the principal tool. This is necessary to determine the character of inflammatory precipitates on the corneal endothelium and to evaluate changes in the iris architecture. A fine or small beam is necessary to quantitate the flare or Tyndall effect of increased protein in the anterior chamber. This should be graded 1 to 4, and at the same time effort should be made to quantitate cells that may be floating in the anterior chamber or fixed there if the chamber appears "frozen."

In posterior uveitis, the indirect ophthalmoscope is often obligatory to see through a hazy vitreous. It is also necessary, along with scleral depression, to visualize the pars plana and to identify the inflammatory foci often called "snowballs," which tend to be chronic in this area.

Slit lamp examination of cellular precipitates (KP) on the corneal endothelium gives a fair guide to the type of inflammation. Polymorphonuclear leukocytes tend to form a very thin cellular layer and may resemble tiny drops before larger volumes of cells gravitate to the inferior chamber angle as hypopyon. Lymphocytes tend to form compact and globular aggregations that are tightly localized. The cells of chronic active uveitis, which are often monocytes, tend to form keratic precipitates that are large, greasy, or mutton-fat in character; these are commonly found in granulomatous inflammations classically related to sarcoidosis, sympathetic ophthalmitis, and possibly tuberculosis.

In very low-grade inflammation such as heterochromic iridocyclitis, the KP's tend to be small, round, and whitish. Precipitates of fibrin in acute and severe uveitis may overlay or obscure the character of the inflammatory cell precipitates and also create extremely turbid or even "frozen" aqueous with the loss of all thermal convexion currents in the anterior chamber. Such dense or plastic exudates generally respond quickly to appropriate treatment, whereas the very low-grade and minor inflammatory reactions may drag on for months and even years, with poor response to anti-inflammatory management.

As the uveitis subsides, KP's tend to thin and the edges become crenated, forming somewhat stellate configurations. Pigmentary deposits, either uveal or fibrinous in origin, are usually the slowest in resolving and may persist weeks after other characteristics of the inflammatory deposits clear.

Roentgenographic examination is also important in diagnostic support of several causative mechanisms. The most obvious is x-ray of the eye for possible retained foreign bodies. Skull x-rays may reveal several important corollaries such as medium-sized cortical calcifications in congenital toxoplasmosis or finer calcific deposits deeper and near the ventricular system in cytomegalic inclusion disease. The same skull x-rays will give an indication of inflammatory clouding of the paranasal sinuses, which may merit treatment in its own right. Chest x-rays are important in parenchymal shadows of tuberculosis or hilar and mediastinal shadows of histoplasmosis. The fingers and long bones may show osteolytic or punched-out areas in the presence of sarcoidosis, and dental x-rays are necessary to reveal the common periapical infection that may be a quiet nidus of intermittent bacteremia.

The diagnostician in uveitis neither throws up his hands in therapeutic nihilism nor spins the prayer wheel of countless laboratory tests and special procedures. He must follow the indications of a penetrating medical history and the leads furnished by the characteristics of the patient and the eye toward a sensible plan of well-oriented studies.

Chapter 9

The lens and its disturbances

The lens is a small, biconvex, and normally transparent focusing component of the optic system of the eye. It is encased in a clear and highly elastic capsule, which in turn is supported by zonular fibers encircling the 360 degrees of its equator and attaching to the ciliary body, generally between the ciliary processes or into the pars plana and ora serrata. The lens normally goes through marked variations in its curvature, softness or moldability, zones of optic discontinuity, and even clarity during the normal lifetime. At birth it tends to be quite spherical and contributes to the shallow anterior chamber of infancy. In the first years of life there is apparent flattening that may be related to increased tension of the zonule and the elastic capsule. Throughout life, new cortical layers of lens fibers continue to be laid down at the periphery or subcapsular portions of the lens. With age, this causes increasing lens thickness, consequent shallowing of the anterior chamber, and, with the swelling that may lead to senile cataractous changes, some "myopic shift" in total refraction.

ZONES OF DISCONTINUITY

Zones of optic discontinuity may be visualized within the lens by careful slit lamp examination. These are variable in relation to (1) age; (2) medical, nutritional, or endocrine disturbances that may be experienced; and (3) individual characteristics of the particular patient under study.

In a high light intensity, narrow slit beam (the "cut" of an optic section in direct or focal illumination), the anterior capsule appears as a distinctly bright or relucent surface layer. The posterior capsule is anatomically thinner as well as somewhat obscured by diffraction of light passing through the lens and is therefore less clearly visible. Beneath the capsule is a less relucent, concentric layer, the cortex, composed of young and superficial fibers. Deep to the cortex, various nuclear zones of optic discontinuity can be identified; these have often been given conflicting names by different observers. The most central and normally the most clear is the embryonic nucleus. A fetal nucleus, commonly seen as areas of slightly greater relucency immediately anterior and posterior to the embryonic nucleus, can usually be identified. Often suture lines, appearing in Y shape anteriorly and in λ shape posteriorly, can be seen in this area or extending to the next most superficial nuclear layer, usually called the infantile nucleus. Superficial to this can be seen various lines of discontinuity representing the adult nucleus, which forms after puberty.

More complex second- and third-order bifurcations of the simple, deep, tripartite suture lines can often be seen extending normally through the adult nuclear layers. Following contusion trauma or early transcapsular fluid imbibition, these may be accentuated or "feathered." In mild injuries this may be reversible by absorption of such fluid, but in more severe trauma (capsular tears, subluxations, intralenticular foreign bodies, angle recession) or with the quiet inroads of maturity this may proceed to major cataractous opacification.

141

Notation of total lens thickness as well as thickness of nuclear and cortical components may furnish vital information concerning impending cataractous changes. This is particularly valuable when comparison can be made with an uninvolved fellow eye. In the juvenile or adolescent lens, interruptions in growth, such as are caused by contusion damage, may be followed in a matter of weeks or a few months by distinct lens thinning. Subsequent thickening seen in the zones of discontinuity is associated with loss of transparency and increased total thickness. In advanced age, the nuclear zone increases excessively and apparently at the expense of cortical thickness. Growth inhibitions in late life primarily affect the thin cortical layers rather than the nuclear zone. Thus an apparently thin nuclear zone in advanced life probably reflects metabolic impairment or contusion injury many years previously. Lenses that remain clear in the presence of other disturbances such as Coats' disease, retinal detachments, or early-onset diabetes tend to be thicker than lenses in the healthy individual (Goldmann, 1968).

POSITION OF THE LENS

Position should be the first element noted in diagnostic examination of the lens. Ordinarily the lens supplies physical support to the iris through its posterior surface. When not uniformly supported in this frontal plane, the lens may be partially dislocated (*subluxated*) or completely freed of its zonular attachments (*luxated*) and moved through the pupillary area (*anterior*) or into the vitreous (*posterior*). Vertical and horizontal directions may also be indicated.

Tremulousness of the iris or iridodonesis suggests posterior subluxation. This may usually be detected with sharp focal light and direct observation while the patient shifts his gaze back and forth between such easily available targets as the right and left ears of the examiner. Infrequently this is noted only with the aid of slit lamp magnification, which may also confirm the positional disturbance of the lens through its

own phakodonesis. If the lens is not seen through the pupil at all, it may be luxated posteriorly or remain hinged below. The posterior subluxation in Marfan's disease is nearly always upward, so that the lower lens equator encroaches on the pupil. Aside from visual distortions, these posterior positions create no acute distress to the patient.

Anterior subluxation is usually marked by lodgment of the lens partially through the iris sphincter with consequent ovalization of the pupil and impaired reactions. With complete positioning of the lens in the anterior chamber (anterior luxation) the iris is behind the lens, but the pupil is again commonly irregular and impaired in its reaction. Lenses encroaching on the anterior chamber commonly evoke a painful secondary glaucoma and require emergency measures to reduce intraocular pressure preparatory to surgical removal of the lens.

PATHOLOGIC ALTERATIONS IN THE LENS

In general the lens has only one major response to any type of insult or injury and that is loss of clarity or the development of opacity. Any opacity occurring within the normally clear lens may be technically called a cataract. A few small, punctate, or eccentric opacities, however, are so commonly uncovered on detailed search of the lens that they may almost be considered normal variations. Indeed, the word "cataract" should not be invoked for small opacities of no visual significance, particularly when they present no symmetric pattern or configuration (such as lamellar separation, subcapsular vacuoles, posterior cupuliform, or the snowflake cataract of diabetes) indicative of progression.

Congenital defects

Many morphologic variations of lens opacities seen in early life may be identified (zonular or lamellar, anterior polar, stellate, centralis pulverulenta). Most of these represent autosomal dominant genetic traits. The anterior capsule often shows small, stellate aggregates of iris pigment (congenital and stationary lens stars), which may at times be connected to the iris collarette by strands of persistent pupillary membrane having the same color as the iris. At times the lens equator will be notched and its suspensory ligaments missing at that point in association with congenital colobomas of the iris or the retina and choroid. Rarely the lens configuration will be quite small and round though completely clear (spherophakia).

Cataract formation other than congenital

Noncongenital cataract formation is one of the most common problems among all the disturbances of the eye. It may be apparently primary, senile, or without cause. At other times it follows injuries such as mechanical contusions, foreign body wounds, electric shock, chemical burns of the anterior segment, x-ray or microwave exposure, and so forth. It may also be associated with other general medical disturbances such as diabetes, tetany, galactosemia, or myotonic dystrophy or with dermatologic conditions such as atopic dermatitis.

The stage of cataractous opacification should be described as incipient, then immature, mature, and hypermature. The many morphologic variations occurring in each stage should be recorded either in descriptive terms or by external photography.

Vision undergoes progressive embarrassment as opacity increases. It is most important, however, to identify the stage of incipient intumescence or approaching hypermaturity because this is associated with increasing lens convexity and thickness. Such changes may shallow the anterior chamber and filtration angle leading to lens-induced glaucoma from mechanical swelling of the lens (phakomorphic glaucoma).

A mature cataract is one that has developed complete opacification throughout. Generally this indicates surgical removal of the lens—particularly if the anterior chamber is shallow—regardless of the clarity of vision in the other eye. This is be-

cause of the threat of acute, secondary glaucoma.

Foreign bodies

Small foreign bodies that penetrate only the anterior and not the posterior capsule of the lens may be tolerated without major cataract formation. This is particularly true if the anterior capsular laceration is so small that the capsule edges tend to fall back onto the lens cortex or into near apposition. The foreign body, of course, must be of an inert material such as glass, aluminum, or stainless steel. Ferrous or copper foreign bodies cause destructive chemical reaction and must be removed except when they are of minute size.

In the presence of an unexplained unilateral cataract it is always essential to make careful slit lamp search for a perforating linear scar through the cornea or a small hole in the iris. Bone-free x-ray studies made with small squares of dental film firmly pressed into the inner canthal area may confirm even low-density material such as glass fragments.

Reexamination of patients with cataracts

Patients with cataracts generally must be reexamined more often than patients without active pathology. Early (incipient or immature) cataracts cause changes in refraction particularly marked by increasing myopia at an age when refraction should either be stable or show increasing hyperopia. Nearly mature lenses, with their threat of maturity and intumescence, also call for frequent examination. In the absence of pain or marked subjective symptoms, cataract patients should probably be reexamined about three times a year. It must also be remembered that senile cataracts occur at a time in life when the incidence of chronic simple glaucoma is increasing. Therefore such cataract patients should be carefully examined for chronic simple or open-angle glaucoma as well as for the state of lens opacification and swelling.

With the diagnosis of cataract—the most

common pathologic alteration encountered in the lens—a morphologic description of the opacities and the areas of involvement should always be noted. An investigation for both local and systemic causes should always be undertaken. One of the most valuable of all diagnostic tools, the subsequent examination, should be scheduled at appropriate intervals of 6 months or less, depending upon the suggestion of progressiveness. Remember, too, that scattered or even localized opacities such as relatively dense nuclear sclerosis generally cause visual distortion that may be ameliorated by spectacle correction. It is important, therefore, to repeat the refractive examination at more frequent intervals than in the noncataractous eye. This may be the greatest contribution made to the patient's visual life.

A record of myopic shift is a documentation of cataract progression and intumescence. This may occur in the diabetic patient (more commonly the young than the old, and more commonly the undiagnosed than the diagnosed) or in the presence of usual senile cataracts. Diabetes and pathology of the lens should be particularly suspected in the adult requiring significant change in spectacle prescription, such as two or three times a year.

Chapter 10

The vitreous and its disturbances

The vitreous body has become of increasing diagnostic importance with improvement in understanding of retinal detachment mechanisms. Refinements in ophthalmoscopy and slit lamp examination of the vitreoretinal interface have also added new clinical significance to examination of the vitreous.

STRUCTURE OF THE VITREOUS

The normal vitreous body is a semisolid, jelly-like mass enveloped within a boundary condensation or "hyaloid surface" variously identified by the anatomic position of its components. Thus the *posterior hyaloid* is generally considered to be the portion in intimate relationship with the internal limiting membrane of the retina from the ora serrata to its generally discrete encirclement of the optic disc. The *base of the vitreous* is a ring varying between 2 and 3 mm. in width and characterized by firm adherence to the ciliary epithelium, with subordinate strands attached to the ciliary processes and some of the zonular fibers.

The *anterior hyaloid* extends forward from the pars plana and almost immediately begins to curve backward, forming a concavity in the phakic eye known as the patellar fossa. A faint and inconstant ring 8 to 9 mm. in diameter, the hyaloideocapsular ligament of Wieger, occurs about the center of this concavity. In youth this constitutes a relatively firm attachment between the posterior capsule and the anterior hyaloid. It is generally difficult or impossible to identify even under optimal conditions of slit lamp examination.

The anterior hyaloid in the aphakic eye generally loses its concavity (patellar fossa) and may variously appear to be flat, convex through the pupil, discontinuous, mushrooming into the anterior chamber, or marked only by irregular fimbria floating forward.

In early life there may be seen a canal of Cloquet of optically less dense or primary vitreous several millimeters in diameter immediately behind the posterior lens capsule. This funnels into a narrower tubular diameter and sags loosely across the main mass of the vitreous to dilate again into the prepapillary space of Martegiani.

Actually the vitreous represents the simplest type of connective tissue and is the largest single specimen of intercellular material that can be found in the body. The vitreous does possess greater relucency than the aqueous when examined in a concentrated light beam. Optically identifiable micellae and fibrillar lines tending to crisscross irregularly are sometimes called "pseudostructures," but they give objective evidence of the physical consistency of the vitreous. When normal gel consistency is preserved, such micellae and vitreous landmarks swirl gently within the vitreous in response to movement of the globe. When the vitreous has undergone liquefaction, these components drift without restraint and fall freely in response to gravity.

PRELIMINARY INSPECTION

Preliminary inspection of the vitreous can be accomplished with either the ophthalmoscope (p. 165) or the slit lamp.

Dilation of the pupil greatly increases the available angle of observation and detection of details away from the visual axis. The high-voltage direct ophthalmoscope, when used in the preliminary position a foot or two from the pupil, immediately reveals the shadows of any vitreous opacities in the line of illumination. The movement of such shadows with or against the direction of rotation of the globe indicates whether the opacities are respectively anterior or posterior to the center of rotation, which is generally 13 to 14 mm. behind the apex of the cornea. The freedom or constraint of movement within the vitreous also indicates whether the vitreous is normal and gel-like or abnormal and liquefied or replaced. With a high plus lens in the ophthalmoscope it is possible to study the size, approximate character, and distribution of the opacities.

The focal beam of the slit lamp also offers a sometimes neglected preliminary view of the vitreous with the unaided eye. Such an initial maneuver establishes the clarity of the media and the presence or absence of gross disturbances. The red color of fresh blood in the vitreous is best identified by this macroscopic technique. Membranous and trabecular formations can also be oriented promptly. With either direct view or use of the biomicroscope, only about the anterior third of the vitreous is accessible to examination.

The indirect ophthalmoscope immediately combines the advantages of high illumination, broad field, and stereopsis. This assists in overcoming impediments of partial opacities in the cornea, lens, and vitreous. The colloquial phrase "to burn through" vitreous haze aptly applies to the advantages of illumination and binocularity in visualizing retinal details through blood, inflammatory cells, or other debris in the vitreous.

DETAILED EXAMINATION

Detailed examination of the vitreous is best done with a modern slit lamp biomicroscope and a lens to overcome the

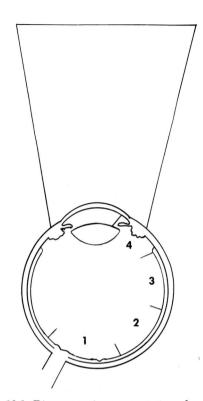

Fig. 10-1. Diagrammatic representation of approximate intraocular areas visualized with aid of Goldmann three-mirror contact lens. *1,* Thirty-degree area of posterior pole seen directly through center of lens face without use of mirror. *2,* Area between posterior pole and equator seen through the wide mirror, which is most nearly parallel to the line of inspection. *3,* Area from equator to near the ora serrata seen through the medium width and medium angulated mirror. *4,* Area including anterior chamber filtration angle, posterior chamber, vitreous base, and pars plana seen through the smallest or semicircular mirror.

strong power of the corneal curvature. The preset Hruby −55-diopter lens mounted on a slit lamp gives good access through the central vitreous and its most posterior portions, including its attachment at the disc and overlying the macula. Because the Hruby lens is not in direct contact with the cornea, however, it affords poor accessibility anterior to the equator and into the peripheral portions of vitreous and retina. It does afford detection of posterior and large detachments of the vitreous.

Contact lenses for vitreous and fundus examination increase the range and angulation of accessibility. The Goldmann fundus lens has a 12-mm. diameter optic surface and will afford inspection of a 30-degree field well into the equator. Similarly the Krieger fundus lens and the Worst Lo-Vac fundus contact lens afford considerably larger areas for examination than can be reached with the present Hruby lens, which is not in contact with the cornea.

More peripheral access to vitreous and fundus with contact lens examination is afforded by the Goldmann (Fig. 10-1) three-mirror contact lens. Through its flat front surface, visualization to the posterior pole is easy; by shifting the lines of illumination and observation, three separate steps or angulations of inspection are available. The smallest and semicircular mirror presents the most angulation and therefore gives visualization not only of the anterior chamber angle but also of the pars plana and ora serrata. Inspection of the vitreous base attachment here is under greater magnification than can be achieved with standard indirect ophthalmoscope lenses. The intermediate width mirror affords visualization from the ora serrata to the equator, and the widest mirror (most closely angulated to the line of inspection) generally bridges the area between the equator and the field of direct observation through the flat front surface. Practice is required in rapidly shifting from one mirror to another, but this technique affords the most information about vitreous attachments to the retina, and specifically their relation to retinal breaks or suspect traction sites.

Scleral depression as an adjunct to examination with the intermediate width mirror sometimes facilitates visualization of the pars plana, ciliary processes, and zonular insertions particularly in the hyperopic, phakic eye. An Eisner funnel (1968) is available as a carrier cone into which the Goldmann three-mirror lens may be placed. The funnel is held between the examiner's thumb and middle finger while the index finger is applied to the near or wide-mouth end of the funnel, at a point corresponding to the region to be indented (Goldmann, 1968).

The unique Lo-Vac Peripheral Fundus Contactlens gives unmirrored or direct (not indirect, as in the Goldmann) view of the region between the equator and the ora. Scleral depression is needed in the farthest periphery, and the lens must be rotated around its axis to reach each quadrant. Though the Lo-Vac series of contact lenses from Holland is of progressive design, actually the question of the lens adhering to the globe presents little need of even finger assistance in most cases. This is because of good corneal curve design and the aid of capillarity.

Posterior detachment of the vitreous may be circumscribed in area, but more commonly the inexperienced examiner is circumscribed in his visualization. Occasionally a large area of posterior cavitation will be mistaken for detachment if the examiner is unable to follow the vitreous boundary. The most resistant sites to vitreous detachment tend to be the base and the optic nerve. Frequently, however, the posterior detachment is well evidenced by a boundary ring configuration (disinsertion from the optic disc) in the posterior hyaloid as it floats in front of the disc.

Though complete detachments may occur in young and nonmyopic individuals without cavitation and disorganization of the vitreous, this type of pathologic change is commonly associated with vitreous collapse and occurs more often in the elderly and the myopic. Funnel-shaped detachment, seen from time to time in old or unsuccessfully treated retinal detachments, is unusual as a type of vitreous detachment. On the other hand, massive vitreous retraction following vitreous hemorrhage, inflammatory complications, fibrosis, and membrane formation is an unfortunately frequent late-stage problem associated with fixed and star folds in the detached retina.

Vitreous opacities may be hemorrhagic, inflammatory (exudative), pigmentary, asteroid, or crystalline (synchysis scintillans). They rarely may be larval invasions, neoplastic cells, or foreign bodies. All complaints of recent or increasing opacities that impose themselves on the patient's awareness *are* significant. The complaint of suddenly-appearing dark spots or floaters in the visual field must be investigated, with particular attention to the peripheral retina and hole formation. These symptoms of opacities are more suggestive of serious retinal traction or tugging when accompanied by flashes of light, lightning streaks, or "sparklers." The early identification of a retinal break or hole may afford an opportunity for relatively simple measures such as cryotherapy and thus avoid more complex surgery that would be needed for a major retinal detachment.

Opacities incidentally discovered during ophthalmoscopy and appearing as small spheres suspended in semifluid vitreous are usually unilateral and without serious significance. They are commonly found in the mature age group and are designated "asteroid bodies." At times their quantity and density will surprise the examiner who anticipates visual handicap from them.

Current advances in understanding of vitreous structure and interpretation of vitreous symptoms have brought entirely new and greatly increased significance to alterations in this body. The examiner now possesses instruments and understanding that did not exist a decade ago; with this armamentarium he may preside over distinctly lessened morbidity from vitreous and retinal disturbances.

Chapter 11

The lacrimal system and its disturbances

Complaints relating to the lacrimal system primarily concern insufficiency of tear secretion or epiphora (excessive tearing caused by inadequacy or blockage of the tear drainage passages). Less commonly there are complaints of enlargement or tumor involving either the tear gland or the drainage passages, and least frequently there is hyperlacrimation or hypersecretion. The last is often psychic, voluntary, or hysterical in origin, though it may be neurogenic from trigeminal or facial nerve irritation.

Examination of the lacrimal system should first assess the anatomy of the lids and lacrimal details without any traction or digital manipulation. This affords notation of tear flow over the lid borders, positioning of the lids, cilia, and puncta, and any disturbance or enlargement of the tear gland (tumors, inflammations, or, rarely, foreign bodies) or tear passages (inflammation, foreign bodies, or tumors). The most common foreign body of the lacrimal system is a broken cilium lodged painfully in the punctum and scratching the bulbar conjunctiva. Its diagnosis is aided by a history of abrupt onset, pain, and hyperlacrimation, with redness confined to the inner canthal area. Direct inspection confirms the diagnosis and immediate relief follows by lifting out the cilium.

The two major areas of functional examination, then, relate to inadequacy of tear secretion and inadequacy of drainage.

Observation, acute and astute, as in every area of diagnosis, spearheads the examination of the lacrimal system.

EXAMINATION OF TEAR SECRETION

A series of progressively quantitative techniques is available for the study of tear flow:

1. Preliminary inspection
2. Slit lamp examination of tear film
3. Vital staining (fluorescein and rose bengal)
4. Schirmer tests (I and II)
5. Provocative tests (irritative and drying)
6. Tear analysis
7. Gelatin rod test
8. Biopsy of the lacrimal gland

Preliminary inspection. As in all areas of examination, preliminary inspection should precede more detailed study. In focused oblique light, the cornea, conjunctiva, and lid borders should be inspected for brightness and the quality of a moist glistening surface. A dull or dry-looking cornea is immediate but gross evidence of tear deficiency. Ropy or stringy secretions on the cornea, in the cul-de-sac, or on the lid borders also suggest deficiency of tears.

Slit lamp examination. More subtle and early changes in the precorneal film are revealed by slit lamp examination. Small round to oval areas of interruption in the normal layering of the precorneal film of-

ten precede actual staining and major reduction in lacrimal fluid formation. Similarly, one may note loss of the "prism" or
meniscus of lacrimal fluid that normally
forms on the lid borders posterior to the
meibomian orifices and curves to the bulbar
conjunctiva (J. E. McDonald, 1968).

Vital staining. Vital staining is best done
either with the familiar sodium fluorescein
on sterile dry paper strips or with 1%
aqueous rose bengal solution. Impregnated
sterile papers eliminate the previously
tragic problem of *Pseudomonas aeruginosa*
contamination and growth in fluorescein
solutions (this is curbed by incorporating
1% chlorobutanol as is done commercially
in "Fluress" solution,* which contains the
topical anesthetic 0.4% benoxinate). With
brief application of a dry or moistened
strip to the upper outer bulbar conjunctiva,
it is not necessary to remove excess fluorescein by irrigation. Devitalized or desqua-
mated epithelial areas on the cornea show
greenish staining with this dye, whereas
similar areas on the conjunctiva show a
yellowish hue.

Rose bengal is not available in sterile
strips, and the aqueous solution presents a
threat of bacterial contamination similar to
that of fluorescein solutions. It is available,
however, in 5-ml. bottles.† A small drop
should be placed on the upper bulbar conjunctiva and permitted to course downward
over the cornea and lower conjunctiva with
the aid of a few blinks. Excess dye must
be promptly irrigated away. Positive reaction is shown by small, round, point-to-dot–
like, rose colored areas, particularly in the
lower corneal epithelium and inferior bulbar conjunctiva. The rose hue is essentially
the same over both cornea and conjunctiva.
This will often be positive before there is
definite fluorescein staining. In more advanced stages of drying, strands or fila-
mentary coils of devitalized epithelium

hang downward from these staining areas
of epithelial damage.

Schirmer test. The Schirmer test (1903)
is the most quantitative clinical procedure
available. No. 41 Whatman filter paper is
cut into strips 5 × 35 mm. in size,* with
the distal 5 mm. at one end folded into an
angulation that may be engaged over the
lower lid border. Care must be taken not
to irritate the conjunctiva or touch the
cornea as the folded end of the strip is put
over the ciliary border of the lower lid. The
eye should be kept open but without restraint of normal blinking movements. After
5 minutes, the strip is removed and the
linear distance of wetting from the fold
measured. The results are crudely quantitative, with normal young adults dampening 15 to the entire 30 mm. of strip. This is
a few millimeters less in males and less with
advancing decades of life. Dampening of
only 10 to 15 mm. is suspect deficiency,
and dampening of less than 10 mm. is distinctly indicative of deficiency. Dampening
of 5 mm. or less is almost invariably accompanied by significant symptoms (Fig.
11-1).

The preceding standard procedure is
sometimes referred to as "Schirmer I," to
differentiate it from a modified technique
called "Schirmer II" (Sexton; Wilson). In
this modification a topical anesthetic is instilled, the lower conjunctival cul-de-sac is
wiped dry with a cotton-tipped applicator,
and then the standard strip of Whatman
filter paper is engaged over the lower lid
border. A 5-minute reading under these
conditions may demonstrate surprisingly
distinct deficiency of tear formation in an
eye that appears clinically *wet* due to irritation of the mucous glands or goblet cells
of the conjunctiva. These unicellular mucous glands are destroyed in xerosis of
the conjunctiva, but in the presence of
chronic inflammation their mucin production, which forms the deep or mucoid com-

---

*Barnes-Hind Ophthalmic Products, Sunnyvale,
California 94086.
†Tilden-Yates Laboratories, Inc., Wayne, New Jer-
sey 07470.

*Available in sterile commercial packets of five
strips from Tilden-Yates Laboratories, Inc.,
Wayne, New Jersey 07470.

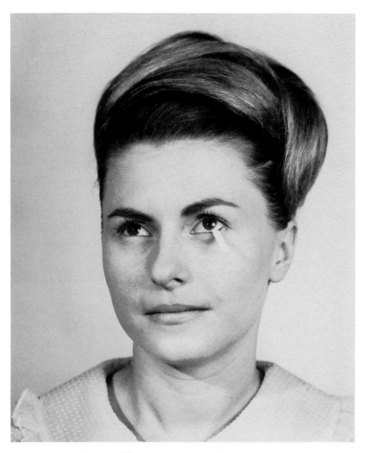

Fig. 11-1. Schirmer test showing filter paper properly engaged over lower lid border at junction of medial and temporal third in order to avoid corneal irritation.

ponent of the tear film, is much increased.

Provocative testing. When the results of Schirmer testing are uncertain or indicate apparent inadequacy of flow, the findings may be verified and amplified by stimulation of the nasal mucosa. Any irritating chemical such as ammonia or the lowly onion may be used to evoke tear flow. In the absence of such agents, touching the nasal mucosa with a cotton-tipped applicator has similar evocative power. These procedures are nonquantitative but, when failing to produce any added tear flow, may be taken as a reliable index of lacrimal gland impairment.

Tear analysis. Tear analysis for deficient lysozyme, which is an early finding in the Gougerot-Sjögren syndrome (deficiency of tears, saliva, and synovial fluid), may be done conveniently by two methods. First,

the dampened filter paper obtained by Schirmer testing can be transmitted to the laboratory in a moist chamber (Fig. 11-2) and used directly for electrophoretic analysis of the protein content of the tears. Second, a 5-mm. section of the tear-moistened filter paper may be placed on a standard blood agar culture plate previously streaked with a known culture of a common pathogen such as *Staphylococcus aureus.* In the presence of significant concentration of lysozyme in the tears, there should be a surrounding zone of bacterial growth inhibition. Complete absence of inhibition is strong evidence of lysozyme deficiency. Contamination may be introduced with the moist filter paper and its localized growth distinguished from the more uniform plating with the known bacteria.

Gelatin rod test. The gelatin rod test

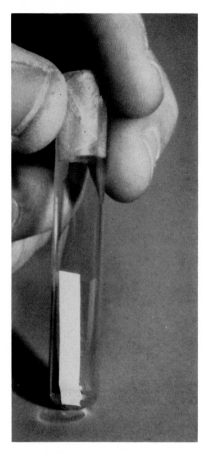

Fig. 11-2. Moistened paper from Schirmer test sealed in glass test tube for direct transmission to laboratory for electrophoretic analysis of protein content.

procedure is infrequently indicated in established deficiency of tears when patient comfort has not been achieved after successive trials of various artificial tear solutions. The test is done in contemplation of elective surgical occlusion of the lacrimal puncta. Small gelatin rods (Foulds, 1961) about 0.5 to 1 mm. in diameter and 1 cm. long are inserted with forceps through each punctum of the eye under examination and positioned within the canaliculi. These provide a test period of about 10 days to evaluate lacrimal fluid conservation and patient comfort before they are spontaneously absorbed. Even when the results are gratifying to patient and examiner, subsequent surgical obliteration of the puncta still must be evaluated thoughtfully because of the

tendency for Sjögren's syndrome to undergo remission after a period of years.

Biopsy of the lacrimal gland. Biopsy is frequently necessary to establish the nature of tear deficiency in the presence of enlargement. This can be done easily under local infiltration anesthesia. If the gland is easily prolapsed on eversion of the lid with the aid of the patient looking down and to the opposite side, it is best to biopsy the smaller or palpebral lobe through a conjunctival incision above the outer fourth of the tarsal plate. If the gland cannot be easily seen in this fashion, and if the orbital or superior lobe can be palpated, it is then permissible to biopsy through a horizontal skin incision. Because of occasional bleeding, these procedures are done most wisely in an ophthalmic operating room.

Should a malignancy such as mixed tumor or adenocarcinoma be suspected, it is wise to have a frozen section read by a pathologist familiar with the lacrimal gland (or the almost identical pathologic variations that occur in the salivary glands). If the findings on frozen section are questionable, then the incision should be closed until a satisfactory reading is obtained from paraffin or other permanent sections.

EXAMINATION OF LACRIMAL DRAINAGE
Preliminary inspection

Preliminary inspection of the drainage apparatus should be both ocular and intranasal. Ocular inspection is done first and in strong oblique light, with the aid of magnification and without touching the patient or lids. Observation should be made for (1) actual spillage of tears over the lid border, (2) maceration fissuring of the skin at the canthi or below the lower lid, (3) secretions on the lid border (ropy debris suggests keratoconjunctivitis sicca; frothy material suggests noninfectious oily meibomianitis; drying yellow debris suggests infectious conjunctivitis; oily scales suggest squamous blepharitis; collarettes about the lash bases suggest chronic staphylococcic blepharitis; and so on), (4) position of

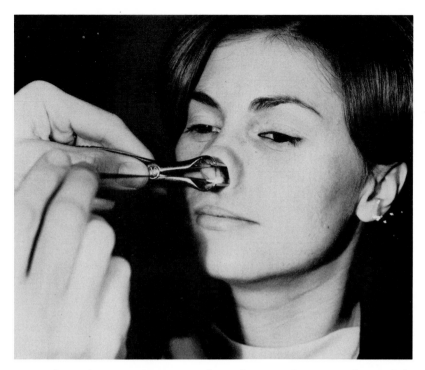

Fig. 11-3. Nasal speculum in position to visualize inferior nasal meatus and site of drainage from nasolacrimal duct. Excellent illumination may be obtained with standard indirect binocular ophthalmoscope.

the lid border, (5) position and configuration of the lacrimal puncta, and (6) action of the lids for frequency of blinking and adequacy of both normal and forced closure.

In all cases of epiphora, there must also be evaluation for nasal disease, particularly allergy, polyps, injuries, or surgery. Every ophthalmologist should have a nasal speculum (Fig. 11-3) and should be comfortable in evaluating normal and altered intranasal anatomy. Any binocular, indirect ophthalmoscope is an excellent illumination source for this purpose. The best dacryocystorhinostomy is doomed to failure in the presence of nasal polyposis, and it may be a lethal error in the presence of carcinoma of the antrum or ethmoids.

Functional testing

Functional testing of the nasolacrimal passages should proceed through the following steps:

1. Dye passage without assistance or force
2. Irrigation of the passages
3. Probing of the passages
4. Roentgenographic examination
   a. Orbital and paranasal sinuses
   b. Dacryocystogram

Dye passage. A strip of tear fluid roughly triangular or prismatic in cross section is normally present along the posterior edge of both upper and lower lid borders. The normal punctum angulates posteriorly at about 45 degrees to dip into this meniscus of fluid rather than opening vertically, into air, or directly posteriorly, into physiologic occlusion by the bulbar conjunctiva. Normally both capillarity and siphoning action (Horner's muscle and the orbicularis oculi [pars lacrimalis]), aspirate tears into the lacrimal passages. Thus fluorescein, when instilled into the lacrimal lake, should appear within a minute or two beneath the inferior turbinate. This is best determined by

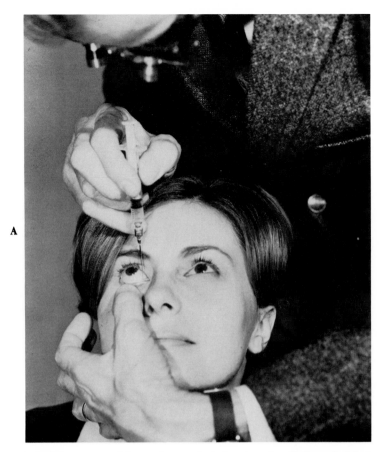

Fig. 11-4. **A,** Initial position of lacrimal cannula being introduced through inferior punctum into vertical segment of the canaliculus. Note slight eversion of the lower lid by thumb of examiner's opposite hand. **B,** Second position of lacrimal cannula, following passage through punctum and vertical segment of canaliculus. Cannula is now being advanced through horizontal canaliculus into the sac. Note gentle downward and lateral tension on lower lid from thumb of examiner's opposite hand.

direct visualization with the nasal speculum and indirect ophthalmoscope (the cobalt blue filter, if available over the light source, helps to reveal minute amounts of fluorescein). If nasal deformity makes direct inspection difficult, a malleable wire applicator carrying a small roll of cotton moistened in any topical anesthetic may be inserted for a depth of an inch or an inch and a half along the lateral nasal wall beneath the inferior turbinate. This can be used to wipe up or recover the fluorescein if it has traversed the passages.

If fluorescein cannot be found in the nose, the passages may be blocked, or the siphoning action may be inefficient.

Irrigation. Irrigation of the lacrimal passages should be done after instillation of a topical anesthetic. This is best accomplished with a plain, straight lacrimal cannula (these are traditionally gold-plated, for no apparent reason) attached to a 2-ml. syringe filled with sterile normal saline. If the puncta appear very small or tight, a sharp, pointed dilator (Simpson size 1 or 2; Ziegler size 1; Ruedemann; or a small safety pin) may be inserted before the cannula is used. Care must be exercised to avoid tearing the lacrimal papillae with large instruments or stretching maneuvers. Because such lacerations are functionally more incapacitating at the lower than the

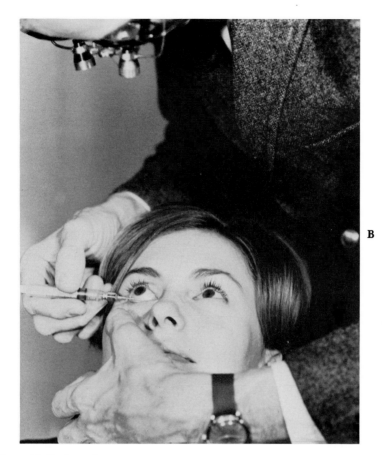

B

Fig. 11-4, cont'd. For legend see opposite page.

upper punctum, many physicians prefer to use the upper for routine access to the nasolacrimal duct.

In examination of canalicular impairments or conjunctivitis secondary to lacrimal disease, it is necessary to enter *both* the upper and lower passages. The irrigating tip is advanced vertically into the canaliculus 1 or 2 mm. into the lower lid (Fig. 11-4, *A*) and slightly less in the upper lid. The syringe and cannula are then rotated laterally about 90 degrees to a horizontal position for traversing the principal length of this passage into the lacrimal sac (Fig. 11-4, *B*). Gentle lateral traction on the lid reduces any tendency for the canaliculus to invaginate or corrugate in front of the tip. Slight injection of saline should accompany the advance of the cannula just as during injection of local anesthetic. The

examiner also palpates for roughness, strictures, or concretions as the cannula is advanced.

Diagnostic irrigation may be made with the tip at any point along the horizontal canaliculus, but if the cannula is a shouldered model, the added proximal diameter may be used to occlude the punctum and reduce any tendency for reflux. When more hydrostatic pressure appears needed and when there is normal, open communication between the upper and lower canaliculi, it may be necessary to occlude the opposite punctum with firm digital pressure against the orbital bone. If irrigating fluid cannot be delivered into the nose even with pressure sufficient to cause firm distension of the sac, it will be necessary to probe the passage.

Probing. Probing of the passages should

be done with a fine malleable probe of small diameter such as the Bowman 0 or 00 or the Williams 0 or 00. Entrance through the punctum and canaliculus should be with the same two-stage maneuver as with the irrigating cannula, but the tip is advanced farther horizontally until obstruction is palpated or the bony wall of the lacrimal fossa is felt. Manipulations should be made to slip through or angle by moderate density obstructions, but heavy-handed pressure can easily cause additional damage to the epithelial lining of the passages. Pain is an indication that potentially damaging pressure is being applied. If the tip of the probe has reached the bone of the lacrimal fossa, a slight withdrawal should be made, and then the end of the probe in the examiner's hand should be rotated upward 90 degrees to a ver-

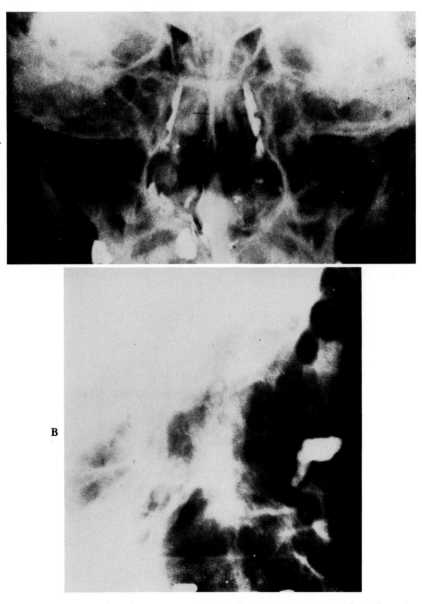

Fig. 11-5. Roentgenographic dacryocystograms in **A**, posteroanterior, and **B**, lateral views showing Lipiodol filling immediately after injection.

tical position. In this alignment, it is advanced downward for passage through the duct into the inferior nasal meatus. A sudden fading of tissue resistance or a small amount of blood into the nose indicates completeness of passage, or unhappily a false passage if too much pressure was applied. In the infant, one or two passages such as this may entirely clear incomplete lumenization of the passages. In the adult with acquired stenosis, however, this may serve only to identify the level of cicatrization or to give temporary patency.

Probing or repeated attempts should not be done with the injection of regional block anesthesia. If the pain evoked on attempted probing is this severe, it is likely that probing will cause more disturbance than it will relieve.

Roentgenographic examination. Examination in a posteroanterior view such as the Waters view will identify areas of osteitis, traumatic bone compaction, or neoplastic involvement that can occlude the nasolacrimal passages.

Dacryocystograms of the membranous passages with the aid of contrast media can be more helpful. Emptying of secretions from the sac by digital compression should be attempted before instillation of contrast media. Injection of 1 to 2 ml. of slightly warmed 40% iodized oil (Lipiodol) should be done with the patient positioned at the unit for skull x-rays. Iophendylate (Pantopaque), with slightly lower viscosity, may be instilled more easily but tends to drain more rapidly. Films should be taken immediately after injection (Fig. 11-5).

Normally, the sac is 10 to 12 mm. in length and the nasolacrimal duct extends 12 to 16 mm. below this. The most common area of obstruction, either congenital (caused by imperforation or incomplete lumenization) or acquired (resulting from infection or trauma) is below the sac or in the nasolacrimal duct. Proximal distension is then usually limited to the sac area because of relatively little constraining tissue resistance to expansion outward or upward between the anterior and posterior bony lacrimal crests. The tightness of lid tissues about the canaliculi and the firm constraints of bone about the membranous nasolacrimal duct preclude these levels from simple hydrostatic or nonmalignant enlargements. Infrequently, in the adult, there can be neoplastic growth producing obstruction in the canaliculi, the sac, or the duct.

Water soluble, more liquid, or lower viscosity contrast substances (such as iodopyracet [diodone, Umbradil, Oparenol]) approach the conditions of normal drainage physiology with lower injection pressures than are needed for the oily contrast media. They give slightly less contrast but are adequate to outline the passages.

Roentgenograms taken in the posteroanterior and lateral positions reveal any pathologic distensions and also visualize levels of obstruction.

This spread of examining procedures should always be confined to the fewest and simplest that will produce desired information concerning tear secretion or the nature and site of lacrimal obstruction.

Part three

Diagnostic procedures relating to multiple disturbances

Chapter 12

Ophthalmoscopy

Ophthalmoscopy, the inspection of the interior of the living eye, fundamentally requires that a source of illumination and the observer's visual axis be brought into a straight line through the patient's pupil. This problem was first solved by the English mathematician Charles Babbage, who demonstrated his fenestrated reflecting glass to the distinguished London ophthalmologist Wharton Jones in 1847. The Jones-Babbage description, however, was not published until October, 1854, *(British and Foreign Medico-Chirurgie Review)* and in the meantime the modest but monumental German physiologist and physicist Herman von Helmholtz published his 1851 landmark description of *Augenspiegels.* Helmholtz's ophthalmoscope was essentially a series of superimposed glass plates angulated at 45 degrees both to his source of light and to the visual axis between his and his patient's pupils.

Within a year C. G. T. Ruete, Director of the Eye Infirmary of Leipzig, Germany, evolved the indirect ophthalmoscope. By 1853 essentially all of the major components of the direct ophthalmoscope as used today were developed.

The first binocular instrument was developed by the Parisian ophthalmologist M. A. L. F. Giraud-Teulon. Hundreds of variations in design were devised, eponymically christened, and committed to musty print during the next century. The incorporation of small electric bulbs into instrument design by William S. Dennett of New York led to development of other electric instruments during the twentieth century.

BASIC TYPES OF MODERN OPHTHALMOSCOPES

Two basic instrumental variations, which supplement one another, are currently available in many modifications. These are the direct and the indirect ophthalmoscopes.

Direct ophthalmoscopes

Direct ophthalmoscopes (Fig. 12-1) use the refractive components of the patient's eye as a magnifying system. A small, erect, and uninverted image is obtained under magnification of about 15× when the examiner and the patient are emmetropic. The hyperopic eye affords a larger area of visualization but under less magnification, whereas the myopic eye yields a more magnified image and a correspondingly smaller area of visualization. The fundal area in view at any particular moment, however, is increased as the examiner comes closer to the patient's pupil; this is similar to the principle of looking through a keyhole, in which the area of view is increased by coming as close as possible to the opening. Moderate degrees of hyperopia or myopia in either patient or examiner can be neutralized by interposing lenses in the ophthalmoscope that, in effect, represent the net difference in spherical error between the patient's and examiner's eyes. Astigmatic errors yield axial distortion of the fundus image and cannot be compensated for by lenses in the ophthalmoscope; if these are of high order, as is also the case in extremely high spherical errors, the ap-

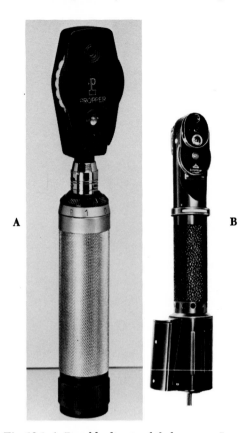

A   B

Fig. 12-1. **A,** Portable direct ophthalmoscope. Long-life, zinc-cadmium battery in handle may be recharged hundreds of times. (Courtesy Propper Manufacturing Co., Long Island City, New York, and Heine designs by Optotechnik G.M.B.H., Herrsching, Federal Republic of Germany.) **B,** Euthyscope of Cuppers (improved model) may be used as a direct ophthalmoscope with large (30-degree) or small (7-degree) field. An auxiliary high intensity light source is included for use in amblyopia and afterimage testing (6 volts; 15 watts). (Courtesy Oculus Products, Dutenhofen, Federal Republic of Germany.)

are available.* The nickel-cadmium battery offers much brighter and better sustained illumination. These instruments should generally be free of graticules, slits, and color filters, which only complicate their design and have little place in the small portable ophthalmoscopes. The major or giant direct ophthalmoscope[†] with high intensity bulbs and transformer current supply are less portable but more versatile for precise office use and can be fitted with filters, grids, or polarizing discs of occasional value.

Direct ophthalmoscopy yields less clarity of details than indirect as examination moves from the posterior pole to the far periphery. This is caused by increasing distortion of oblique pencils of light passing successively through equatorial portions of the lens and peripheral portions of the cornea. It is practically impossible to visualize the ora serrata and totally impossible to visualize the pars plana with direct ophthalmoscopes.

Indirect ophthalmoscopes

Indirect ophthalmoscopy utilizes a supplementary, convex lens (+13 to +30 diopters aspheric) held a few inches in front of the patient's eye to focus the light reflected from the retina into a real, inverted, and laterally reversed aerial image between the lens and the examiner's eye. Though under less magnification, this affords a much larger field of view, distinctly less distortion in examination of the retinal periphery, and access (with the aid of scleral depression) to the pars plana and ora serrata. With progressively stronger condensing lenses the area of visualization is increased and magnification of details is reduced.

Much greater light intensity is required for indirect than for direct ophthalmoscopy.

propriate spectacle or contact lens correction should be worn. Most ametropic examiners and all astigmatic examiners are wise to wear their own correction during ophthalmoscopy to obtain (1) a clear focus with fewer changes in the lens disc of the ophthalmoscope and (2) a qualitative estimate of the patient's spherical and cylindrical errors.

Many good hand ophthalmoscopes (Fig. 12-1) with battery or rechargeable handles

---

*Keeler Practitioner; Welch Allyn; A-O Ful-Vue; Propper; and others.
[†]Keeler Pantoscope; A-O Vistadial Giantscope; Bausch and Lomb Professional Ophthalmoscope; Oculus Visuscope.

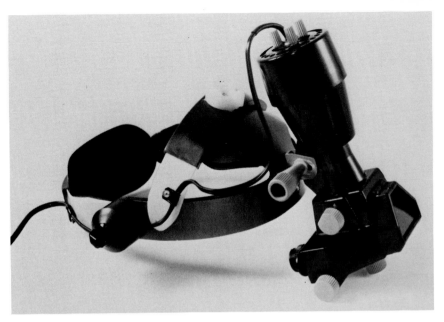

Fig. 12-2. Schepens design small pupil indirect ophthalmoscope made by MIRA, Boston, Massachusetts 02114. Rheostatic control of illumination is mounted on right side of head band. Infrared filter removes light rays of 800 to 1,400 mμ. Weight: 20 oz.

Probably the most contributing refinement in this technique has been development of the high light intensity head-mounted instrument by Charles Schepens of Boston (1947).

Schepens' refinements have also made true stereoscopic examination practical and valuable both at the posterior pole and the far periphery. This requires optic positioning of the observer's two pupils within the pupil of the patient by prisms or paired mirrors in front of each eye of the examiner. This is to be distinguished from older, table-model, binocular ophthalmoscopes with single objective lenses that present identical images to both of the examiner's eyes but do not afford the slightly disparate imagery necessary for true stereopsis.

Pupillary dilatation greatly aids stereoscopic indirect ophthalmoscopy by (1) affording a more easily accessible field, (2) displacing the dazzling effects of corneal light reflections, and (3) increasing the amount of stereopsis in proportion to the available width of the patient's pupil (that is, maximum separation of the examiner's

pupils). The Schepens improvements necessitate good pupillary dilatation. Introduction of the Small Pupil Ophthalmoscope (Fig. 12-2) in 1967[*] made possible some, though reduced, stereopsis with pupillary diameters as small as 1.5 mm. The new Schepens instruments incorporate infrared filters over the high-intensity light source to reduce photic heating effects within the eye.

A newly modified, lightweight, and efficiently cool binocular indirect ophthalmoscope was introduced by the Keeler Optical Company[†] in 1969. This study instrument has a pleasantly simplified headband. Mirror optics eliminate the weight of prisms and a Bi-Mirror viewing attachment is easily fitted so that a student or second observer may see the fundus simultaneously with the examiner wearing the instrument. This is the result of refinement in design by L. G. Fison of London. Lambert and

---

[*]Medical Instrument Research Associates, Boston, Massachusetts 02114.
[†]London, W1, England.

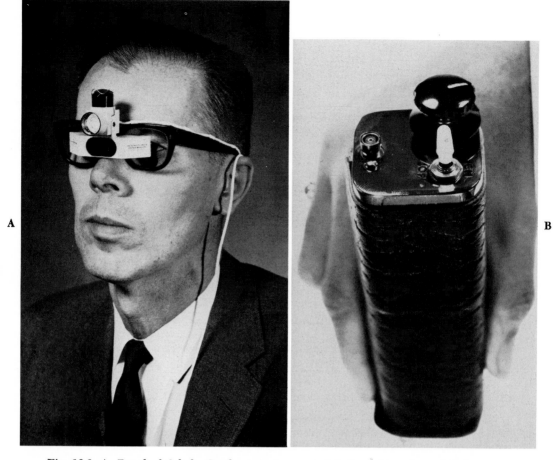

Fig. 12-3. A, Detail of Schultz-Crock spectacle-mounted indirect binocular ophthalmoscope. Two models are made with mean interpupillary distances of 64 and 68 mm., which will accept examiner's variances of ± 3 mm. Weight: 4⅛ oz. (Manufactured by Sola International Pty. Ltd., Adelaide, South Australia 5035.) **B,** Compact or pocket-size, rechargeable battery power (6 volts) supply for Schultz-Crock spectacle-mounted binocular indirect ophthalmoscope. Three-position toggle switch provides for operation, charging, or off. Rheostat controls intensity of light. (Manufactured by Sola International, Pty. Ltd., Adelaide, South Australia 5035.)

Cohen have also introduced (1970) a lighter and somewhat simplified instrument of shock-resistant materials that appears to be very durable. This is manufactured by Xonix Incorporated and distributed by Bausch and Lomb, of Rochester, New York.

The Australian-made Sola spectacle-mounted binocular indirect ophthalmoscope offers a new concept in lightness and portability with the maintenance of high intensity illumination. The unit utilizes front surface mirrors instead of prisms, and angulation of the light beam is directly ad-justed by vertical movement of the light housing (Fig. 12-3).

CONTRAST DYES AND VITAL STAINS TO AID FUNDUS EXAMINATION

Relatively nontoxic intravenous dyes* to aid in differentiation of fundus lesions have been explored for several decades, but not until the 1961 introduction (Novotny and

---

*Kiton fast green; Geigy blue; merbromin (Mercurochrome); and others.

Alvis) of modern intravenous fluorescein retinal angiography have any of these attempts yielded practical and useful information (pp. 225-228).

TECHNIQUE OF DIRECT OPHTHALMOSCOPIC EXAMINATION
The pupils

Direct ophthalmoscopy, like indirect ophthalmoscopy or looking through a keyhole, is best done with the largest possible aperture or maximum pupillary dilatation. Principal reasons for not attaining good dilatation are (1) shallow anterior chamber or narrow iridocorneal angle predisposed to acute angle-closure glaucoma by mydriasis, (2) constriction or displacement of the pupil by adhesions, scars, or congenital iris anomalies, and (3) iris fibrosis of advanced years or chronic miotic instillations. Inexcusable rationalization for not dilating the pupil are (1) visual acuity better than 20/20 and peephole glimpses of a normal posterior pole, leading to the hazardous assumption that "the rest of the fundus is probably OK," (2) insufficient time, (3) "I looked at the fundus on her last examination 2 years ago," or (4) the self-assuaging note appended to the end of an office examination record: "Check fundus on next visit."

The drops

Mydriatics for ophthalmoscopy should be rapid in onset, short in duration, and as free as possible from impairment of accommodation (cycloplegia). A drop or two of topical anesthetic facilitates corneal penetration and accelerates dilatation. One percent tropicamide (Mydriacyl) or 2.5% phenylephrine (Neo-Synephrine) are generally quite satisfactory with normal and light-colored irides. Darker irides may require a second or third instillation and sometimes a stronger drug such as 10% Neo-Synephrine. After examination, a drop of 1% pilocarpine should be instilled. If there is any question concerning marginal chamber depth, the physician should have the patient remain in the office until miosis is achieved, thus removing the threat of induced angle-closure glaucoma.

The position

Patient and examiner are preferably seated with their eyes at similar heights. Room light should be very subdued, particularly in the presence of any opacities in the media; these cause irregular reflections of ambient light and distressing diffraction of the ophthalmoscope light in proportion to their number and density. Holders for ophthalmoscopes should turn on the electricity when the instrument is lifted up and may be wired to turn off room lights at the same time. Generally, in binocular patients and examiners, the *right first* rule is extended to *all* right first. Thus the scope is held in the examiner's *right* hand before the examiner's *right* eye to examine the patient's *right* eye. The *right* index finger is positioned on the lens disc for rapid changes in lens power, and the examiner is a bit to the *right* of the patient who is fixing straight ahead. Initially, the aperture (zero) opening of the lens disc is rotated into position, the light intensity set at or near maximum, and the area of illumination adjusted to small or medium.

The steps
Initial examination

Initial inspection is accomplished with the examiner 1 to 2 ft. away from the patient and the ophthalmoscope light directed into the pupil. The examiner should see a homogeneous or uniformly red reflection of light from the fundus. Any opacities from the cornea to the retina will appear as dark spots impairing this red reflection. A nuclear cataract appears as a central dark spot and cortical lens spokes appear as dark radial streaks toward the edge of the pupil. Corneal or vitreous opacities are distributed in the red reflection just as they are distributed in the pupillary axis. A bright and even reflection is general assurance of no significant opacities of the media that might impair acuity.

The location or depth of opacities can

usually be quickly determined at this inspection by asking the patient to rotate his eyes up and down. The geometric center of rotation of the eye is usually just behind the posterior surface of the lens. Thus opacities in front of this center of rotation (lens, anterior chamber, and cornea) move upward with upward rotation of the eyes, and opacities behind the center of rotation (vitreous and sometimes posterior lens pole) move downward as the line of sight is rotated upward. An estimate of the freedom of such opacities or the fluidity of the medium in which they are contained is gained from their activity with eye movement. Opacities in a liquified vitreous thus are seen to drift or swirl when movement of the eye is stopped. Asteroid bodies in a normally gel-like vitreous recover their position in a somewhat spring-like manner, or as ornaments stop bobbing on a Christmas tree.

Fundus examination

Following inspection of the fundus reflex and identification of opacities in the media,

the examiner then brings his ophthalmoscope and his eye quite close to the patient by approaching along the path of the bright red fundus reflection (Fig. 12-4). Details of the fundus are brought into optimal focus by rotating the lens disc to bring between the patient and examiner the suitable dioptric lens to compensate for the net difference in their ametropia. With an emmetropic examiner and patient, no lens power may be needed. Commonly, however, the mere nearness of the examiner to the patient evokes accommodation and therefore the prepresbyopic examiner may need to interpose a −2 or −3 diopter lens.

The presbyopic examiner is spared the need for this extra maneuver and, if emmetropic or wearing his proper distance correction, can actually measure the patient's refractive error on the basis of the needed interpositional lens more precisely than can the prepresbyopic examiner. If either the examiner or patient is significantly nearsighted, then the appropriate minus sphere must be rotated into position. Similarly, if the patient is significantly far-

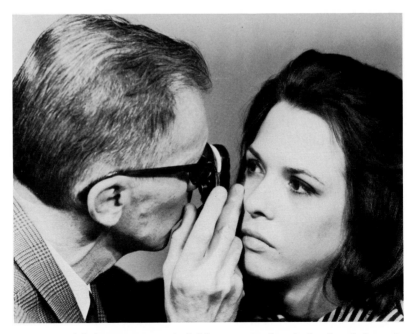

Fig. 12-4. Direct ophthalmoscope properly held in examiner's right hand with his index finger on lens disc and approaching patient's right pupil for detailed examination of the posterior pole.

sighted or aphakic, the compensating plus sphere must be rotated into position.

If the patient is steady in maintaining straight-ahead fixation, the examiner usually will come somewhat directly onto the optic nerve head. If it is not immediately in focus, the examiner must follow progressive enlargement of the retinal vessels to the nerve head or rotate the lens disc of the ophthalmoscope to achieve clear focus.

Major ophthalmoscopic landmarks

With direct ophthalmoscopy the major points to be observed systematically are in the posterior pole and extend to the midperiphery. Indirect techniques are preferable for examination of the far periphery, and scleral indentation is usually needed in the nonaphakic eye to visualize the ora serrata and the pars plana.

Optic disc

The optic disc is the first and most conspicuous landmark. Its basic configuration and apparent distortions are closely dependent upon structural characteristics of the eye. Thus in a small and hyperopic globe, the posterior scleral foramen through which the optic nerve passes is generally small. This crowds the several hundred thousand axons of the retinal ganglion cells and tends to obscure the definition of the disc borders, reduce or eliminate the physiologic cup or depression commonly occurring in the center of the disc, and give a somewhat hyperemic appearance to the disc.

Conversely, in a large, myopic globe the posterior scleral foramen may be large and the axon fibers may thereby be distributed over a greater disc circumference. This yields sharper definition of the disc borders, a large and sometimes saucer-shaped physiologic cup, and relatively less intense capillarity of the disc with the hazardous potential of diagnosing "myopic pallor."

Moderate to large amounts of astigmatism make the disc appear ovalized or elongated in proportion to the degree of astigmatism. Like every other structure in the body, the optic disc is subject to nu-

merous congenital irregularities or anomalies that may (coloboma; congenital pits; large or multiple drusen; extensive medullation of the axons; inversion of the disc) or may not (oblique insertion of the optic nerve; small drusen; mild medullation of the axons; persistent Bergmeister's papilla or proximal segment of the hyaloid artery; congenital epipapillary veils) cause disturbances in vision.

Components of the optic disc that should be evaluated are the rim, the cup, the color, and the border. The *rim* is the healthy neural tissue between the physiologic cup or its excavation and the disc border. Normally this rim is somewhat narrower temporally than nasally and shows slightly less capillarity in the temporal portion. This is related to the crowding of large numbers of axons over the nasal half of the rim, whereas the temporal half serves almost exclusively the axons coming from the macular area. Even in the presence of myopia with normal intraocular pressure or of a documented and stationary large physiologic cup, there should be a healthy rim of normally colored disc.

The *cup* varies widely within physiologic limits, tending to be small in the hyperopic eye and large in the myopic eye. Its base is the sieve-like lamina cribrosa through which the axons pass into the optic nerve. This is mechanically a weak area of the sclera and yields to increased intraocular pressure by bowing posteriorly. This commonly is more marked in the temporal and inferior portions of the cup as it yields to pressure, and therefore nasal and superior field defects are among the earliest perimetric findings of nerve head damage. Except in moderate to highly myopic eyes, the lamina is normally not conspicuous. It does become more distinctly checkered in appearance, though, with the inroad of pressure.

The reddish *color* of the disc is normally somewhat more intense nasally than temporally. The *border* also tends to vary from usually clear definition temporally to slightly less definition nasally. Thus early changes of papillary congestion may appear as slight hyperemia or blurring nasally, whereas early changes of atrophy appear as pallor temporally.

Blood vessels

The vessels seen in the fundus are preponderantly of the *small* classification. Components of this arterial system are properly considered to be arterioles, except for the central retinal artery, its first bifurcation into superior and inferior papillary arteries, and occasionally proximal portions of the second degree (second bifurcation), which may be minimal examples of medium-sized arteries. Thus pathologic processes of medium or large arteries such as medial hypertrophy and atherosclerosis are generally confined to vessels on or near the disc or hidden proximal to the lamina cribrosa. Changes manifest in the vast majority of the arterial tree throughout the fundus are perforce the diseases striking arterioles (vessels without an internal elastic lamella and without a continuous muscular coat), such as arteriolosclerosis with its visibly conspicuous hyalinization and its close association with hypertension. Similarly, components of the vascular drainage system are properly considered venules and, in respect to the direction of blood flow, the lesser ones are tributaries rather than branches.

Vessel distribution and quantitation on the nerve head. Divisions and arrangements of blood vessels at the disc are highly varied, though striking similarity is seen in the majority of identical twins. Normally the largest vessels are positioned slightly nasalward on the disc. Kestenbaum (1946) introduced a reliable quantitation of these vessels by grossly dividing them into large or small and counting their numbers as they cross the disc border. The larger vessels normally number eight to ten and are rarely reduced, even in optic atrophy. The smaller vessels normally number a few more and are lost to visualization in atrophic processes (Kestenbaum count).

Vessel changes associated with papil-

ledema. The reverse of atrophic changes and insufficiency in these vessels is seen in papilledema (congestion of the optic nerve head) or acute inflammatory disturbances (optic neuritis). The full-blown pictures of these conditions with the long preservation of central acuity in papilledema and the early loss of it in optic neuritis present little diagnostic challenge compared to the far more important identification of papilledema in its earliest stages. The ophthalmoscopic signs of papilledema in order of their appearance are:
1. Venous fullness and tortuosity
2. Hyperemia of the disc
3. Slight blurring of the disc borders, vertically or nasally
4. Accentuated striations from the disc along the major vessels
5. Loss of venous pulsations, particularly in the presence of mild digital compression applied to the globe
6. Filling in of the physiologic cup
7. Blurring of the temporal disc border
8. Peripapillary edema and hemorrhages

In papilledema, tangent screen studies of the visual field show enlargement of the blind spot roughly proportional to the duration and intensity of the congestion.

Vessel changes associated with hypertension and sclerosis. Retinal vessels should be evaluated not only for their relation to optic nerve head pathology but also in terms of their general characteristics throughout the fundus. Particularly the changes of hypertension (spasm, narrowing, straightening, wider angulations at bifurcations) should be distinguished from those of arteriolosclerosis (increased light reflex, sheathing, arteriovenous compression, tortuosity, copper wire appearance, silver wire appearance) and each graded 1 to 4 in accordance with severity of the vascular changes and associated disturbances such as hemorrhages, exudates, and secondary papilledema.

Examination for grading of vascular changes must differentiate the hypertensive signs from those of arteriolosclerosis and must be based upon the most marked manifestations of each. Some vessels in the fundus may show distinctly less involvement than others, but it would be false assurance to base the quantitation on the least involved area. The following are usual grading criteria in arteriolosclerosis:

Grade 1 Early compression of vein at arteriovenous crossing; some limited disappearance of venule at either side of arteriole; slight increase in arteriolar light reflex

Grade 2 Similar crossing phenomenon as grade 1 and with early copperish light streak on arteriole

Grade 3 Distinct tapering, humping, or depression of vein at arteriovenous crossing; marked copper wire light reflex; early sheathing of arterioles; increased tortuosity

Grade 4 Pipestem sheathing and silver wire arterioles; blood column not apparent in most severely involved vessels; deflection of venules (Salus sign) at crossing sites; stasis in vein peripheral to crossing changes; marked tortuosity

The following are usual grading criteria in hypertensive changes:

Grade 1 Diffuse mild arteriolar constriction with infrequent area of focal constriction

Grade 2 Distinct generalized arteriolar constriction with scattered areas of severe focal narrowing; arteriovenous ratio of vessel diameters about 1:3

Grade 3 All of the above plus some straightening of the arterioles; scattered flame-shaped hemorrhages; small to medium-sized cotton-wool patches (small infarcts); some edema and edema residues

Grade 4 Vascular changes as above plus some areas of apparent obliteration of the arteriolar blood column; small and large flame-shaped hemorrhages; scattered areas of retinal edema and edema residues; many cotton-wool spots; papilledema from mild to massive

Vessel changes associated with diabetes mellitus and diabetic retinopathy. Ophthalmoscopy also offers a unique capability to diagnose and to quantitate the vascular concomitants of diabetes mellitus as revealed in early retinal changes and established diabetic retinopathy. Improved approaches to therapy of this retinopathy (such as pituitary surgery, photocoagula-tion, and laser coagulation) demand careful notation of these changes with widely acceptable grading. To this end, the Airlie Classification of Diabetic Retinopathy (Davis, Norton, and Myers, 1969) represents the most widely based and comprehensive approach thus far evolved. Details of this classification require not only direct ophthalmoscopy of the posterior pole but also the assistance of (1) binocular indirect ophthalmoscopy to evaluate peripheral and proliferative changes, (2) slit lamp biomicroscopy with a Hruby or similar corneal contact lens to detect early retinopathy and disturbances in the vitreoretinal relationship, and (3) fluorescein fundus angiography to evaluate intraretinal microvascular abnormalities as well as early nonproliferative and early proliferative changes.

This classification emphasizes photographic grading in relation to five specific fields of approximately 30 degrees each: *1*, centered on optic disc; *2*, centered on macula; *3*, temporal to macula or nasal limit tangent to macula; *4*, above disc with nasal limit tangent to perpendicular line through center of disc; and *5*, below disc with nasal limit tangent to perpendicular through center of disc.

Each fundus photograph roughly equates in area with the view obtained with indirect ophthalmoscopy using a +14-diopter lens. By either technique this is considered a standard measuring area. Severity is specified in only three grades: *0*, no changes; *1*, mild to moderate; and *2*, moderate to severe.

Characteristics are graded under the following four headings as applicable:

A. Nonproliferative phase
1. Hemorrhages and/or microaneurysms by number in a standard area
2. Hard exudates by extent of fundus area involved
3. Soft exudates by number in the total fundus
4. Venous dilatation, beading, sausaging, or other abnormalities
5. Intraretinal microvascular abnormalities as shunt vessels and dilated capillaries
6. Macular edema by severity and area of extent

B. Fluorescein angiographic findings
  1. Changes seen in arteriovenous phase 15 to 25 seconds after injection (microaneurysmal changes)
  2. Changes seen in late phase 3 to 5 minutes after injection (leakage)
C. Proliferative phase
  1. Neovascularization within one disc diameter of the disc
  2. Neovascularization in areas other than centered on the disc
  3. Fibrous proliferation within one disc diameter of the disc
  4. Fibrous proliferation in areas other than centered on the disc
  5. Plane or forward extension of proliferation from normal level of retina
  6. Retinal detachment and elevation by extent of area
D. Vitreous hemorrhage
  1. Preretinal hemorrhage by severity
  2. Vitreous hemorrhage by severity
  3. History of previous vitreous hemorrhage by number of episodes in past year

Even though present therapy may carry disappointments, this is no excuse for the clinician to avoid some functional classification or grading of the disease process. Certainly many individuals and many institutions render good and adequate care, both clinical and research, with simpler methods than this evaluation. The clinician, however, must have some landmarks for overall evaluation of progress or failure and may add other and even more specific notations in areas where he has investigated interest.

The macular area

After studying details of the disc and vessels, the macula should routinely be examined. This vessel-free concavity normally appears slightly darker than the surrounding retina and in younger life presents a distinct yellowish center. This darkens and becomes less conspicuous with age. The radiating axons from the fovea constitute the nerve fiber layer of Henle. Because of their precise regularity of geographic arrangement, these axons have a polarizing effect on light and also tend to confine exudates (macular star) and hemorrhages into a radiate pattern when they present in this area. The prefoveal reflex normally is a pinpoint of light reflected from the ophthalmoscope by the concavity of the fovea interna. When this is bright and distinct, it indicates essentially no disturbance in the internal limiting membrane that lines this shallow concavity; loss or distortion of the prefoveal reflex is an early ophthalmoscopic sign of macular edema or distortion and should be studied further by slit lamp examination with the aid of a Hruby or contact lens. Pathologic elevations here, when nondestructive, give rise to an acquired hyperopia that may range from 0.5 to 2.5 diopters. When caused by edema or similar transient insult, the artificial hyperopia subsides with resolution of the disease process.

The macular area has a very high metabolic rate and is quite vulnerable to minor vascular insufficiencies, contusion insults, or the induced gliosis of even minute amounts of retinal hemorrhage. Lipid deposits are a common cause of central visual loss in adult life, and patients with such macular deposits should have careful study of their serum cholesterol and lipid fractions.

The periphery

Even with good pupillary dilatation, direct ophthalmoscopy of the far periphery is distorted and that of the ora serrata and pars plana is precluded. These areas, which are vitally important in the problems of retinal detachment, sickle cell disease retinopathy, retinoblastoma of infants, the chronic inflammations of pars planitis, and contusion injuries, must be inspected by indirect binocular ophthalmoscope.

BINOCULAR INDIRECT OPHTHALMOSCOPY

L. K. SARIN, M.B.B.S.

In addition to direct ophthalmoscopy, a complete fundus examination requires binocular indirect ophthalmoscopy and slit lamp examination using the Goldmann or similar contact lens. The binocular indirect ophthalmoscope offers advantages of (1) true stereopsis, (2) a larger field, up to 42 degrees in diameter with a +30-diopter lens, (3) clearer visualization through hazy

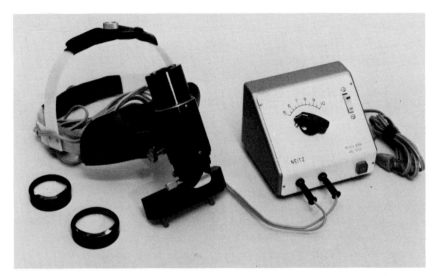

Fig. 12-5. Conventional head-mounted binocular indirect ophthalmoscope with transformer power supply and two strengths of condensing lenses. Observer's pupils are brought to interpupillary distance of about 3.5 mm. within patient's pupil. (Courtesy Neitz Instruments Co. Ltd., Tokyo, Japan.)

media, (4) easier access to infants and children because of the more remote position of the examiner, (5) less distortion and larger field when examining the high myopic patient, (6) better access to the peripheral fundus, and (7) reduced distortion in examining the far periphery of any eye. Its greatest advantage is achieved in combination with scleral depression both to bring the far periphery into view and to differentiate, by pressure or manipulation, the true retinal hole from confusing lesions such as cysts, small hemorrhages, or pigment disturbances. Disadvantages include the vertically inverted and laterally reversed image and the high light intensity that most patients endure unhappily (Figs. 12-2, 12-3, and 12-5).

The major optic accomplishment of the ophthalmoscope design is effectively to position both pupils or visual axes of the observer within the pupil of the patient. This is done by paired mirrors or prisms before each of the observer's eyes. Since stereopsis is proportional to the interpupillary distance, it is essential to have maximum pupillary dilatation, not only to gain widest access to the fundus but also to attain the maximum degree of stereopsis. The ophthalmoscope must be properly and securely adjusted with most of its weight supported from the strap over the crown of the examiner's head rather than by poorly endured tightness of the encircling head band. The oculars should be as close as possible to the examiner's eyes and centered for comfortable binocularity with gaze directed slightly downward and at a focal plane 14 to 18 in. away. The illumination mirror must be angulated to center the light in the upper half of the field of view or away from the line uniting the entrance images of the observer's pupils in the patient's pupil. The patient's pupil is the pivotal and fixed center of rotation for the examining axis on which the fundus point of regard, the examiner's eyes, and the condensing lens must always be kept centered.

The room should be dark and the patient supine. It is essentially impossible to attain adequate peripheral examination in the vertical meridian if the patient is in the seated position. There must be access of about 270 degrees around the patient's head to align the 360 degrees necessary for inspection.

The condensing lens

The light reflected from the fundus must be brought to a real focus in front of the patient's eye and at a convenient anterior focal plane for the examiner's eye. This is done with a condensing lens held about 2 to 5 in. anterior to the patient's eye, depending upon the converging power of the lens. Generally, there are three ranges of powers to choose among: (1) a low diopterage of about +13 to +16, which usually is made as a large diameter (52-mm.) lens, gives high magnification of about 4×, presents a relatively small area of fundus view, and must be held farthest from the pupil (about 5 in.); (2) a high diopterage of about +26 to +30, which must be made as a small diameter (28- to 34-mm.) lens, gives low magnification of 2× or slightly more, shows the largest useful area of fundus view, and is held closest to the pupil (about 2 in.); and (3) an intermediate diopterage of about +18 to +22, which falls between the characteristics of the preceding lenses. The real, aerial image of the fundus is formed toward the examiner, at the focal length of the condensing lens—for example, at 4 cm. from a +25-diopter lens. Moderate latitude is available between the image and the observer to adjust his arm length, accommodative status, and slight gains in magnification afforded by approaching the image more closely.

For optimal clarity of imaging, the lens surfaces are preferably aspheric or constructed of unequal front and back curves to reduce optic aberrations such as pincushion effect, coma, and astigmatism of oblique pencils. So-called "crossed lenses," as designated by English terminology of the previous century, are combinations of inexpensive spheric rather than aspheric lenses in which the radius of curvature on one surface is about six times greater than the radius of curvature on the other. This is scant improvement over the even cheaper plano-convex lens to reduce spheric aberration, and this method cannot be recommended in preference to condensing lenses, which add aspheric or conoid surfaces to the unequal powers of the two sides. The constant user will find the durability and scratch resistance of such lenses in glass preferable to the lighter weight plastic.

The lenses may be ground from crown glass, which has the disadvantage of weight and the high cost of hand-lapping aspheric surfaces. Lenses made of optical plastic (usually allyl diglycol carbonate, CR-39) have the advantage of lightness and the reduced expense of being injection-molded. The plastic lenses scratch much more easily than glass and can have their usefulness grossly impaired by careless surface scratches. In all events, the lens must be handled only by its mounting rim and kept carefully free of finger smudges or dirt.

Fundus sketching or drawing

In addition to mere inspection of the fundus, the examiner planning treatment of retinal disease should sketch with color-coded pencils the vascular details (landmarks) and pathologic changes. This promotes a discipline of thoroughness and exactness. A beginner will find the 30-diopter lens convenient because of minimal distortion in peripheral examination and because of the larger field it provides in comparison to lenses in the midteen or low twenty diopter ranges. Its low magnification and short working distance make for easy control. In small pupil ophthalmoscopy, the high power lens of small diameter advantageously restrains tendencies to move the lens beyond its correct position, though it does restrict the available ophthalmoscopic field.

In changing the area of fundus under examination, the observer's head and the condensing lens always move in the same direction and *to* the side of the fundus image toward which one wishes to shift.

The patient lies on a narrow, padded stretcher,* table, or fully reclining chair without a pillow and with his chin slightly elevated. The examiner begins from a standing position or seated on a high stool at the

---

*Da-Laur, Inc. Ophthalmic Examining Table, West Roxbury, Massachusetts 02132.

head of the table. The patient is instructed first to look straight up at the ceiling. The examiner holds the selected condensing lens in his nonwriting hand between the first two fingers and the thumb. The ring finger is used for retracting the lid and the little finger may be rested on the patient's face to assist in maintaining proper lens distance. The writing hand is kept free for scleral depression and drawing. The drawing chart on a clipboard may be placed on the chest of the patient, on the stretcher by his head, or on a small caster-based podium. The 12 o'clock position of the chart is toward the patient's feet.

The light from the scope is directed into the fundus while the patient is reminded (sometimes frequently) to keep both eyes open. There is a natural tendency to close the other eye. The condensing lens is first brought into the light path close to the patient's eye and then moved toward the examiner until the fundus image fills the entire lens. The annoying light reflections from both surfaces of the condensing lens can be avoided by slight tilting of the lens.

Excessive tilting of the spherical power condensing lens induces cylindric effects or astigmatic distortion similar to that interposed by the normal cornea and crystalline lens when attempting to see peripheral details with a direct ophthalmoscope. Fortunately, planned tilting of the condensing lens can create a compensatory spherocylinder of variable strength and any axis. The lens must always be tilted or rotated about an axis at right angles to the axis of rotation of the eye in order to achieve this effect.

The inherent prismatic power of the lens can also be utilized (at a sacrifice of part of the field of view) by sliding the lens in its plane so that only the peripheral lens overlaps the pupil. This affords more angulation or peripheral view.

The examiner focuses critically on the aerial image only and draws it on the chart as he sees it. The inverted image drawn on the reversed chart yields normal anatomic correspondence when the drawing is righted and attached to the patient's chart. Initially, 2 to 3 hours may be required to draw all the retinal blood vessels of one eye. However, with practice this can be accomplished in less than half an hour, and when no pathology is discovered such detailed drawing is unnecessary.

All fundus details and pathology are drawn in relation to careful plotting of the retinal blood vessels. Landmarks like pigment deposits, nevi, and retinal folds should be drawn in proper relationships to facilitate later relocation of pathologic areas easily and quickly.

Use of the scleral depressor

Variously designed smooth, metal contact tips mounted on gently curved but rigid shafts are great aids to thorough examination. The scleral depressor, if thimble-mounted, is usually placed on the index finger of the writing hand with the remaining fingers kept flexed. It may also be used by grasping the thimble between the thumb and first two fingers. The latter hold has a slight advantage, especially if the thimble does not fit the finger snugly. The middle finger is actually the fine control finger in indentation, guarding against excessive wrist or hand pressure. The shaft and tip are kept tangential to the sclera with pressure applied only to the area of the globe that coincides with the examining axis through the patient's pupil, the condensing lens, and the examiner's eye.

If the area of scleral pressure is not seen, then the depressor tip is not in the axis of observation. The tyro examiner must resist the temptation to press harder—which the patient will find distinctly painful—and instead make corrective movement of the tip without interposition of the condensing lens.

The scleral depressor of Hovland, Tanenbaum, and Schepens (1968) has a hinged depressor shaft mounted with a spring action on a small stainless steel cylinder. The serrated and slightly concave ends of the cylinder may be held between the thumb and index finger, using the middle finger to

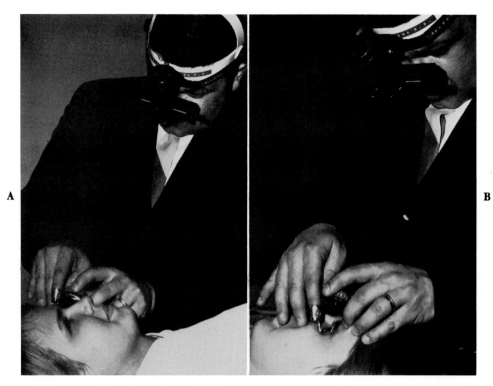

Fig. 12-6. A, Indirect binocular ophthalmoscopic examination of superior retinal periphery. Patient must be recumbent and examiner positioned below the ocular plane. Low magnification, high dioptric condensing lens is steadied close to patient's pupil, which is fixed fulcrum of examining axis. **B,** Indirect binocular ophthalmoscopic examination of inferior retinal periphery. Scleral depressor is thimble-mounted on tip of index finger; it may be steadied by thumb and middle finger as needed. Depressor tip is positioned below lower edge of inferior tarsal plate and pressing against sclera in 6 o'clock periphery. Note axis of observation uniting site of depressor tip, retinal area of regard, patient's pupil, condensing lens, and examiner's point of reduced interpupillary distance beneath light source.

press on a small post perpendicular to the depressor shaft in its proximal third. Any tendency to exceed the slight scleral pressure required to bring the ora into view is called to the examiner's attention by mild discomfort in the pulp tip of his second finger as applied to this post. Length of the depressor shaft has been increased beyond that of the Keeler (large or small) or Schepens American Optical Company's thimble and is an advantage in deep-set eyes.

To visualize the superior ora, the examiner moves beside the patient's midbody position; the patient looks slightly down, and the depressor tip is applied through the lid just above the tarsal plate. Pressure cannot be applied through the thickness of

the tarsal plate because this is painful and because the pressure effects become unacceptably diffused. The patient is then asked to look up and at the same time the depressor tip is carried posteriorly, still tangential to the globe. The examiner looks into the fundus without the condensing lens and usually can see slight graying of the retina at the site of depression. The high-power condensing lens is again introduced close to the cornea and then brought toward the examiner approximately 2 in. or as needed to produce a sharp focus. Once the observer has noticed the position of scleral depression in the fundus, the depressor tip is moved anteriorly to bring the ora serrata in view. Only minimal pressure is needed to visualize the periphery. The depressor tip should hug the edge of the tarsal plate and not be applied too far above the upper tarsal border or the lid will drop over the upper cornea when the patient looks up and thus frustrate visualization of the upper pole (Fig. 12-6, *A*).

To examine the inferior ora, the examiner moves to the head of the table. The technique is similar to that for examination of the superior ora but is facilitated if the patient's chin is well elevated (away from his chest). A common mistake is to have the patient look too far down (Fig. 12-6, *B*).

The temporal periphery is most easily studied from across the patient's head.

The nasal periphery should be done last because the depressor tip must be applied to the bulbar conjunctiva and because topical anesthetics with their adverse effects of epithelial drying and hazing are usually needed.

Scleral depression to visualize any quadrant of the equatorial region can be done with the patient looking straight up (not away from the examiner), or at times slightly toward the examiner. The new and sometimes heavy-handed examiner should avoid scleral depression in patients who have had retinal detachment or cataract surgery within 4 or 6 months because of possible mechanical opening of the wound. Remember that only the most gentle pressure is needed, never more than that required for tactile estimation of ocular tension.

Examination of immediate postoperative retina cases

The side of the patient to which the examiner stands is usually in accordance with the eye operated upon or the quadrant under particular study. The examiner rests one hand on the forehead of the patient and uses that thumb gently to retract the lid against the bony orbital rim. The condensing lens is held in the other hand. A common mistake is attempting to retract the lid with the middle finger of the hand holding the lens. Without good support of the hand, the extended finger can slide over the globe and cause discomfort to the patient.

Monocular indirect ophthalmoscopy

Monocular indirect ophthalmoscopy has recently been given instrumental attention by some manufacturers on the heels of increased interest in binocular techniques and use of the monocular indirect system in fundus cameras. The Lozano monocular indirect ophthalmoscope (1966) by Rossbach, Mexico City, Mexico, requires a fully dilated pupil. The American Optical Company's Monocular Indirect Ophthalmoscope (1968), Buffalo, New York, affords fundus screening information through an undilated pupil. A possible justification for such an instrument is the one-eyed examiner, though a field of about 20 degrees and an erect (aerial) image are lauded by some of the producers.

The Cardona Indirect Ophthalmoscope* (1970) is a hand-held, single-unit optic system that presents a real and erect fundus image through either monocular or binocular eyepieces. It contains a heavy hexagonal prism in its lighting system that transmits from a fiber optic source, two bundles of light directed as semicircles on the fundus. The image returns through a 4-mm. diaphragm in the center of this illuminating prism. The objectives can be changed to provide high magnification in a 35-degree field or low magnification in a 55-degree field. The erect and uninverted image is an advantage to the new user of indirect ophthalmoscopy, but the mechanical restraint of a stand or hand-held unit a foot or two from the examiner creates limitations.

Landmarks: physiologic and anatomic features seen by indirect ophthalmoscopy (Fig. 12-7)

The long ciliary vessels and nerves conspicuously divide the fundus horizontally. These can be recognized in the 3 and 9 o'clock meridians as yellow strips bounded

*Edward Weck & Co., New York, New York 10021.

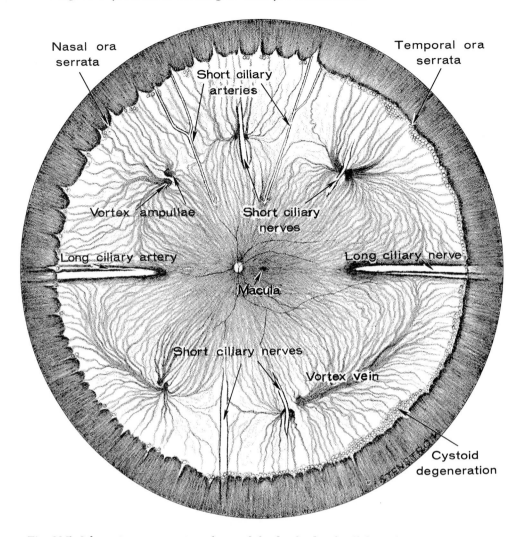

Fig. 12-7. Schematic representation of normal fundus landmarks (left eye) as seen with the indirect ophthalmoscope and the aid of scleral depression. (By Stenstrom and Tilden of the Retina Foundation; courtesy MIRA, Inc., Boston, Massachusetts 02114.)

by pigment on either side extending from midway in the fundus to the mid–pars plana. The short ciliary vessels are considerably more difficult to see, particularly in brunettes, and are located near 6 and 12 o'clock positions, well anterior to the equator.

The scleral exits of the vortex veins form the best clinical landmarks for the equator. They are particularly conspicious in blondes.

The equatorial region extends approximately two disc diameters on either side of the anatomic equator. The posterior

limit of the equatorial region is formed by an imaginary circle passing through the posterior edge of the scleral exits of each vortex vein. The anatomic equator is difficult to identify clinically but is approximately two disc diameters anterior to this circle. The vortex veins usually number four, but at times as many as seven may be seen. The peripheral fundus clinically is the area anterior to the exits of the vortex veins.

The ora is marked by distinct, peripherally pointing retinal extensions or teeth separated by variously wide oral bays nasally, but these are generally smoothed

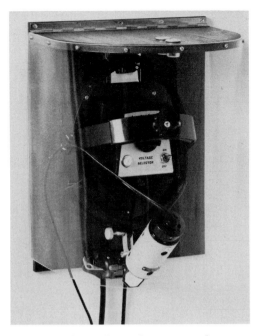

Fig. 12-8. Plastic front dustcover and support bracket for indirect ophthalmoscope. Tight closure is secured by magnetic catch. Raising hinged dustcover and top gives immediate access. Lifting ophthalmoscope from suspension hook turns on current. (Jenkel-Davidson Optical Co., San Francisco, California 94119.)

out in a more even ora temporally. There are about forty-eight teeth per fundus and they correspond approximately to intervals between the ciliary processes. The teeth are often the sites of peripheral termination of congenital meridional folds, and in about 10% of autopsy eyes zonuloid traction tufts 0.25 to 1 mm. long are found here. The clinical importance of these meridional folds and zonuloid traction tufts lies in the fact that holes can form at their posterior tips. Meridional folds are more common nasally than temporally. The bays are finely

irregular and wavy convexities found directly posteriorly between two teeth. In many patients neither bays nor teeth appear in the temporal periphery. Cystoid degeneration is almost always located in the retina adjacent to the ora serrata and is seen more frequently in the temporal periphery. Appearance of "white-with-pressure" seen on scleral depression represents cystoid degeneration of the retina, which in most eyes is a normal finding, especially in mature years. When cystoid areas of degeneration become confluent they form a senile type of retinoschisis that also appears white-with-pressure on scleral depression, but which in advanced cases is white-without-pressure. White-with-pressure is also seen in flat retinal detachment. However, it is almost always seen in Negro eyes where it may not represent any pathologic change.

The occasional user will find indirect ophthalmoscopy frustrating. Only perseverance and constant use will make one a proficient indirect ophthalmoscopist.

Only frequency of use and intimate familiarity with technique will bring the indirect binocular ophthalmoscope into the widespread use it merits in protection of eyesight entrusted to each ophthalmic examiner. With its use, peripheral retinal breaks will be detected early and many patients will be spared later, more hazardous scleroplastic retinal repairs. Also, peripheral fundus malignancies will be detected while they are small and before metastatic hazards increase.

The instrument should be connected at all times and immediately convenient to the examiner. A dust-free plastic front cover and holder such as Fig. 12-8 is therefore very valuable in facilitating frequent use.

Chapter 13

Visual field examination

> "Examining a visual field is as personal a matter as any other form of clinical examination; if full benefit is to be obtained the tests must be carried out by oneself and not delegated to an assistant."
>
> BRODIE HUGHES, 1954

Perimetry, the investigation of indirect vision or visual fields, has been subject to countless refinements of instrumentation, but from its Hippocratic beginning in the fifth century B.C. has been shackled by its subjective nature and dependence on the alertness, mentality, and cooperation of the patient. Simplicity of procedure plus direct observation of examinee by examiner are therefore vital to validity. The nearly 100 years of "morphologic ophthalmology" that characterized the nineteenth century were replete with ingenious devices to examine the outlines or periphery of the photosensitive area. Only at the end of that century did Bjerrum of Copenhagen discover that he could evoke more detailed and informative data from a black cloth stretched over a pair of large doors in his office. Thus evolved the valuable Bjerrum (tangent) screen, campimetry, and scotometry. Esoteric techniques of autoperimetry and afterimage perimetry have led to many publications by scotomatous ophthalmologists but are of almost no practical clinical value.

Examining techniques may be divided according to whether the target stimulus moves (kinetic method) or whether it increases in luminosity (static method). Office examination of the visual fields is conventionally a kinetic or topographic method in which fixed-brightness targets are moved from nonseeing to seeing areas. Light-sense or static (profile) methods, contrariwise, measure thresholds directly at various locations within the visual field; these are more particularly laboratory or research techniques requiring preadaptation, precisely controlled background brightness and target illumination, and much more time.

Only in the 1960's has the objective technique of visual field examination by visually evoked (occipital) responses or electroperimetry offered a laboratory approach to refreshing freedom from subjective methods. Such potentials are in the range of only a few microvolts and ordinarily are overshadowed by other electric activity in the brain and about the skull. Equipment requires all the components of electroencephalography, plus countless varieties of photostimuli and computerized averaging equipment to sift gestalt from the grass of higher voltage background noise. Compact and practical, though inescapably expensive, models of such equipment may soon be available for hospitals and medical centers where many ophthalmic and neurologic patients are to be examined. Completely shielded rooms are necessary.

In the primary effort to prevent blindness from ocular disease or ocular manifestations of systemic disease, visual field examination is a vital step. This follows closely on the heels of preliminary inspection, the establishment of optimal visual acuity with refractive correction as needed, and ophthalmoscopy. Qualitative or preliminary perimetry is an important diagnostic step after the above procedures when acuity cannot be corrected to full

20/20 in each eye or when there is disparity between the two eyes, as 20/20 in one eye and 20/12 in the other, without firmly demonstrated reason. Perimetry is also needed for its diagnostic *and* localizing value when specific headaches, menstrual deficiencies, hemiparetic disturbances, papilledema, or other allied findings suggest central nervous system pathology encroaching somewhere on the long visual pathways from the orbits to the occiput. Perimetry may further be the only reliable measure of progression or control in chronic open-angle glaucoma or the elusive complex sometimes called "low-tension glaucoma."

No individual assuming responsibility for the sight of a fellow human being can meet this obligation without a thorough working knowledge of at least one accurate and standard perimetry method. The 1-meter tangent screen is the recommended minimum.

Visual field studies are particularly suitable on the basis of instrumentation for division into qualitative and quantitative tests, or preliminary and screening test versus detailed examinations.

A. Qualitative or preliminary procedures
   1. Autoperimetry (patient sketches)
      a. Amsler grids (1947)
      b. Afterimage projections
      c. Auto-ophthalmoscopic perimetry
   2. Tests administered by an office aide
      a. Harrington-Flocks (1954) ten-pattern tachistoscopic test
      b. Horizontal field of vision screener
      c. Automated or self-administered spherical perimetry and blind spot campimetry
   3. Tests conducted by the practitioner
      a. Confrontation or comparison test—simultaneous double confrontation (extinction, inattention, or suppression fields)
      b. Tangent (Bjerrum) screen tests; Auto Plot; Pantographic aids
B. Quantitative or detailed tests
   1. Arc perimetry
   2. Spherical projection perimetry: Goldmann; Harms
   3. Color perimetry
   4. Flicker fusion frequency fields
   5. Dark adaptation perimetry
   6. Stereocampimetry
   7. Angioscotometry
C. Scoring of visual fields

QUALITATIVE OR PRELIMINARY PROCEDURES
Autoperimetry

Autoperimetry is principally the patient's notation or informal sketching of his own field loss. This is usually evoked by sudden and major field losses and is often unnoticed in minor or slowly progressive losses. The patient's delineation of defect may afford lucid understanding of occupational handicaps, as for example the judge of thoroughbred horses or other animals who is completely incapacitated by a fixed homonymous hemianopia even though retaining 20/20 in each eye. The engineer patient may present himself with a detailed drawing of field impairment (or distortion in the specific axis of his astigmatism).

Amsler grids (1947-1949) have formalized such notations for the central 20 degrees of field by plates containing patterns of white lines each 1 degree apart when viewed at a distance of 30 cm. Distortions of these lines reveal and quantitate macular disturbances causing micropsia and metamorphopsia, but they have largely been superseded by slit lamp examination of the fundus and fundus photographs for both diagnosis and follow-ups. The advent of fluorescein fundus angiography since the early 1960's has added identification of vascular leaks and pathologic mechanisms amenable to photocoagulation therapy, further exceeding the almost negligible patient aid obtainable from Amsler chart demonstrations.

Afterimage fields may be evoked following timed exposure to bold, intensely transilluminated patterns (Williamson, 1945). In a darkened room, positive afterimages of the same color or bright configuration can be seen. Against a bright background, negative or dark afterimages will be seen. Both positive and negative afterimages undergo a succession of changes influenced by secondary stimuli and colors but apparently related to retinal or photochemical alterations. An intelligent patient can describe and sketch these afterimages and defects in them indicating retinal disturbances, particularly from tumors, exudates, vascular occlusions, and similar locally destructive pathology.

Auto-ophthalmoscopic perimetry is an entopic phenomenon evoked with closed eyes in a dark room by continuously moving an electric light source to and fro across the lower lid with gentle pressure against the globe. Soon a magnified and inverted image of the retina appears in space before the patient. The network of branching vessels is usually identified first and then a perceptive patient may describe the optic nerve head area and the avascular macular area. Retinal lesions appear as dark or negative defects in this pattern. Contracted fields or quadrantic or sector defects can be identified, particularly if the patient has a good fellow eye with which to compare. This method is useful in the presence of opaque media, in order to assess the function of the posterior segment.

Tests administered by an office aide

Although an office aide is distinctly valuable in the conduct of preliminary screening or survey visual field examination, the ophthalmologist himself generally can evoke the most informative and diagnostic data with desirably minimum fatigue. This

is because the ophthalmologist knows the areas in which there is possible trouble. He therefore concentrates immediately on the areas of significance and brings to bear the most appropriate stimulus and test distance. Thus in the presence of an enlarged pituitary fossa or menstrual impairments suggesting pituitary tumor, he examines particularly the bitemporal outer isopters and gives only brief survey attention to the blind spot. Conversely, in suspect or early glaucoma, he carefully seeks arcuate defects, minimal enlargements of the blind spot, or early nasal steps (Roenne) and gives only brief survey attention to the temporal isopters. In the presence of hazy or clouded media such as corneal dystrophies, early cataracts, or old vitreous hemorrhage, he avoids the small 2- or 3-mm. test objects and immediately turns to the larger 5- or 10-mm. objects.

Harrington-Flocks screening. The aide or technologist can easily accomplish specified techniques on first visit (preliminary) examination with the Harrington-Flocks (1954) campimeter screener.* This tabletop unit is self-contained (Fig. 13-1), with

---

*Jenkel-Davidson Optical Co., San Francisco, California 94119.

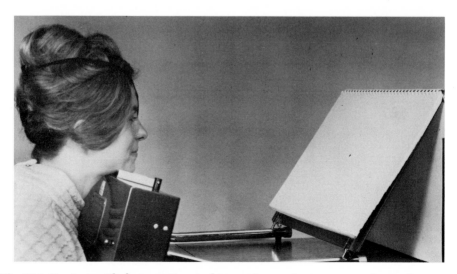

Fig. 13-1. Harrington-Flocks ten-pattern tachistoscopic campimeter screener in use. Instrument is placed on table top, and ultraviolet light source is concealed beneath the patient's chinrest to left. Cards are hinged above.

an ultraviolet light source shielded beneath the chinrest. Ten different cards, hinged at one edge, may be flipped open consecutively as a campimeter field and present abstract patterns of three to four dots and crosses.

The patterns are printed in white fluorescent sulfide ink on white cards so that in ordinary room light only a central 5-mm. black fixation point is visible. At the fixed testing distance of ⅓ meter, these cards, which are 12 × 17 in. in size, cover a field of approximately 25 degrees. Controlled test exposure of ¼ second is achieved by a fixed duration flash of ultraviolet light, which is adequate for visualization and registration of the stimuli on each card but too short to allow a shift of fixation. Errors are checked off on record charts that indicate the composite thirty-three stimuli of the ten charts. By removing the white cards, the dull gray supporting surface may be used as a ⅓-meter tangent screen; a fluorescent fixation spot is incorporated centrally so that wand-mounted fluorescent targets can easily be used with the ultraviolet light source. The complete ten-pattern screening test can be accomplished in 4 or 5 minutes and is desirable as part of general eye examinations, routine physical examination, driver license examinations, moving equipment operator examinations, armed forces personnel examinations, and mass surveys.

Children under the age of 8 or 9 commonly present major difficulties in classical tangent screen, arc, or spherical perimetry. Often, however, the child of 6 or over will respond reliably to the Harrington-Flocks screener either verbally or by pointing.

Horizontal field screening. Driver testing is creating increased need for quick and simple screening devices for horizontal form fields as well as other visual functions necessary in transportation. The American Automobile Association* has for more than 20 years been developing about eight sturdy and inexpensive devices for visual screening

to be operated by vision technologists or police personnel. Their table model Field of Vision screener* is 20 in. in diameter and encompasses approximately 220 degrees horizontally within a steel band finished on its interior surface in flat black. Under shielded illumination sources, black and white segmented disc targets rotate as they are moved from peripheral to central under lever control hidden from the subject. The subject, while looking straight ahead, advises the examiner as soon as he becomes aware of a target approaching from either the right or the left. Calibration of the arc in degrees is easily read immediately in front of the examiner. Only the horizontal meridian can be examined, but this type of information meets model criteria suggested by the American Committee on Optics and Visual Physiology as well as by the Department of Health, Education and Welfare (1969).

Automated or self-administered spherical perimetry and blind spot campimetry.† Beginning with prototype perimeters and preliminary publications in 1962, J. A. Gans has evolved a practical and patient-operated visual field test system that frees both professional examiners and aides from physical presence during this part of ocular study. The Ocutron Automatic Electronic Perimeter in its 1970 model (Fig. 13-2) continues as a conveniently compact 30-cm. radius hemisphere. The number of sequentially illuminated targets has been reduced to ninety-one and these are placed every 10 degrees along twelve major axes. Targets are 1.5 mm. in diameter and white. Neutral density or colored filter sets are supplied to place before the patient's eye when such reductions in stimulus are desired. Constant fixation illumination is provided centrally and is monitored by a blind spot illumination, which is recorded as unseen so long as the patient maintains proper fixation.

Target illumination is sequentially pulsed

---

*Washington, D. C. 20006

*No. 3535.
†Ocutron Co., Shaker Heights, Ohio 44122.

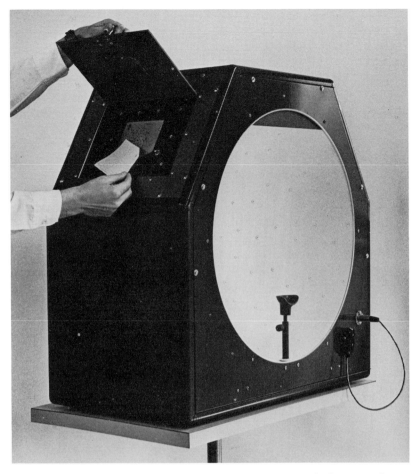

Fig. 13-2. Ocutron Automatic Electronic Perimeter showing special electronconductive chart being inserted at left side for marking by recorder. Pushbutton indicator at lower right side of instrument face is held in patient's hand during self-administered field examination. Control unit is built into self-contained cabinetry of this table model equipment.

at adjustable intervals of 1 to 4 seconds. The patient registers his awareness of the individual targets by pressing a hand-held button. This automatically makes a mark on the recording chart to correspond with the stimulus position in the visual field. Programmed stimuli directed into the blind spot, of course, will not be acknowledged by pressing the button and thus serve to verify fixation. When the machine has completed the cycle for one eye, it turns itself off and sounds a gentle alarm for the operator to return, transfer the patch to the opposite eye, or remove the patient.

The Ocutron uses no pantographs or mechanical linkage that may require ad-

justment. Special electroconductive chart paper 4×5 in. in size is necessary for recording (Figs. 13-3 and 13-4). Electronic components are solid-state transistors and integrated circuits capable of years of trouble-free operation. The control panel is built into the table-model design.

Though the instrument is sufficiently simple to be used as a time-saving screener, it does produce conventional type field charts entirely by the patient without supervision. Patients needing serial fields over several years, such as those with chronic glaucoma, learn in a couple of visits not only to use the push-button recorder but also to seat themselves in proper position

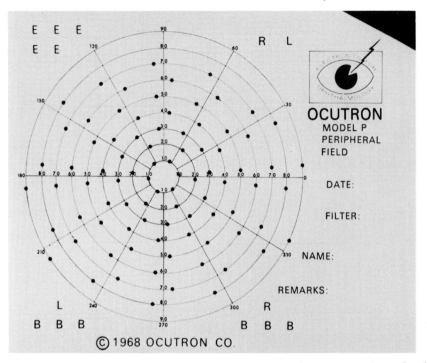

Fig. 13-3. Ocutron Perimeter Chart, 4 × 5 in., made of electroconductive paper shows distribution of the ninety-one sequentially presented test stimuli and gives a conventional portrayal of visual field.

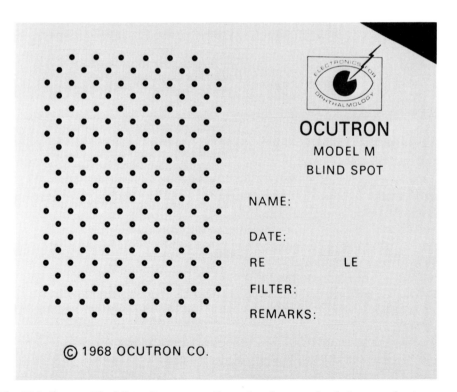

Fig. 13-4. Ocutron Blind Spot Campimeter Chart, 4 × 5 in., made of electroconductive paper shows distribution of the 154 sequentially presented test stimuli.

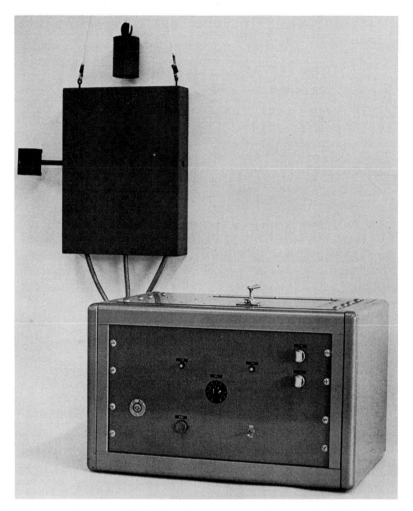

Fig. 13-5. Ocutron Automatic Blind Spot Campimeter is shown in suspended position with fixation light inserted to left for use with right eye. Control cabinet, shown below, is kept out of view of patient.

and place the patch over each eye successively.

Because the spherical perimeter does not analyze the blind spots in detail, Gans has more recently devised an Automatic Blind Spot Campimeter on identical operating principles. This is a rectangular plate 25 × 36 cm. in size and when used at a distance of 1 meter subtends 14 × 20 arc degrees. One hundred fifty-four target positions are presented in a diamond grid pattern. The unit should be suspended against a wall and adjusted in height by a counterbalanced lead weight on nylon cords. A fixation light is plugged into either the right or left side of the campimeter to test the left or the right eye respectively. A control cabinet 23 × 14 × 16 in. may be placed at any convenient location within cable distance connection to the campimeter (Fig. 13-5).

Tests used by the practioner
Confrontation or comparison

The confrontation screening technique should be familiar to the ophthalmic as well as the neurologic examiner and the general physician. It is useful in handling young children of 4, 5, or 6 years as well as in emergency room situations and bedside examinations. Confrontation compares the (previously established) normal field of the examiner with the suspect field of the examinee, who should be seated or facing the examiner at a distance of about 1 meter.

Preferably the examiner is in front of a homogenous and dull surface. Diffuse light comes from behind the patient. One eye at a time is tested; it is best to tie or tape an eyepatch over the eye not being tested rather than to rely on the patient to occlude manually this eye. The examiner similarly must close one of his eyes; initially this should be the right so that he is using his left eye, which is positioned directly in front of the patient's right eye. The patient and examiner maintain fixation on one another's eye.

The test object is brought, as usual, from the nonseeing area or periphery toward the center, testing each quadrant successively and checking such additional radii as the suspect defect indicates. The examiner's fingertip or a cotton-tipped applicator are the most ubiquitous test objects; asking the patient to note whether one or two fingers are displayed adds a rough estimate of peripheral acuity. A semiquantitative aspect to the test is added by a suitably sized white target ball (5, 10, or 15 mm. in diameter, commonly) mounted on a handle. When vision is extremely poor, the exposed bulb of a small flashlight or hand ophthalmoscope may be used with crude validity. With an alert patient, it is even possible to identify the physiologic blind spot a few inches temporal to the imaginary line connecting the fovea of the examiner and examinee; it is essentially impossible, however, by this technique to estimate enlargement of the blind spot.

Failure to demonstrate a defect on confrontation must never be interpreted as a "normal field" but rather as "no defect to finger confrontation" (or to 5- or 10-mm. white confrontation, and so on). Defects of considerable size and density can be missed by this technique.

In the child of 4 to 6 or 7, the most useful field examination is generally the confrontation procedure. An activational accom-modative target hooked over the bridge of the examiner's spectacles as in near-range motility examinations will often secure the child's fixation. Confrontation testing in various quadrants may then be accomplished engagingly with small toys or figures mounted on wands. The self-contained fluorescent Lumiwand (Fig. 13-6) also is often attractive to the child patient. Most department stores carry a variety of small figures or toys incorporating activity components; these should be part of the ophthalmic office equipment.

Extinction, inattention, or suppression techniques. Confrontation lends itself particularly to the eliciting of extinction (or inattention or suppression) fields by simultaneous double confrontation. With this variation, relative or early defects may be uncovered or exaggerated. The technique may be used in monocular or binocular testing, and again patient and examiner face each other directly. Two identical stimulus targets (Fig. 13-7) are exposed briefly in diametrically opposite portions of the field, or they may be advanced from the periphery centrally. Depending on the patient's level of acuity and alertness, the targets may be as gross as the examiner's two index fingers or as subtle as 2-mm. white discs.

Better localization in degrees from fixation may be gained by displaying two targets against the background of an arc perimeter. If a tangent screen is used for display of the two stimuli, rather than as background for the physician, then two examiners are required to present the targets from opposite directions.

The physiologic effect (Bender, 1952) is such that distinct perception evoked through one part of the visual field causes a similar stimulus in another part of the visual field to become imperceptible. In certain cases, when the stimulus is removed from the perceptual field, then the previously undetected stimulus is perceived. In some pathologic conditions, particularly neurologic disturbances of the cortex, extinction fields may reveal homonymous de-

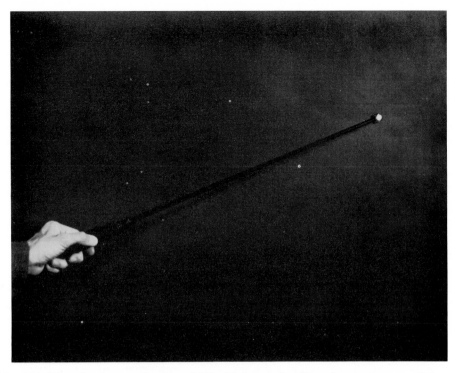

Fig. 13-6. Electroluminescent Lumiwand III with battery handle and activating control button under examiner's thumb. Ten-millimeter diameter stimulus (shown) covers reduced stimulus diameters to 6, 4, 2, and 1 mm. Wand is 22 in. long.

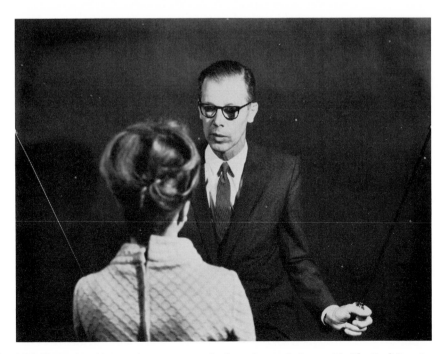

Fig. 13-7. Extinction (inattention or suppression) testing technique with identical Lumiwands in each hand of examiner.

fects that cannot be elicited on single target examination.

Tangent (Bjerrum) screen tests. The tangent screen is the most essential, most flexible, most practical, most diagnostic, and least expensive of all available instrumentalities in visual field examination. The same screen may serve as a highly efficient preliminary inspection device or as a detailed and subtle verification tool. In the decades of retinal surgery before introduction of the binocular, self-illuminated indirect ophthalmoscope, the perimeter was hauled into service to outline areas of gross detachment and to plot holes. However, perimetry is no longer desirable in the study of detachments and even as an academic exercise is at best an incomplete one. A 1-meter distance screen (Fig. 13-8) (64 to 65 in. square) is the most practical, though the larger screen, useful at 2 meters,

gives greater magnification of central details. The greatest usefulness—and with minimal edge distortion—is within 30 degrees from fixation. Practically any peripheral field defect extends to within 30 degrees of fixation, and therefore probably less than 0.25% of neurologic patients will present with such a minute and early defect as to elude tangent screen detection, particularly if the small 1- or 2-mm. white test objects are used. The same screen can be used for (1) any size test object, (2) fluorescent techniques, (3) flicker fusion methods, (4) dark adaptation studies, or (5) examination with colored stimuli.

For individual adaptation, space, economy, and understanding of tangent screen mathematics it is well to construct your own tangent screen. Black felt is commercially available in rolls 50 in. wide. This slightly exceeds the needed width

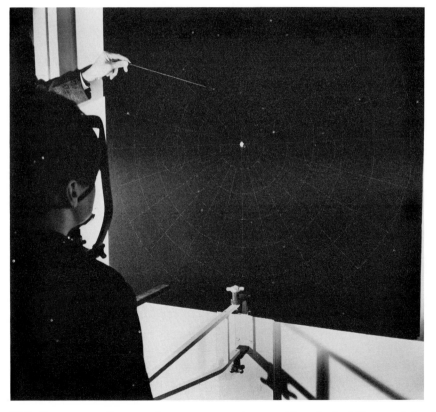

Fig. 13-8. One-meter wall-mounted tangent screen in use with author's folding steel bracket and chinrest preset for test distance.

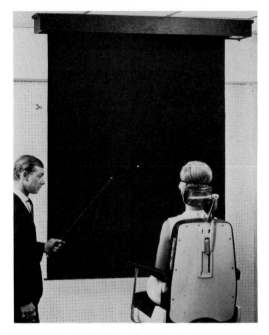

Fig. 13-9. Jenkel-Davidson motorized tangent screen suspended from ceiling at preselected test distance in front of patient seated in examining chair.

for a screen subtending 30 degrees at 1 meter and therefore allows a small amount of felt on either edge for hemming or tacking to a wooden frame. A commercial windowshade roller in this width will serve well if the screen is to be retractable above another wall testing background, as for the Lancaster red-green test. Motorized 1- and 2-meter tangent screens for ceiling (8 ft.) mounting directly in front of the examining chair are available from Jenkel-Davidson Optical Company (Fig. 13-9) to drop or to elevate silently in 4 seconds.

The technique of tangent screen examination is essentially the same as for confrontation, arc, sphere, and other instrumental methods. Basic principles are:

1. Equipment should be as close and accessible as possible to the patient to minimize patient movement or the setting up of equipment.

2. The patient should be seated as comfortably as possible, adjusting the equipment to him.

3. Explanations (like equipment) should be simple and should be tendered as the patient is moved into position.

4. The eye not under examination (remember, the right eye is traditionally examined first) is occluded.

5. Test objects should be the smallest practical size based on preliminary evaluation of retinal function and mental agility. With near normal acuity, most intelligent patients from childhood to late life can recognize a 2-mm. white object, which makes a broadly suitable examining target. In the presence of moderate corneal- or lens opacity–reducing retinal resolution throughout, a 5- or 10-mm. white target may be necessary. Marked loss of central vision from a circumscribed macular lesion, however, may not affect the extramacular retina and in such cases, even with best central acuity below 20/200, the small target size should be used.

6. Test distance should be practical and adaptable to usual office floor space, though larger screens (2 meters) and spheres (1 meter radius) give greater magnification of field defects. A 1-meter working distance is excellent for most tangent screen diagnostic and follow-up studies. (Similarly ⅓ meter or 33 cm. has become the standard radius for office types of arc and sphere perimeters.)

7. Surrounding illumination should be low; distracting movements, light colors, and reflecting surfaces should be excluded to avoid dazzling and disturbing light.

8. Spectacles generally should not be worn during field studies because (a) the frames create a positive ring scotoma; (b) high plus lenses create both "pincushion" distortion of the field and, from their edges, a negative ring scotoma that widens in proportion to increasing dioptric power; (c) high minus lenses cause peripheral doubling or target jump; and (d) high-power lenses incorporate optic distortions such as marginal astigmatism and chromatic aberration. Bifocals add inferior field confusion and "target jump" in their area. High dioptric prescriptions, however, may have to be worn at times to study the central 10 or

15 degrees when a small target is required to elicit details. Contact lenses have very little effect on the central field and should be worn if the patient is generally adapted to them. Small diameter contact lenses, particularly in young or myopic patients with large pupils, may create aberration rings at their edges or in relation to peripheral bevels and may have to be removed under these circumstances. Rarely is it desirable to map out the ring scotoma from spectacles or high power lenses in order to demonstrate its hazard to a patient.

9. Pupillary size does not have major effects on kinetic (topographic) field studies, but dilated pupils tend to increase apparent field size by affording better light admission. Conversely, very small pupils tend to reduce apparent field size by reduction of light access to the retina and by excluding a few of the most peripheral rays by virtue of the large (opaque) iris diaphragm.

10. Fixation must be maintained by the eye under examination on an easily identified central marker and monitored by the examiner. When central acuity is grossly reduced, several methods are available to secure fixation:

  a. Vertical and horizontal strips of ½-in. white adhesive tape may be placed on the screen intersecting at the fixation center. Even though the central portion of these strips may not be seen by a patient with a central scotoma, he can project their intersectional point by completion or "gestalt." This is suitable even for a one-eyed patient.

  b. Where the opposite eye can be used, the simplest technique is to roll up a short paper funnel or cone 5 or 6 in. long and big enough in diameter at the large end to cover the eye not being examined. The patient holds this with one hand over the eye not being examined and maintains alignment on the fixation marker while the other eye is being tested.

  c. Finger fixation can be used when acuity is extremely poor in both eyes

and when testing is being done with 10- or 20-mm. diameter targets or a small light source.

  d. More complicated procedures are (1) fixation through a mirror angulated at 45 degrees before the eye not being tested; (2) use of polarized light and polarizing glasses with axes at 90 degrees from one another over each eye; or (3) employing red-green glasses with a red fixation light for one eye and green test light for the other. These three methods, however, use not widely available office equipment, except for the last, which can be easily made from Lancaster red-green test equipment used in motility examination. The flashlights can be modified by a cap or opaque paper diaphragm to convert their streak image to a spot of known size.

11. Movement of the test object should proceed from a less sighted or sightless area to the visible area. It is best to make one or two introductory advances of the target from the periphery toward the center to demonstrate the outer isopter and the target size. The patient is instructed to report his first "awareness" of the "white" rather than waiting until the target outline can be clearly described. Similarly, if colored targets are used, the patient reports his first awareness of the *hue* or *color*—he may actually discern a form or colorless target before the color is recognized. The physiologic blind spot and all pathologic scotomata must be outlined by moving the test target from within the defect to the seeing area.

12. Blind spot outlining should be done immediately after eliciting the first point on the outer isopter. It is wise, in the absence of known temporal field impairment, to initiate the examination of each eye from the temporal periphery so that the examiner is in physical position to proceed to the blind spot. Outlining the physiologic blind spot (Mariotte) will (a) provide a sharp or steep edge of transition for the patient to identify, (b) instruct the patient in the

appearance-disappearance behavior of the target, (c) give an index of the patient's mental alertness or responsiveness, and (d) accomplish an important element of the tangent screen examination, which is generally unreliable on a 33-cm. radius perimeter. If the patient cannot identify the blind spot disappearance of the 2-mm. white target at 1 meter, then for demonstration purposes the examiner should switch to a gross 10- or 20-mm. target, which will, of course, completely disappear within the blind spot. This dramatic illustration enables the examiner to compliment and encourage the hesitant performer. The optimally small target should then be resumed.

13. Radial exploration should proceed in an orderly fashion at intervals of about 45 degrees. This is reduced in keeping with suspect areas of pathology and for the verification or elucidation of defects (contracture, depression, quadrantic, altitudinal, homonymous). After identifying the outer isopter, advancement of the target should be continued steadily on to the fixation point, looking for scotomatous defects (peripheral, central, paracentral, centrocecal, winging, arcuate, annular, junctional, or sector).

Pantographic aids. Pantographs are devices generally using mechanical, electric, optic, or magnetic components to move targets by remote control, coupled with a recording device to automate a precise outline map of patient responses. A simple and serviceable pantographic apparatus is manufactured for each of the three basic types of field testing equipment: (1) for the tangent screen, the Bausch and Lomb Auto-Plot projection device, (2) for the spherical or bowl perimeter, the Goldmann projection pantograph, and (3) for the arc perimeter, the AIMARK or Bausch and Lomb table-model, cable-driven projection unit.

Other pantographs for the tangent screen

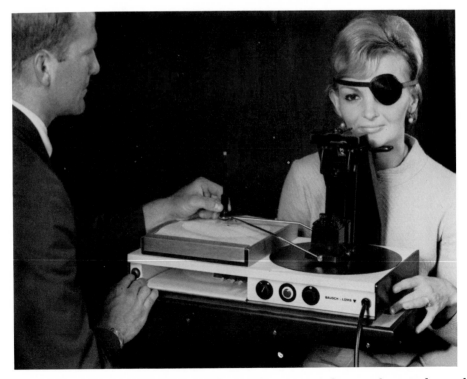

Fig. 13-10. Bausch and Lomb table-mounted Auto-Plot projection device with unitized control of projection light and recording stylus in examiner's hand. Examiner faces away from tangent screen to obtain constant observation of patient's fixation.

include the Gunkel wall-mounted screen and pantograph; the Allied Ophthalmic Corporations tripod mounted Photo Field Plotting Unit, using multiple exposures on Polaroid film; the Guist magnetically controlled test object; and others. For the spherical perimeters, a mechanical pantograph is incorporated in the 2-meter diameter behemoth of Donaldson and Norton. For the arc perimeter there have been many self-recording and semi–self-recording devices led by the Maggiore and the Ferree-Rand.

Auto-Plot. The Auto-Plot projection device introduced by Bausch and Lomb in 1965 reduced projection equipment and pantographic charting to a small unit (12 × 21 in. base; 13 in. high) that eliminates extraneous optic or acoustical cues to the target. The unit is solidly built of welded steel. Though distraction of the examiner's arms and carrying devices are eliminated in common with all projection systems, this table-top unit allows the examiner to sit quietly at the patient's right, removing him totally from movements that could be disturbing and yet allowing necessary observation of the patient directly and without instrumental aid.

The Auto-Plot is fixed to the practical 1-meter test distance and provides finger control of the projection aperture to give targets of 0.5, 1, 2, 3, 6, 12, and 15 mm. in white, red, green, or blue light. A short, mechanical pantographic arm links the projection head to a pencil holder over the record paper. A completely unmarked gray vinyl plastic screen is furnished for consistent brightness and procedural uniformity, though a similarly light wall surface may be substituted. Room light should be low. In use the patient's chin is placed on a movable rest behind the projection light and adjusted vertically until the eye under examination centers behind the eye ring (which is folded down during testing). A magnet and ferrous fixation target may be held on either side of the vinyl screen. The eye not under examination is occluded. Testing is rapid because the target stimulus

is moved by the examiner's hand as it holds the pencil in the pantoscopic arm on the record chart; thus control and record marking are with the same fingertip movements (Fig. 13-10).

QUANTITATIVE OR DETAILED TESTS
Arc perimetry

Arc perimetry is mechanically simpler than spherical perimetry and offers some operational advantages:
1. Less complex and less expensive equipment
2. Easy, direct observation of the patient for fixation, alertness, and so on
3. Smaller equipment requiring less physical space and amenable to wall mounting (Fig. 13-11), stand suspension (Fig. 13-12), or fold-up unit on caster-based floor stand*
4. Complete freedom and interchangeability of projection targets, mechanical target carriers, or hand-controlled targets

The disadvantages of arc perimetry in comparison to spherical or bowl perimetry are (1) less uniformity of background conditions and illumination, (2) difficulty of controlling preadaptation when desired, (3) more conflicting and distracting stimuli from both the examiner and the surrounding area, and (4) less certain relation of target to background intensity. However, for practical clinical screening of the peripheral fields between 30 and 100 degrees from fixation, the arc instrument affords an adequate working answer to most diagnostic problems.

Modern arc perimeters have been standardized with (1) radius of 33 cm., (2) arc exceeding 180 degrees, (3) rotation of 360 degrees, (4) uniform or coordinated rotating light source providing approximately 7 foot candles of illumination, (5) uniform matte black or dark gray finish for the arc surface, and (6) minimal arc width

*Harrington 33-cm. cold cathode and ultraviolet illumination unit; formerly made by Jenkel-Davidson Optical Co.

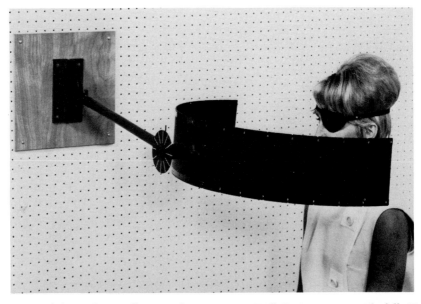

Fig. 13-11. Jenkel-Davidson wall-mounted swing away Wall Perimeter arc with full 33-cm. radius.

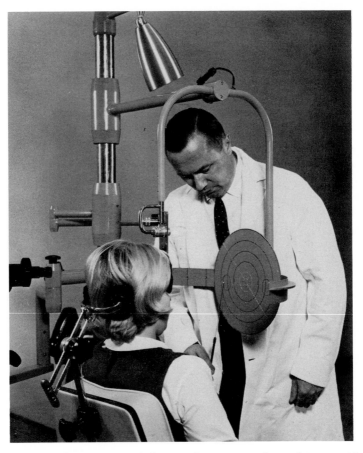

Fig. 13-12. Guyton-Carlson 33-cm. unified arc and campimeter lowered into position in front of patient.

of 3 in. Much of the basic understanding of perimetric findings in the modern context of ocular disease was derived by H. Roenne of Copenhagen, as was much of the understanding of field changes in neurology by C. B. Walker of Boston. The practical and still simple perimeters of today's office have evolved from dozens of prototypes but largely from combined work on instrument and technique as accomplished by Walker, by C. E. Ferree with Gertrude Rand, and by the Italian ophthalmologist Maggiore.

The most useful and rugged arc perimeter commonly available today was designed by the Allied Instrument Manufacturing Company of England and called AIMARK. It is also built in New York for the Bausch and Lomb Optical Company and sold under the designation Projection Perimeter. This ingeniously uses one light bulb to produce the target (variable in size, intensity, and color), the fixation point, and illumination for the recording form. Hand rotation of a control knob simultaneously moves the projected light stimulus and a recording punch stylus, without any sound or movement of the examiner's arm—operational advantages not afforded by the Bausch and Lomb Ferree-Rand perimeter.

In use, instrument height must be adjusted comfortably to the seated position of the patient and then the chinrest elevated or lowered so that the eye under examination is directly centered on the fixation target or light. The eye not under examination is occluded. Distracting lights, sounds, and other stimuli must be excluded from the area and the examiner must be in position to observe the patient's maintenance of fixation.

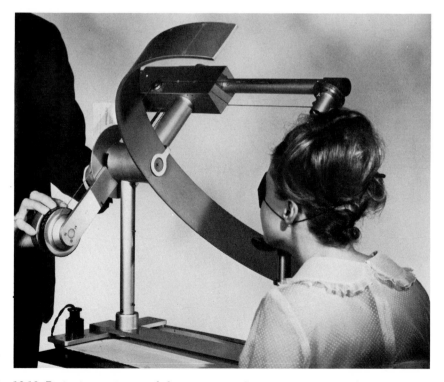

Fig. 13-13. Projection perimeter of the arc type with semiautomatic recording device. Patient is shown with right eye fixing. Fold-down auxiliary fixation ring surrounds the smaller illuminated fixation cross. Examiner's right hand is on rotating drum that controls the projection light and the marking stylus with same endless cord drive. Three knurled rings in bulb housing and control box at top permit adjustment of stimulus diameter, intensity, and color. (Distributed by Instrumedic, Ltd. and by Bausch and Lomb.)

Perimetric fields are traditionally outlined with the patient frontally aligned to the fixation point. This produces a variable nasal obscuration artifact because of the relative prominence of the nose to the globe. Similarly a superior field artifact may be created by a protruding brow or deep-set globe. Studies made in this position should be designated *relative perimetric fields.* Fuller analysis of the outer isopters is obtained by turning the face approximately 30 degrees to the opposite side and slightly extending the chin, if needed, to see beneath a massive brow. (This may require the examiner, as with a ptosis patient, to elevate the patient's upper lid with his finger or a cotton-tipped applicator while exploring the upper field quadrants.) This may be called a *maximum perimetric field.* In the presence of marked latent nystagmus, strabismus fixus, bilateral nerve VI paralysis or in motor transport driver examination, practical evaluation of the func-

tion field may require perimetry with both eyes open. For this examination, the midline of the face should be centered on the fixation point and findings designated as *binocular perimetric field.*

The patient must not be involved in conversation during testing and should make only the simplest possible responses such as "yes," "no," or a tap on the table to advise the examiner. A few verification or confirmation runs are necessary to check consistency of response; all projection perimeters have a silent flicker or extinguishing device that may also be used to check the patient's accuracy of responses. Eight meridians usually constitute a maximum test unless specific defects require further exploration. The examination should be kept as brief as possible consistent with securing minimally adequate data. Fatigue of either patient or examiner greatly reduces accuracy of field findings.

For bedside, emergency room, or home

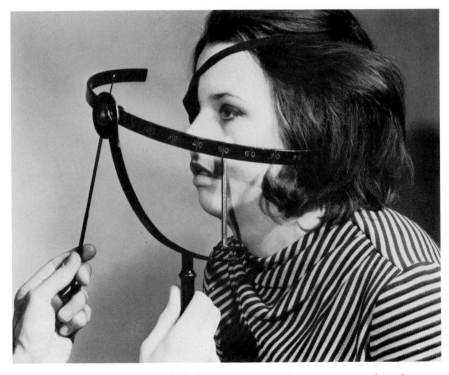

Fig. 13-14. Schweigger or Spiller bedside arc perimeter showing patient aligned on mirror fixation device for her left eye. Patient holds perimeter in left hand with cheek support resting on lower orbital rim.

examinations the 15-cm. radius Schweigger or Spiller hand perimeter (Fig. 13-14) is quite serviceable, easy to carry, and provides testing meridians through 360 degrees. In use the patient (or the examiner) holds the instrument by its handle with its cheekrest against the inferior orbital rim. Fixation is maintained on the reflected image of the patient's own eye in a small central mirror. A short, wand-mounted test object 3 to 5 mm. in diameter is desirable, but a cotton-tipped applicator may be used for less exacting or urgent diagnostic steps. This instrument affords better observation of the patient and manipulation of the test object than can be achieved with any of the collapsing umbrella-type bedside devices.

Spherical projection perimetry
Goldmann Perimeter (Fig. 13-15)*

The Goldmann Perimeter, a rather imposing though table-top instrument, was introduced in 1945 and has undergone only minor modifications, which are incorporated into the current Model 940. It is uniquely accurate for both dynamic and static perimetric techniques and affords unusual speed of operation for the familiar examiner. When the patient can maintain fixation with the eye under examination, the observer merely watches the patient's pupil through a telescopic observation tube immediately above the illuminated recording

---

*Manufactured by Haag-Streit Co., Berne, Switzerland.

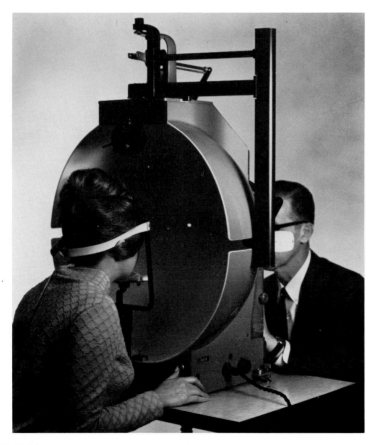

Fig. 13-15. Goldmann spherical projection perimeter made by Haag-Streit; pantographic arm is shown projecting stimulus to left of dark fixation spot. Examiner monitors patient fixation in primary position. Electric buzzer operated by patient's right thumb is used to indicate appearance of target.

surface. The examiner, who is seated behind the bowl, has complete control of the silent recording pantograph, movement of the target, and adjustment of its size ($\frac{1}{16}$ to 64 mm. in diameter) and brightness (1.0 to 0.0001).

Auxiliary color filters are not incorporated but can be supplied on request. The radius is 30 cm., and theoretically a patient under examination should have ametropia corrected for this distance (a supplemental lens holder is provided). Diffuse background illumination of the bowl provides excellent control both of preadaptation and surrounding light conditions during actual examination.

A central scotoma device may be added to increase the area of display and accuracy of plotting minute central defects. The patient is freed from necessity of talking (and moving his head) by an electric buzzer system under his fingertip control with which he notifies the examiner of his target awareness.

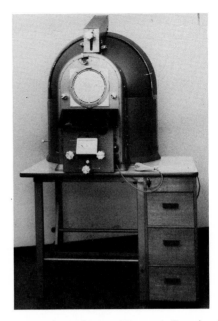

Fig. 13-16. The Tubinger (Harms-Aulhorn) spherical projection perimeter is shown from the examiner's side. Table-model unit may be placed on any convenient height stand.

Harms (Tubinger) Perimeter*

The somewhat massive Harms Perimeter console unit (Fig. 13-16) was introduced by H. Harms and Aulhorn in the mid-1950's and is particularly useful in elaboration of static (light-sense or profile) perimetry. Moreover, it also has full capacity for conventional kinetic or topographic examinations. It has a unique facility in examination of the foveal area, because the observation system enabling the examiner to monitor the patient's fixation comes through the area of the normal blind spot rather than centrally as in the Goldmann instrument. The blind spot area is also used to introduce dazzle or glare for simulation of testing of night-driving conditions. This instrument affords capacity for special testing of (1) dark adaptation curves, (2) central and peripheral visual acuity, (3) flicker fusion frequency, (4) motor sensitivity of the pupil, and (5) color perimetry. With this

*Manufactured by Oculus Products, Dutenhofen, Federal Republic of Germany.

equipment and a careful technologist, it may be possible to diagnose such disease processes as primary pigmentary degeneration of the retina (retinitis pigmentosa) before ERG reductions or ophthalmoscopic manifestations appear.

Color perimetry

A controversial aspect of perimetry, color perimetry reflects much difficulty in achieving standardized color test objects (both pigment and light), maintaining their color values, controlling preadaptation, obtaining proper background illumination, establishing absolute luminous flux values for targets, and ensuring proper recognition responses by the patient. The peripheral retina normally has a dyschromatic zone of variable width in which a patient may detect the presence of a colored test object before detecting its hue or color.

Color fields are generally a function of stimulus intensity, but they do present a method for reducing stimulus brightness or simulating a type of mesopic testing without other luminance variables. Harrington and Hoyt (1955) reported careful identification of a normal, minute central scotoma for monochromatic blue light (450 to 475 mμ) when testing with a stimulus under 2 mm. in diameter.

Most careful perimetrists feel that any type of defect elicited with colored test objects can be demonstrated with small and carefully controlled white test objects. As a matter of convenience, however, when ambient and stimulus light cannot be as well controlled as in a Goldmann spherical perimeter, the use of a large red test object 15 or 20 mm. in diameter (preferably Heidelberg red paper) may at times elicit a conduction defect before it is demonstrated by the conventional 2-mm. white object at 1 meter.

Generally in clinical testing, precision and repeatable findings with color perimetry are more difficult to obtain than with white perimetry. Therefore color testing is usually an adjunctive procedure.

Flicker fusion frequency (FFF) perimetry

FFF perimetry is a static technique of plotting sensitivity at various areas in the visual field on the basis of the latent period between the light stimulus and response, plus the time required for groups of percipient cells to recover from the inhibitory phase following a stimulus and thus to become sensitive to a subsequent stimulus. Individual sites in the field are quantitated numerically on the number of flashes per second required to make flickering light appear continuous. For practical purposes of testing, this method has only been in use since the early 1930's.

Equipment for the background commonly is the 1-meter tangent screen, though larger screens and large bowl perimeters may be used. A small, portable stroboscope* is an easily adaptable stim-

ulus source. The strobe flashbulb is modified and covered with opaque black paper, conventionally leaving open a target area of 3 to 5 cm. in diameter. Latitude of several degrees in target size will not alter clinical findings, but FFF does increase with the log of the stimulus area (Granit-Harper law).

The exposed target area should be covered with white translucent paper as used for typing so that the light is diffused. The four-wire electrical cable connecting the flash tube is passed through a rigid steel or aluminum tube 2 or 3 ft. long, which constitutes the supporting wand. This should be covered with black felt matching the tangent screen, or at least painted dull black. A conventional outline chart for noting tangent screen findings is used for record purposes, and the numbers in flashes per second representing FFF are written in for the macula and at appropriate locations corresponding to each site tested. The eyes are tested separately, and normally a few flashes per second difference may be found between the two eyes, particularly in the macular area. Testing may well be confined within the central 30 degrees from fixation because (1) most pathologic depressions appear within this area, (2) testing beyond 30 degrees is mechanically difficult except with a major spherical perimeter manufactured to include flicker, and (3) findings in the far periphery tend to be variable and less reliable.

FFF testing, like auto-ophthalmoscopic perimetry (p. 180), is particularly indicated in the presence of opacities in the media, poor vision, high refractive abnormalities, and suppression amblyopia. It may also present an advantage in testing patients with limited intelligence or poorly sustained attention. The technique is suited to detection of early or subtle field depressions, which may be widespread. Small scotomata, however, may be easily missed.

Macular or central fusion frequencies normally tend to be quite consistent at about 42 flashes per second. The midperiphery, however, has greater sensitivity to

*Strobotac, manufactured by General Radio Co., West Concord, Massachusetts 01742; or Photo Stimulator, manufactured by Grass Medical Instruments, Quincy, Massachusetts 02169.

flicker and therefore rates in this area normally climb to 50 or 55 flashes per second, with slightly lower frequencies temporally. Beyond 20 degrees from fixation, the FFF drops progressively through the midforties at 30 degrees and to frequencies as low as 20 in the extreme periphery. Minor variations from these normal frequencies are physiologic, but pathologically reduced frequencies are usually distinct. The FFF rate or the "end point" in testing may be determined either from ascending or descending changes in frequencies, with some questionable variation in significance. Therefore the selected alternative in technique should be noted on the record. Changes in rate of flicker (ascending or descending) during the examining run at each test site should be just slow enough for patient awareness and fast enough to avoid fatigue.

Angioscotometry

From the 1890's through the 1930's, many morphologic studies and plots were made of the vascular shadows radiating from the optic nerve head, particularly about the posterior pole and macula. In the United States, however, John Evans went beyond academic interest in these minute shadows to describe (1926-1938) pathologic widening phenomena of angioscotomata under such conditions as increased intraocular pressure, increased jugular pressure, fright, extraocular congestion, and cervical sympathetic irritation. The technique is laborious, requires excellent fixation, and needs minute silver bead targets 0.25 and 0.50 mm. in diameter. A 1-meter tangent screen can be used for demonstration of these vascular shadows, but rigidly solid "short range" (190-mm.) instruments with appropriate aspheric collimating lenses (+5.25 diopters) are much more efficient.*

Improvements in tonometry and tonography have superseded the particular role of angioscotometry in detecting widening of

---

*Lloyd Stereocampimeter, American Optical Co., Instrument Division, Buffalo, New York.

the vessel shadows as a sign of early open-angle glaucoma or inadequate control.

SCORING OF VISUAL FIELDS (TANGENT SCREEN AND PERIMETRIC)

Attempts at scoring visual fields quantitatively by some numerical or percentage system are as old as this century and generally have relied upon comparing serial fields, hopefully obtained under similar conditions, in order to assess improvement or loss. Increasing needs for accuracy in establishing compensation for permanent loss, or establishing criteria for transport licensure, led Ben Esterman* to develop and validate (1967-1968) two scoring grids, one for tangent screen and one for perimetric studies, each of 100 units. Component units, however, are of unequal size and unequal distribution, recognizing the unequal functional value of different parts of the field. Though each unit is valued at 1% and therefore a simple count of included units yields the functional score in percent, this relative value scale weighs central units above peripheral units, inferior units above superior units, and horizontal units above those in other meridians (Fig. 13-17).

In use, the outer isopter is first recorded in the standard fashion (2-mm. white test object at 1 meter for the tangent screen; 3-mm. or 0.5-degree white test object at 33-cm. radius for the perimeter). The grid, printed on transparent Mylar, is superimposed on the field record; alternatively, the field outline may be transferred by carbon paper to the appropriate grid. A central dot is printed in each of the 100 grid squares. The dots within (not touching) the field outline are merely counted in order to obtain the score. The percentage score thus derived (1) eliminates guesswork of significance, (2) reduces total calculations to be made in determining field

---

*Esterman, B.: Grid for scoring visual fields, Arch. Ophthal. 77:780-786, 1967; ibid. 79:400-406, 1968. Approved by the American Committee on Optics and Visual Physiology, October 27, 1968.

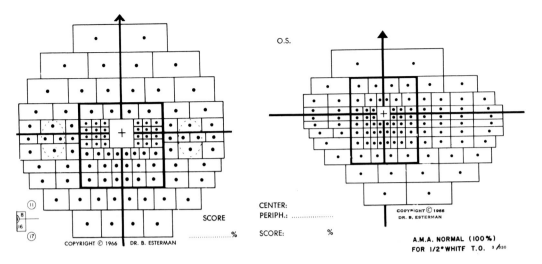

Fig. 13-17. Esterman 100-unit scoring grid for tangent screen (left) and for arc perimeter (right) in "relative perimetric position." (Courtesy Benjamin Esterman, M.D.)

efficiency, and (3) yields a numerical expression that is computer-compatible.

FINAL RESPONSIBILITY

The conscientious examiner will maintain an easily accessible tangent screen or other favorite perimetric device for frequent and quick use both in clinical diagnosis and in follow-up evaluation. All perimetric findings must be interpreted in the light of ophthalmoscopic findings. The examiner must recognize normal variations and pathologic changes in the fundus that alter the visual fields. In the absence of fundus pathology he should be prepared to make appropriate central or neurologic interpretations, see that the patient has proper neurologic studies (examination, skull x-rays, electroencephalogram, spinal tap, or air studies as indicated), and interpret the localizing specifics of visual field defects to the neurologist or neurosurgeon planning definitive care.

Chapter 14

*Tests of color vision**

Color depends upon hue (wavelength of light), brightness (intensity of light), and saturation or chroma (homogeneity). When either the intensity of light is reduced or the specific spectral components are missing, coloration disappears. Thus when the amount of white light (a mixture of radiant energies of all the visible wavelengths or approximately 400 to 750 mμ) is reduced or when, for example, wavelengths for red (650 to 750 mμ) are excluded from the light, it will not be possible to perceive the color red. Testing for color vision must be done with fully adequate illumination and with full spectral representation in the light used.

High filament temperature of about 6,750° K. may be used to produce illumination that simulates the full spectral range derived from the sun. More economically and with longer filament life, a conventional 100-watt light bulb (which operates at a tungsten filament temperature of about 2,854° K.) may be used if provided with the bluish appearing "C" filter of C.I.E. (Commission Internationale de l'Eclairage) illuminant standards. This filter removes a disproportionate amount of the long or red wavelengths. A New London Easel Lamp of table base design and yielding a desirable 15 to 35 foot candles of illumination[†]

has been made particularly to meet these specifications for color vision testing. If resort is made to fluorescent bulbs of the "daylight" type, care should be taken to ensure that full and proportioned spectral representation is present. The Duro-Test Corporation[*] produces a Vitalite tube that yields unusually full representation in the short (violet) wavelength end of the spectrum.

A useful and preliminary inspection of color vision is accomplished by a self-testing procedure such as the Rosner "Do-it-Yourself" wall-mounted color test. This 24 × 30 in. walnut-framed display of sixteen pseudoisochromatic plates can be hung—possibly—in some area of the office where it may attract the patient's attention. Two legend areas within the bottom portion of the frame give interpretation for the patient. (Though solid and substantial, it will tax a decorator's ingenuity to work this into attractive office appointments.)

Of more immediate usefulness is the unlearnable Hardy-Rand-Rittler[†] (HRR) (Fig. 14-1) booklet of twenty-four plates of gray versus color-confusable dots. The introductory four plates demonstrate, even to the color defective, the three types of colored test figures (O, X, and △) immersed within the field pattern of gray dots. These are followed by six plates specifically for preliminary screening to separate the red-green defectives, the blue-yellow defectives, and the normal trichromates. Ten further test plates

---

[*]Lewis, M. F., and Ashby, F. Y.: Diagnostic tests of color defective vision, annotated bibliography, 1955-1966, Washington, D. C., May, 1967, Federal Aviation Administration Office of Aviation Medicine.

[†]Manufactured by the Macbeth Corp., Newburg, New York 12550.

[*]North Bergen, New Jersey.

[†]American Optical Co., revised 1957.

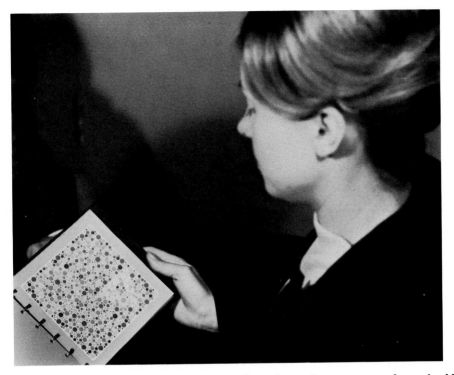

Fig. 14-1. Hardy-Rand-Rittler booklet of twenty-four plates of gray versus color-confusable dots. Patient is requested to identify only three test figures: O, X, and △.

quantitate the red-green failures and four final plates evaluate the blue-yellow failures, thus yielding qualitative classification of the defect and quantitative degree of impairment as mild, medium, or severe. Scoring and interpretation sheets are supplied with the booklet of test plates. The older Stilling (1883), Ishihara (1925, thirty-eight plates; 1968, twenty-four plates), Dvorine (1953, twenty-one plates; revised 1955), and similar sets of plates are based on pseudoisochromatic dots but are less specific in their differential capability and, by using learnable series of Arabic numbers, are subject to the disadvantage of memorization.

Because the precise physical basis for color perception remains obscure, and because nonspectral cues and psychologic factors affect testing procedures, visual literature contains dozens of other color tests based on spectroscopic matching (Helmholtz; Abney; Nagel), pigment or dye matching (Wilson; Holmgren; Jeffries;

Farnsworth), or lantern identification (Donders; Edridge-Green, 1920; Williams, 1903).

For critical accuracy and quantitation, the spectral matching technique as utilized in the Nagel anomaloscope (1899-1907) continues as the most definitive instrument.* This consists essentially of a telescopic tube directed at a light source. The lower half of the field of view is filled with a sodium yellow color that can be adjusted by the examiner both in brightness and in components of red and green. The subject then attempts to match the yellow of the lower field as preset by the examiner with the upper field where he may adjust the proportions of red, green, and yellow. Settings of the subject's controls then indicate the relative amounts of red, green, or yellow that he needs to match the test setting.

The time-consuming Nagel precision test

---

*Manufactured by Schmidt and Haensch, West Berlin, Federal Republic of Germany.

is of less ready practicality than a good lantern test such as that of F. W. Edridge-Green. Twenty-one variously colored glass filters on three rotating discs can be combined in front of a standard luminance source. A fourth rotating disc contains seven variously sized apertures that can be used as diaphragms to reduce the stimulus intensity. The fifth rotating disc contains modifiers such as ground glass to simulate mist, ribbed glass to simulate rain, or neutral densities to simulate fog. For usual requirements in the transport industry, examining is restricted to the control colors of yellow, red (A or B), and signal green. The compact unit takes considerably less table space than does a Macbeth easel lamp.

Less subtle tests to identify patients with functionally limiting color deficiencies are lead by such pigment matching tests as the practical Farnsworth D-15 test (1943). This test does not identify minor degrees of anomalous trichromatism but does identify significant anomalous trichromatism and true dichromatism (protanopia or deuteranopia). The D-15 test is simple, inexpensive, and easily accomplished by children or those with reduced acuity. Illumination requirements are less exact than with the HRR and Ishihara dots. A fixed reference chip of color is presented along with fifteen movable and numbered chips of hue progression. The subject is asked to align the fifteen movable chips in an order of color progression, matching their colors to that of the fixed reference chips. Scoring sheets as provided identify handicapping degrees of anomalous trichromatism or dichromatism but neither separate the two nor identify the quite rare blue-yellow defective. Patients may fail the HRR or Ishihara plates but, if able to pass

the Farnsworth D-15 test, may be considered functionally color adequate.

This test is to be differentiated from the more time-consuming, costly, and complex Farnsworth-Munsell 100-hue test (1943), which is not dependable for classification on a quantitative basis.

Color vision testing has not been a routine facet of eye examination in many clinics and offices because there is essentially no treatment for color defects after they are diagnosed. Industry, the military, and public carriers, however, maintain various standards of color perception that must be met by individuals in these fields. Distress at the time of a later request for such information may be avoided by incorporating some simple color screening into usual routine. Having such information in a diagnostic form will also avoid embarrassment at the end of an eye examination when a patient inquires about the significance of his previously unmentioned difficulty with colors.

Identification of deficiency in color vision will occasionally aid greatly in the diagnosis of specific congenital defects such as the nystagmus accompanying congenital achromatopsia. Notation of color defects in family members will be of frequent value in genetic counseling and in career planning for young individuals.

The exacting or compulsive examiner in this field can invest much time in complex testing systems that are of both research and genetic importance. Only rarely are such tests of value in identification of toxic damage to the retina. For usual purposes, however, the HRR or Ishihara test plates presented in proper light give secure diagnoses or clinical data and should be an easy working part of most eye examinations.

Chapter 15

Light sensitivity and dark adaptometry (mesopic and scotopic vision)

Evaluations of vision under reduced illumination fall into four sets of contrasting conditions:

1. Laboratory versus clinical
2. Absolute minimum thresholds versus practical levels for seeing in dim light
3. Minimum threshold of appearance versus course of dark adaptation
4. Objective versus subjective techniques

Complicated tests requiring preconditioning, such as for absolute minimum thresholds and minimum light differences, like quantum physics of the light-sense, are time-consuming labors primarily of the pure or laboratory-oriented examiner. They have suffered from insufficient control of the many variables that affect such examinations. Similarly, diagnostic attempts oriented to practical needs of assessing working vision under dim light (as a watch at sea) or under variable low intensities (as in night driving) are largely empirical, do not yield absolute values, and are subject to considerable latitude in reproducibility.

McFarland (1960) has disquietingly quantitated what most presbyopic examiners know, that man needs essentially doubled amounts of illumination every 13 years of life in order for objects to be seen under dim light. Thus presbyopia not only calls for a quantitative addition of plus spherical diopterage for near acuity but also presents a quantifiable need for progressively increasing illumination. The grandparent who puts larger bulbs in his reading light understandably remonstrates with the young teen-ager who reads happily and healthily in "poor" light that would be impossible for the oldster.

Finally, there is a peculiar lack of correlation between performance of an individual under mesopic illumination (0.01 to 0.5 foot lambert) and his tests of dark adaptation. This is a curious result of psychology, fatigue, motivation, alertness, and technique of visual use at night.

Empirically, there are three factors of night vision that are clinically important and amenable to some practical quantitation: (1) mesopic acuity or acuity under reduced illumination, (2) glare tolerance, and (3) glare recovery time, which is usually expressed in seconds. Preadaptation (photostressing) for standardized periods of 10 seconds to 3 minutes, followed by 10 to 40 minutes of dark adaptation, adds an element of laboratory quantitation to any of these procedures. Similarly, the use of repeated pilocarpine instillation to fix the pupillary diameter and to reduce this great variable makes test results more comparable, but these steps introduce abnormal conditions that will not be present in actual working or environmental situations.

Several practical devices are available to

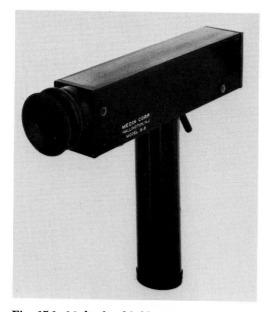

Fig. 15-1. Medin hand-held scotometer with optically simulated distance Snellen type and built-in dazzle source.

the practitioner for office testing of mesopic functions. The Feldman adaptometer (1937) has been produced by the American Optical Company in several compact, table-model versions, but essentially it permits only a measurement in minutes between standardized photostressing (3 minutes) and recognition of a dimly illuminated bar. The scotometer of Henkind and Siegel (1967)[*] is a smaller, hand-held, monocular instrument that affords an optically simulated distance Snellen reading followed by 10 seconds of dazzling glare. After extinguishing the glare, the patient continues fixation on the reduced Snellen chart (through the fading afterimage) until attaining his preglare level of Snellen recognition. Under these conditions, glare recovery time in normal individuals under age 40 should be less than 40 seconds, but this may be prolonged by age or disease to 180 seconds or more. This self-contained instrument also may serve as a bedside test for visual acuity (Fig. 15-1).

A screening instrument widely used by driver license examiners in North Amer-

ica is the table-model Night Sight Meter[*] (1953) (Fig. 15-2). This unit is built in a light-tight box 30 × 10 × 7 in. Below the viewing point is an illumination source that may be reduced by rotation of two sheets of Polaroid film over it. At the far end of the box, a motor-driven target wheel presents Landolt C's at the rate of 45 per minute (angular displacement of 18 degrees per second), requiring the patient to identify the direction of the opening in the C and announce one of four possible positions (up, down, right, or left) every second and a half. The size of the C's simulates 20/300 acuity. In use, the patient is asked to report the direction of the openings as the illumination is reduced under dial control. At the lowest level where he recognizes the openings, an empirical unit reading from the dial is recorded as mesopic acuity. Two glare sources (approximately 1 foot candle) are then presented at an angle 9 degrees to the left of the targets, thus simulating a car approaching on the left side of a 20-ft. wide pavement at a distance of 150 ft. Target illumination is then increased to a level necessary for recognition again of the Landolt C's; the dial reading is now a measure of glare tolerance.

For the third phase of the test, the glare source is extinguished and target illumination simultaneously decreased to the last visible level as determined in the first part of the test. The patient maintains fixation on the target area, and the examiner watches the interval timer reading in seconds. When ability to see the moving targets under his previously established mesopic acuity illumination is just regained, the elapsed seconds are recorded as glare recovery time.

These three procedures can be done by an office aide in 5 minutes with no more preconditioning than exposure to usual indoor ambient illumination. Results are generally repeatable, though a small percentage of patients, even with apparently normal

[*]Medin Corp., Wallington, New Jersey 07055.

[*]Manufactured by the American Automobile Association, Washington, D.C.

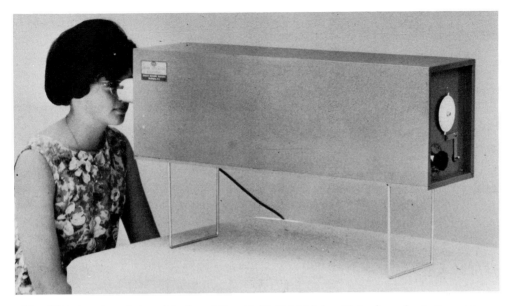

Fig. 15-2. American Automobile Association Night Sight Meter, 30 in. long, for testing vision under reduced illumination, glare tolerance, and glare recovery.

eyes and a few pretest runs, seem too slow in interpretive ability to report the necessary discriminations.

About a dozen sophisticated modern test instruments for testing minimal thresholds are available. The French Jayle-Blet adaptoperimeter (1955) is almost as large as a Link trainer and also capable of flicker, chromatic, and glare testing. At the other end of the size scale is the small, compact Comberg nyctometer with only a preadapting lamp and a 25-cm. diameter sphere in which test letters are exhibited after photostressing. Intermediate in size are projection devices to give controlled target stimuli (Beyne, 1952) or to present full cinemas of actual environmental conditions (Jayle, 1957).

Of the modern, absolute value type instruments the Goldmann-Weekers adaptometer (1950)[*] is the most accurate compromise between research laboratory equipment and office devices. This hemispheric instrument, though elaborate and only slightly smaller than the Goldmann table-model spherical perimeter, is uniquely flexible and simple to use. Determinations can

[*]Haag-Streit, Berne, Switzerland.

be made of minimal thresholds, differential thresholds, visual acuity at any level of adaptation, sensitivity to dazzle, response to color, and time course of light adaptation, both through the rapid alpha phase (measured in tenths of a second) and the slower beta phase (measured in seconds and minutes). Brightness steps are controlled in logarithmic units. Both subjective and objective measurements, with automatic drum recording of data, and examination of all or any portion of the retina, either central or peripheral, are possible (Fig. 15-3).

Though most adaptometry relies on subjective responses of the patient,[*] objective

[*]The Hartinger Recording Adaptometer, built on the basis of two Ulbricht spheres, and the simpler Recording Nyctometer, which automatically proceeds through a four-phase test cycle, are manufactured by Carl Zeiss of Jena, Democratic Republic of Germany. The Aulhorn projection mesoptometer, made by Oculus Products of Tubingen, Federal Republic of Germany, is designed for a 3-meter test distance in a totally dark room and is therefore cumbersome and space-consuming. It utilizes Landolt ring optotypes to quantitate (1) acuity at nine preset luminances, (2) night myopic shift, (3) glare recovery time after a 10-second stimulation of oncoming headlights, and (4) acuity in the presence of glare.

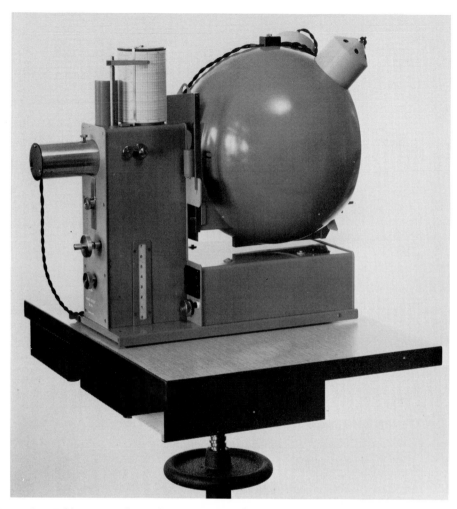

Fig. 15-3. Goldmann-Weekers adaptometer manufactured by Haag-Streit. Hemispheric bowl is shown from the rear (to the right), and automatic drum recorder is shown to the left.

methods (including electroretinography) are adaptable and commercially available. The Rieken principle (1941-1943) of utilizing opticokinetic nystagmus is incorporated in the Goldmann-Weekers and also the Jonkers (1947) adaptometer. Deviating from the precontrolling technique of fixing pupillary size with topical pilocarpine, Alpern (1959) incorporated pupillometry as an objective index, recording the intensity of light required to keep the pupil at a given diameter during an initial 12 minutes of dark adaptation. The relationship between sensory response and pupillary diameter becomes less correlated after the first 12 minutes of adaptation as the visual process becomes mediated primarily by rods (below the level of 0.1 meter candle [lux]). This objective technique, however, requires an infrared viewing or photographing system and is not easily integrated into office routines.

In general, test equipment for dark adaptation and mesopic vision is usually very complex and expensive or empirical and less reproducible in results. Compared to equipment for visual field studies or color discrimination, it is relatively unavailable in the offices of most eye practitioners. Therefore, as recently as 1969, both the American Committee on Optics and Visual Physiology as well as the A.M.A. Committee on Medical Aspects of Automotive Safety advised that practitioners evaluating night vision capabilities place primary reliance on detecting the disease entities and morphologic variations known to reduce visual capability in low illumination. Those especially reducing mesopic acuity and glare recovery are glaucoma (particularly when requiring miotic therapy), primary pigmentary degeneration of the retina (retinitis pigmentosa), retinal and choroidal arteriolosclerosis, retinal abiotrophies, retinitis punctata albescens, choroideremia, diabetic retinopathy, aphakia, degeneration of the macula, optic atrophy, Oguchi's disease

and other forms of familial or congenital night blindness, chronic hepatic disease, and avitaminosis A. Reduced glare tolerance or increased dazzling may similarly be predicted in the presence of opacities or diffraction alterations in the media such as corneal irregularities, scars, opacities or dystrophies (particularly affecting the central portion), lens opacities or vacuoles, and vitreous floaters. Dirty, pitted, and scratched spectacle lenses or windshields create similar effects and present a further handicap compounding any pathology in the patient's eye.

Chapter 16

Exophthalmometry

Instrumental exophthalmometry need not be performed as a routine on every patient; rather, it should be done in keeping with the patient's complaints, ocular history, and preliminary findings. Every examiner should also remember that the complaint of exophthalmos on one side may actually be enophthalmos on the other. Critical attention should therefore be given also to the possibly normal or relatively enophthalmic fellow globe. Sometimes the concealed history of a blow or the omitted diagnosis of a previous orbital floor fracture initiates orbital fat atrophy or herniation and possible incarceration of extrabulbar soft tissues. At times all the clinical wit of the examiner plus x-rays, ultrasound, ear, nose, and throat examination, medical studies, and even biopsy are needed to attain a satisfactory diagnosis in exophthalmos.

Preliminary inspection should evaluate each eye in relation to the other eye (orthophoria to heterotrophia) and also in relation to other facial landmarks (exophthalmos, enophthalmos, displacement). This inspection should not only be in frontal view of the patient but also by examination from above (Fig. 16-1), where it is easier to note the relative position of the lateral orbital rims and the relative position of the zygomatic arches (Fig. 16-2). The examiner should palpate the orbital rims with equal pressure in the pulp tips of each index finger. Holding the fingers in straight extension augments, by aligning power, the ability to discriminate small differences in anteroposterior position. Similar position-

ing of the fingers over the zygomatic arch indicates their relative anteroposterior position. This physical inspection can be supplemented with a submentovertex x-ray view (Fig. 16-3), which displays the angulations and relative depths of the orbits.

It is important to record any relative anteroposterior asymmetry of either lateral orbital rim in reference to the other, because these sites are reference points for essentially all exophthalmometers, except for the Mutch proptometer, which compares a plunger depth setting on the closed lid over the corneal apex, with vertical reference points on the orbital rim at 12 and 6 o'clock.

The simplest exophthalmometer is the Luedde rule (Fig. 16-4), made of transparent acrylic and vertically etched in millimeters from zero at a notch on one end. The observer places the notch firmly against the lateral orbital rim and, from his lateral position, aligns the etch marks on both sides of the rule with the anterior-most limit of the corneal curvature while the patient fixes straight ahead. Usually it is necessary to direct a bright penlight beam onto the cornea from below with the other hand or else this essential distal line is lost in the shadows of the inner canthal recess. Ordinarily the Luedde measurement ranges from 16 to 20 mm., but scale markings extend to 40 mm.

Recently this instrument has been made available in double form by mounting two of the single Luedde rules onto a connecting crossbar of similar plastic.* Each rule

---

*Instrumedic, Ltd., London W1, England.

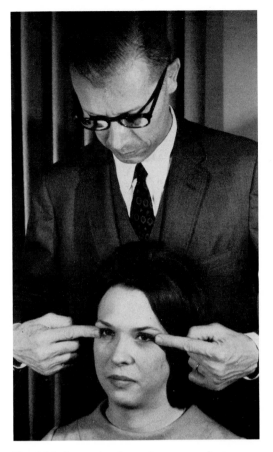

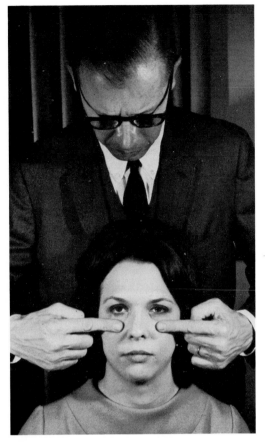

Fig. 16-1. Inspection from above to evaluate symmetric position of lateral orbital rims. Direct extension of examiner's fingers gives added assistance of aligning power to differentiate small irregularities.

Fig. 16-2. Examination from above to evaluate symmetry of zygomatic arches. Examiner uses equal pressure of fingertips against midpoint of lower orbital rim. Extended fingers again afford advantage of aligning power in estimating small differences.

can be moved laterally or medially on the ungraduated crossbar in order to position the notched ends of the exophthalmometer scales on the lateral orbital rims. When viewed from above, this arrangement helps to identify symmetry or asymmetry of the anteroposterior position of the lateral orbital rims.

More complex instruments with right and left prisms (Rodenstock), or right and left double mirrors (Hertel) (Fig. 16-5), enable the observer to make readings of each corneal limit while maintaining a frontal position to the patient. The design of these instruments is based on an assumed mean distance (usually 20 mm.) between the cor-

neal apex and the lateral orbital rim. In small children or broad-faced individuals accuracy of reading may be compromised. A scale measuring the distance of separation between right and left units of these exophthalmometers is etched on the carrier bar; this figure has no bearing on the exophthalmos reading but should be noted in order to set the reading surfaces in the same relative position on subsequent examinations.

The Copper* orbital tonometer (1948) (Fig. 16-6) is an elaboration of exophthal-

---

*Lameris Instrumentum, Utrecht, The Netherlands.

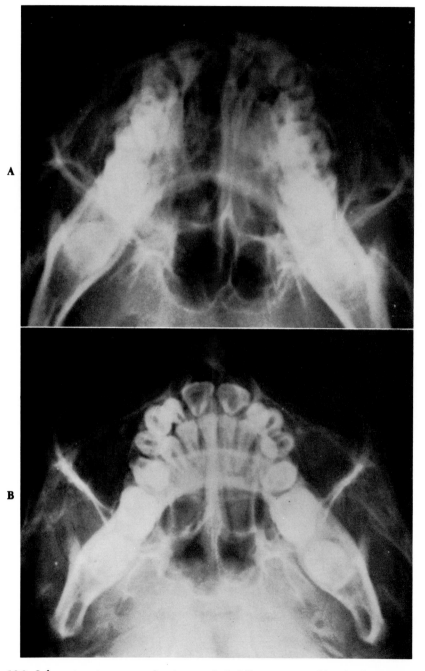

Fig. 16-3. Submentovertex x-rays showing marked difference in width of orbital angles and position of lateral orbital rim. **A** shows broad or flat facial configuration; **B** shows narrow or slender facial configuration.

mometry using a slotted aluminum bridge with fixed height-supporting legs against each lateral orbital rim and a third or center leg adjusted in height to the glabella. The patient must be recumbent. The unit is secured by an elastic band adjusted to stay around the occiput with minimum tension. Topical anesthetic is instilled and a clear plastic contact shell bearing a female receptacle on its convex surface is inserted between the lids onto the cornea. A spring-loaded dynamometer is then introduced through the slot in the aluminum bridge while the patient steadily fixates through the slotted bridge with the other eye.

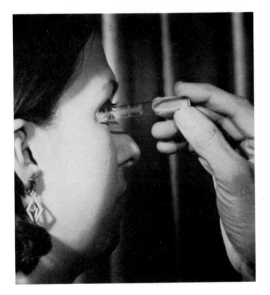

Fig. 16-4. Luedde exophthalmometer placed on right lateral orbital rim to measure linear distance from rim to corneal apex.

For the initial or base reading, the tip of the dynamometer is rested in the receptacle of the contact lens. The position of the cornea is read in millimeters from the point where an etched scale on the plunger of the dynamometer appears above the bridge. This figure should be recorded by an aide and then successive readings made with plunger loads of 100, 200, 300, and finally 400 gm. If the readings are done quickly, most patients do not find this uncomfortable, except for the maximum or 400-gm. pressure. A compression curve should then be plotted on the patient's record to indicate the reduction in exophthalmos in relation to increasing pressure. Expression of blood or soft edema fluid in the first 100 or 200 gm. of compressions usually accounts for a proportionately greater initial reduction in exophthalmos than is achieved with succeeding weights. In the presence of scirrhous orbital neoplasm, the compressibility curve may be quite flat from 0 to 400 gm.

The Copper instrument is a very accurate exophthalmometer and, as a piezometer, may theoretically aid in the differentiation of soft or vascular retrobulbar lesions (showing early, steep drop in the orbital compressibility curve) from hard neoplastic or infectious processes (showing flattening of the orbital compressibility curve). Thus a cavernous hemangioma or thyrotoxic exophthalmos might be expected to show distinct retrodisplacement of the globe with light pressure of 100 and 200 gm., whereas a meningioma, thyrotropic

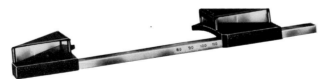

Fig. 16-5. Hertel reflecting exophthalmometer. Millimeter marks apparent on front surface of horizontal carrier bar should be noted after contact points of instrument are adjusted to lateral orbital rims; this facilitates same separation of reflecting mirrors on subsequent examinations. Millimeter scale indicating actual position of corneal surface anterior to orbital rim is read on sighting through the mirrors at each side.

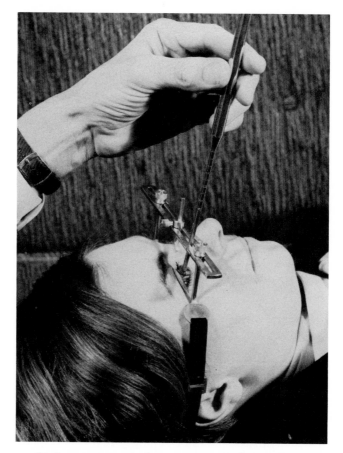

Fig. 16-6. Copper orbital tonometer secured in position with elastic strap around occiput. Right contact lens is in place, and spring-loaded dynamometer is inserted through slot in bridge to engage in receptacle of contact lens.

exophthalmos, or orbital cellulitis might show relatively less retrodisplacement (flattening of the curve) with the 100- and 200-gm. forces. However, just as in Mulvany's effort (1943) to categorize thyrotropic and thyrotoxic forms of Graves' disease, there are transitional or unclear cases both to clinical and to orbitometric evaluation.

In diagnosing very slight or questionably pathologic exophthalmos, it can be helpful to make measurements in the recumbent position in addition to the seated position (Hauer, 1969). A slightly prominent globe in the absence of orbital pathology will normally show a bit less exophthalmos in the recumbent than in the sitting position. In the presence of endocrine ophthalmop-athy or orbital infiltration, such reduction does not occur.

The conscientious though sometimes puzzled diagnostician must be prepared from time to time to defer diagnosis and recommend reexamination in a few weeks. Repeating detailed measurements and studies may then yield far more information as to both basic nature and activity of a suspect process. Exploratory orbitotomy, differing from the more flexible confines of exploratory laparotomy, is a hazardous and significantly traumatic procedure. Generally it will not clear up deep enigmas unless they have been localized preoperatively to specific orbital depths, quadrants, and relationships to such structures as the extraocular muscle cone.

Chapter 17

Ophthalmodynamometry and the diagnosis of carotid artery insufficiency

In the presence of amaurosis fugax, occlusion of the central retinal artery or its branches, or suspect carotid artery system impairments, it is diagnostically important to compare ophthalmic artery pressure on the two sides. Diastolic readings can be made first, but if significant difference (exceeding 20%) is not found, systolic readings should also be made. Other diagnostic evidence of arterial insufficiency disease may be gleaned by (1) palpation of the carotid arteries (Fig. 17-1) in the neck for thickening, reduction of pulsation, or thrill, (2) auscultation for bruit in the ipsilateral neck or over either eye, (3) x-ray examination of the carotids for calcification, (4) carotid system angiograms, (5) studies of the Doppler effect by transcutaneous ultrasound, or (6) thermography (Keeney and Guibor, 1970).

Palpation of the carotid arteries serves not only to compare the strength of pulsation and the vascular firmness or thickening on each side but may also yield tactile evidence of thrill when there is advanced stenosis. A thrill is a vibration or fremitus tactually detected by the fingertips and probably caused by eddies in the bloodstream beyond an area of narrowing. Thrills in carotid impairments are generally synchronous with cardiac systole and become increasingly apparent with increasing degrees of vascular narrowing. The thrill is most commonly related to the carotid system when felt high in the neck; its presence low in the neck may represent transmission from the heart (aortic valve stenosis) or aortic arch (coarctation or patent ductus) (Knox, 1969).

Auscultation of the carotid artery is best done in the lateral aspect of the neck just anterior to the sternomastoid muscle. The patient should be asked to stop breathing briefly during auscultation so that breath sounds do not interfere with the detection of subtle murmurs. Localization is also enhanced by using the open-bell or Ford type fitting of small or pediatric diameter rather than a diaphragm type chest piece on the stethoscope (this instrument, of course, should preferably be called a stetho*phone*).

The absence of any carotid artery bruit means either no encroachment on the lumen or else complete occlusion. If the bruit is best heard high in the neck, this suggests stenosis in the area where the common carotid bifurcates into the internal and external carotid arteries. If the bruit is only heard low in the neck, it may represent transmitted cardiac sounds. Bruits heard primarily in the posterior triangles of the neck generally are not specific for carotid impairments but rather represent vertebral artery stenosis when heard on the right, or subclavian-vertebral artery stenosis when heard on the left.

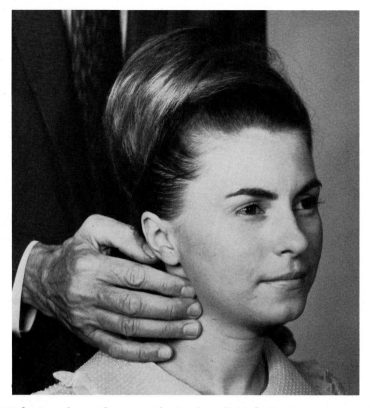

Fig. 17-1. Palpation of carotid artery pulsation from behind, showing correct positioning of examiner's three fingers on the course of the artery. Right and left are compared simultaneously.

Doppler effect or frequency shift studies using ultrasound reflections from moving blood cells detect different velocities within the blood column. These are usually maximal in the center of the column and minimal near the vessel wall. They also detect alterations in blood flow rate as surge characteristics resulting from cardiac action. These compressions and rarefactions of ultrasonic waves are transferred to visual display on an oscilloscope, or the differences between emanated and reflected frequencies may be used as audible signals. The nonpulsed or continuous-wave ultrasound required for Doppler studies necessitates energy delivery at several logarithmic units greater than is used in time-amplitude (A-mode) diagnostic studies and therefore should be used for minimum periods of exposures. Since Doppler studies of vessels beneath soft tissue, such as the carotids, are qualitative rather than quantitative, it is necessary to compare right and left counterparts. Equipment, though simpler than that for time-amplitude ultrasound, is relatively expensive and more readily available in medical center settings than in clinical offices.

Thermographic apparatus* may run into investment of $15,000 to $25,000 and is primarily of investigational status in ocular diagnosis at present. It graphically creates thermal portraits in shades of gray or maps isothermic "contour lines" connecting selected heat levels. Temperature variations over the face commonly range through 10° C. from the cool lashes and tip of the nose to the warm inner canthal area. It will

---

*Manufactured by Barnes Engineering Corp., Stamford, Connecticut; AGA Corp., Secaucus, New Jersey 07094.

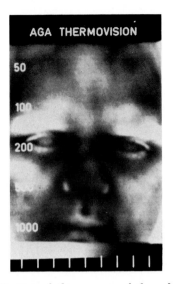

Fig. 17-2. Normal thermogram of the orbits and midface. Relative heat scale shown across the lower edge indicates warmth (represented as darkness) and coolness (represented as lightness). The brows and nares can be seen as white or cool. The lips and inner canthal recesses appear as dark or warm. Corneal surfaces appear as intermediate grayness or coolness. Warm paths of the supraorbital vessels are indicated by dark lines extending upward through the nasal portion of the brow. (Thermogram produced on AGA Thermovision equipment.)

record differences as slight as 0.1° C. and shows both focal and diffuse patterns of thermal increases (uveitis, arteritis, infections, neoplasms) and decreases (hemorrhage, retinal detachments, contusion edema, vascular occlusion) in tissue temperature. Ischemic areas as well as the specific paths of dilating collateral vessels can be quantitatively shown with complete objectivity (Fig. 17-2).

Ophthalmodynamometry produces more dynamic information and has less likelihood of dislodging emboli than either palpation or angiography. It is prerequisite for the patient to have two eyes, each with visible fundi, in order to accomplish this examination. Brachial artery sphygmomanometry should precede ophthalmodynamometry for comparative reference.

Under normal conditions of intraocular pressure and carotid system sufficiency, pulsations are not seen in the retinal arteriolar

tree. Because the retinal vessels, however, are subject to an intraocular or tissue pressure of 15 to 20 mm. Hg rather than the much lower tissue pressure elsewhere in the body, a paradoxic venous pulsation is created during diastole in more than half of all normal persons. When intraocular pressure is increased by digital pressure, compression instruments, or glaucoma, rhythmic constrictions synchronous with cardiac diastole appear in the retinal arterioles. Conversely, when diastolic arterial pressure drops below intraocular pressure because of syncope, peripheral collapse, or aortic valvular insufficiency, pulsations also appear in the retinal arterioles.

These physiologic principles underlie the measurement of ophthalmic artery pressure with the ophthalmodynamometer as developed by Paul Bailliart (1917). In use, a topical anesthetic is instilled and ocular tension measured by indentation or applanation. Dynamometry readings should first be made in the seated position. The patient is instructed to maintain steady fixation. The direct ophthalmoscope may be preferred to the indirect because of its greater magnification. With the ophthalmoscope in the hand corresponding to the patient's eye under examination, the dynamometer in the other hand is aligned with a diameter of the globe. The footplate is brought into contact with the lateral sclera, and pressure is evenly increased at the rate of about 20 gm. per second while the major retinal arterioles on the disc are kept under clear observation. Care must be taken not to angulate the dynamometer away from a position corresponding to a diameter or radius of the globe. This is often helped by steadying the instrument gently against the angulation of the outer canthus (Fig. 17-3).

At the first appearance of pulsation in the retinal arterioles, the *diastolic* readings are taken from the dial or scale on the instrument. Increasing pressure may be continued until the first complete collapse of the retinal arterioles; at this point, *systolic* pressure is read.

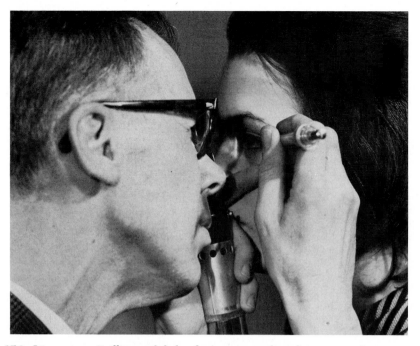

Fig. 17-3. Linear type Bailliart ophthalmodynamometer aligned in use with an equatorial diameter of the globe and steadied against the outer canthus. Examiner watches central retinal artery pulsation as pressure is increased.

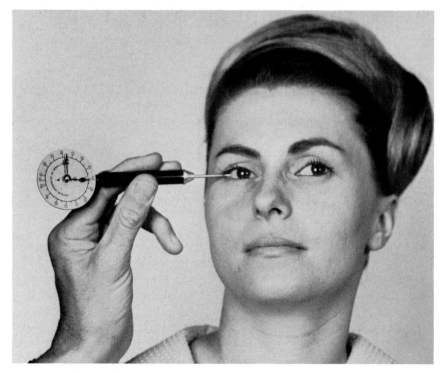

Fig. 17-4. Dial type Bailliart ophthalmodynamometer shown in correct radial position with footplate against right eye. Slave or passive indicator is resting above 80-unit mark and active indicator is shown lower near 40-unit level as pressure is being decreased from systolic to diastolic level.

The Bailliart spring dynamometers come in two designs: dial and linear. The dial type (Fig. 17-4) has two indicators—one active pointer connected to the spring load and equipped with a finger-controlled stop, and one passive or "slave" pointer, which remains at the highest reading. The cylinder or linear registering type reads directly from engravings on its piston and has a single stop button that can hold only one reading after removal from the eye. With either type, if the diastolic or low reading is made first (as the pressure is being increased) it is necessary for an assistant to note the diastolic reading while the examiner watches the retinal artery. The dial model offers an advantage if the systolic (higher) reading is made first; then the slave pointer will remain at this value and, on reduction of dynamometer pressure to the diastolic level (last pulsation), the finger-controlled stop can be engaged to hold the lower value (McLean, 1963). Thus both readings may be retained without the use of a second observer. Some examiners elect only to make diastolic readings, but this will miss a percentage of carotid insufficiencies.

The greatest difficulties in ophthalmodynamometry are maintaining perfectly radial position of the instrument to the eye and avoiding displacement of the eye from ophthalmoscopic observation. Because even slight inclinations of the instrument away from the radial position introduce gross errors, it is customary to make about three separate readings and to record the average.

Direct readings are in grams of pressure, but by plotting them against Schiøtz indentation tensions on the Magitot-Bailliart nomogram (1922), pressure in the ophthalmic artery may be derived in millimeters of mercury.

With Goldmann applanation tonometry values it is necessary to use the Bedavaija nomogram (1960). These figures, however, are subject to errors, and the comparative or relative values are of greater significance. Average normal systolic pressure in the ophthalmic artery as indicated by this technique varies between 60 and 85 mm. Hg. Average normal diastolic pressure varies between 30 and 40 mm. Hg or about one-half of brachial diastolic pressure.

If the diastolic pressure as found in each eye is more than 10 or 15 mm. Hg higher than the brachial diastolic pressure, it suggests increased intracranial pressure. Readings of the two eyes should agree within 10% to 15%. If either systolic or diastolic pressures are reduced by 20% or more on one side, this is excellent evidence of carotid system insufficiency proximal to the origin of the ophthalmic artery. If ophthalmic systolic and diastolic pressures are equal in the two eyes and in balance with brachial pressure, carotid system insufficiency can be excluded almost with certainty.

Slightly higher pressure readings and slightly less marked differential reductions may be found in the supine position, whereas slightly lower pressures and more marked differential reductions may be found in the standing position.

Other procedures, better described as "orbital plethysmography," have been evolved using water-filled goggles ("pulsensors") or latex balloons against the lids and orbits (Hager, 1964) that sense the results of many forces within the eye and orbit. Sometimes their use is referred to as "ophthalmodynamography," but the figures derived are difficult to relate to any single vascular component. Further validation is needed.

A piezoelectric crystal or sensor contained in a liquid silicone–filled sphere approximately the size of a pencil eraser has been designed by Kalb (1969) for direct application to the topically anesthetized globe. This will record the pattern of arterial wave forms concurrently with externally applied pressure. The equipment will transcribe this wave form onto a narrow tape recorder from which can be read systolic and diastolic transitions. This removes the need for direct visualization of the vessels within the globe and furnishes a permanent record tape of the ophthalmodyna-mometry. This equipment is not commercially available at this time.

Suction ophthalmodynamometry is a variation in technique that increases intraocular pressure by the use of a perilimbal suction-cup apparatus of hemispheric configuration attached to the lateral aspect of the globe. By use of a built-in 50-ml. syringe, vacuum force is created and measured within the system. A 14-mm. external diameter suction cup is connected through the suction apparatus by firm plastic tubing. The equipment* is able to attain and measure 600 mm. Hg vacuum pressure. However, a suction of 500 mm. Hg will raise intraocular pressure to approximately 140 mm. Hg. In use, applanation tonometry and brachial artery sphygmomanometry are obtained before application of the suction cup. Withdrawing on the 50-ml. syringe creates suction as recorded on the vacuum gauge.

Under ophthalmoscopic observation, the first frank pulsation of the central retinal artery at the disc is considered to be the diastolic end point, whereas the first completed occlusion of the artery is considered to be the systolic end point. Generally, values obtained by the suction technique are higher than those obtained by the Bailliart method. The range of difference between the two methods, however, is essentially similar. Though this technique is far less well established than is compression ophthalmodynamometry, it avoids the problems of obliquity in compression of the globe, movement of the globe during ophthalmoscopy, and slippage of the footplate (Galin, 1969).

Careful history of arterial occlusive episodes plus physical examination by palpation, auscultation, and ophthalmodynamometry often yield a definitive working diagnosis of insufficiency disease of the arterial supply to the globe or localization to a major carotid arterial component. However,

*Available from Storz Instrument Co., St. Louis, Missouri 63110.

more specific and graphic localization is generally desired by a vascular surgeon before electing to do corrective surgery. The most finite step in diagnosis is carotid angiography by injection of radiopaque contrast medium, usually through the brachial artery. Because there is mild morbidity (conjunctival hemorrhage, transient contralateral weakness in the extremities), or infrequent mortality, the indication for such x-ray studies should be appreciated and organized by the eye examiner. The following general principles should be met (Knox, 1969) before undertaking angiography:

1. The patient should be relatively well, without suffering a major stroke or other life threatening disease.
2. Transient ischemic attacks should correspond to the area of suspect arterial insufficiency.
3. Bruit or thrill should be present in the suspect artery to suggest a pathologic compromise but not complete occlusion of the vascular lumen.
4. Ophthalmodynamometry should be low on the involved side.
5. No other diseases that could explain the symptoms exist.

The increasing numbers of older persons in the population is producing an increasing incidence of vascular insufficiency diseases, arterial occlusions, or ischemic disturbances. With a high coefficient of correlation, such disturbances in the ocular fundus indicate carotid system insufficiencies. As a working dictum, central retinal artery occlusion should be considered carotid system insufficiency disease until proved otherwise, as should the presumptive diagnosis of "ischemic optic neuritis" in a patient of advanced years. Thus ophthalmodynamometry is more frequently needed now than it was a few decades ago in order to achieve optimal interpretative value from fundus findings. With this instrument, the examiner again not only achieves diagnostic information concerning arterial supply of the eye but may also gain lifesaving information from a grossly uninvolved eye.

Chapter 18

Fundus photography and fluorescein angiography

Terrance L. Tomer

Fundus examination in its ophthalmoscopic aspects now benefits from the many advantages of photography such as (1) detailed permanent record, (2) magnification of 2.5× to 10×, (3) recording in monochromatic light for occasional accentuation of aspects that may otherwise be inapparent, (4) optimal study of contrast dye injection angiography, (5) rapid sequence recording of dye passage or active vascular changes, and (6) later and leisurely study of the fundus after the patient's visit.

Ease, economy, and excellence have been introduced into this phase of examination, particularly since World War II, by vast technologic improvements in cameras and light sources, by refinements in speed and detail capacity of both black and white and color film, and by clinical need for fundus information on which to base treatment decisions concerning photocoagulation, laser intervention, or even enucleations in such questions as subretinal hematoma versus malignant melanoma of the choroid.

THE PHOTOGRAPHER

Fundus photography may be particularly beneficial in finding and focusing significant pathology or in bringing out precise details if the clinician makes the pictures himself. More commonly, however, in university centers, schools, or clinics serving several or more examiners, a skilled photographer is given full responsibility for this work including loving, dust-free maintenance of equipment and, at least, supervision in processing of the film. This photographer should be an expert with both the direct and indirect ophthalmoscopes. He must be familiar with the normal topography and landmarks of the fundus as well as the types and characteristics of alterations produced by pathology. Investment of a few moments from time to time by the clinician to demonstrate pathologic changes to the photographer will yield, over the months and years, steadily increased excellence of photographic records and conservation of time for the patient, the clinician, and the photographer.

Incidentally, the clinician must be certain that the photographer has and wears any appropriate refraction correction that he needs. Young and nonpresbyopic photographers, as well as those having even mild or modest refractive errors, will often have marked difficulty in attaining or maintaining maximum focus of the viewing lens. Their spectacles should be prescribed under cycloplegic examination and then the distance correction consistently worn for this work.

The photographer must be intimately familiar with the working controls and variations in the camera settings. He should have a knowledge of basic photographic princi-

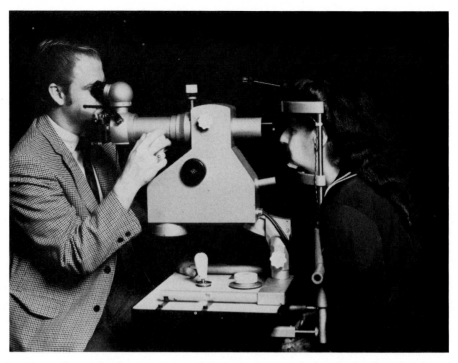

Fig. 18-1. Carl Zeiss fundus camera in use showing photographer's right hand on fine focusing adjustment and patient properly seated with fixation device before her right eye.

ples and a working understanding of the optics of fundus cameras.

High quality and consistency in fundus photographs are determined more by how the camera is maintained and used than by which make of camera is employed. A systematic routine both considerate of the patient and technically complete must be followed.

THE CAMERA

After a few decades of unsuccessful attempts in many countries, the first satisfactory fundus photographs were presented by Friedrich Dimmer of Vienna in 1899 (IX International Congress of Ophthalmology). Unfortunately his apparatus was very cumbersome, being literally as large as a grand piano. Dimmer's technique was not published until 1911 and his process was not functionally repeated.

In 1922 J. W. Nordenson of Uppsala presented his compact table-top camera based on the Gullstrand principles (International Congress of Ophthalmology, Washington,

D. C.). After more than 9 years of refinement, this self-contained, carbon arc camera was marketed in 1926 and was widely acclaimed. The first English language atlas of fundus photography was published in 1928 by Arthur Bedell using one of these cameras.

Another great dimension in fundus photography was added by the introduction of Kodachrome film in the early 1930's. The Bausch and Lomb camera (1950) served to maintain some capability in fundus photography until the modern Carl Zeiss fundus camera (Fig. 18-1) became available with the redevelopment of the West German optical industry after World War II. This camera is now essentially the basic standard of all other instruments in the field, such as Topcon II, Nikon, Mamiya, and Olympus. Two reliable hand-held fundus cameras—the Kowa RC-2 and the Nikon Retinal Hand Camera—are also available.

Details and instructions in this chapter relate primarily to the Carl Zeiss fundus cam-

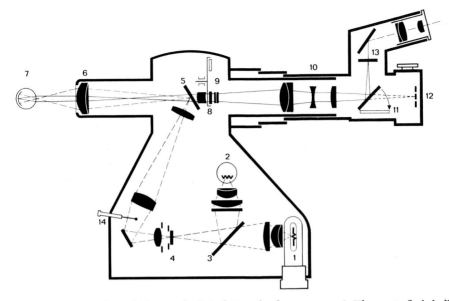

Fig. 18-2. Light path through the standard Carl Zeiss fundus cameras. *1,* Electronic flash bulb; *2,* double filament incandescent illuminating system; *3,* glass plate; *4,* diaphragm disc to rotate different apertures into illuminating beam; *5,* mirror; *6,* aspheric objective lens; *7,* patient's eye; *8,* spherical corrective lenses; *9,* cross cylindrical lenses to compensate for astigmatism in patient's eye; *10,* collecting or focal lens system; *11,* tiltable mirror; *12,* camera back; *13,* eyepiece reticule; *14,* fixation target attachment.

era* (Fig. 18-2), because it has become a standard of excellence, and secondarily to the Kowa RC-2† hand-held camera, because of its excellence and originality in this type of equipment.

ROUTINE TECHNIQUE
Preliminary preparation of patient

As in all procedures requiring patient participation and ocular fixation, it is essential to explain briefly what is to be anticipated and to build confidence with soft, courteous words coupled with sure and direct actions. Topical anesthetics should be avoided before fundus photography since they tend to soften the epithelium or disturb the precorneal tear film and in turn interfere with the necessary corneal clarity for sharp imagery. This precludes manipulations such as retinography, tonography, gonioscopy, lacrimal probing, or corneal staining before photography. Similarly,

*Carl Zeiss, Inc., Oberkochen, Federal Republic of Germany.
†Kowa Co., Ltd., Nagoya, Japan.

protracted examinations by indirect ophthalmoscopy with scleral depression, or even repeated direct ophthalmoscopy by multiple examiners, may cause some drying or subsequent epithelial disturbance and should not be done immediately before photographic sessions.

The pupils must be dilated to at least 7 mm. in diameter (somewhat more if stereoscopic photographs are to be made). Dilatation is necessary to transmit the illuminating ring of light into the fundus, and complete cycloplegia is also necessary to stabilize the position of the image. The Zeiss fundus camera, like most instruments of this type, utilizes indirect ophthalmoscopy and a real aerial image that is focused by the ophthalmoscopic lens of the camera. Thus accommodative action by the patient will shift the aerial image of his fundus forward and backward to the frustration of the photographer trying to maintain a sharp focus.

Cyclopentolate (Cyclogyl) alone gives excellent mydriasis and cycloplegia without undesirable disturbance of the corneal epithelium, but it may take more than a half hour for maximum effect and cause some accommodative impairment for 3 or 4 hours. A more rapidly acting combination of drugs with shorter duration is 1 drop of 1% Mydriacyl repeated in 3 minutes and followed in another 3 minutes by 1 drop of 10% viscous Neo-Synephrine. The viscous solution of Neo-Synephrine should be used instead of the aqueous, which may disturb the epithelial clarity, or the emulsion, which may leave disturbing bubbles in the precorneal film. The usual precautions must be observed in the presence of a shallow anterior chamber or of a history of angle-closure glaucoma. When dilatation is elected in this situation, a weak miotic such as 1% pilocarpine should be instilled several times after photography and the patient retained in the office until miosis is achieved.

The patient should be seated comfortably on a sturdy chair of adequate size. A secretarial posture chair is quite satisfactory. When using the hand fundus camera, better control and patient comfort are secured with the patient lying down.

Preliminary preparation of equipment

Before the patient is brought into the darkened camera room the equipment should be checked. The proper camera back should be attached and contain adequate amounts of the desired film. Kodachrome II (ASA 25) is excellent for color transparencies. High-Speed Ektachrome (ASA 160) is desirable when using the Kowa RC-2 because of its lower flash intensity. Kodak Plus X (ASA 125) is adequate for black and white photography.

The photographer must be sure that the relay circuit or flash synchronization cord is properly inserted on the film holder and should check to see whether or not the 2× accessory lens is in place, depending on the planned use of magnification. This magnification attachment, which locks between the objective lens system and the camera, increases the image size from a standard 22.5-mm. diameter to utilization of the entire 24- × 36-mm. film area. The lower magnification should be used on all initial and survey photographs.

The photographer should focus the eyepiece to bring the cross hairs into maximum sharpness for his own eye. He should set the control knobs on the top of the camera for cross cylinder astigmatic correction to 0 diopters and axis 90 degrees, except for the occasional patient with high astigmatism who requires interposition of compensatory lenses to attain sharp focus throughout the image field. On the right side of the camera, the control knob for the Rekoss disc should be set at the red printed number (−16 to +17 diopters) or alternate spherical diopterage range as needed to compensate for high myopia, hyperopia, or aphakia.

The diaphragm selector knob on the left side of the camera should be set to bring aperture No. 7 (the 14-mm. diameter opening on the older models or the bull's eye opening of newer models) into the light path.

The power supply should be turned on at this time and the focusing light intensity placed at the medium or No. 2 setting. Flash number intensity should be correspondingly set at II when Kodachrome II is being used without the magnification attachment or at IV if the attachment is used. For color Polaroid film type 108 the intermediate flash setting III is used. The photographer must make knowledgeable adjustments in flash intensity for extremely light or dark fundi. In an albino patient or one with a large coloboma of the retina and choroid, flash brightness would be reduced to setting I while using Kodachrome II film. In a Negro or darkly pigmented eye, flash intensity must usually be increased to No. III.

Final positioning of patient

With the patient comfortably seated, elevation of the table and chinrest are adjusted to the height and position of the patient. A few moments of adjustment here will gen-

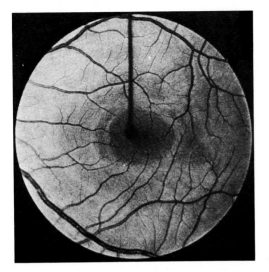

Fig. 18-3. Fundus photograph of posterior pole with Carl Zeiss fundus camera showing fixation target. This auxiliary device is particularly helpful in securing fixation of the one-eyed patient or the individual with poor vision in the other eye. It also serves to document the pattern of monocular fixation.

erally yield both a shorter and a more successful photographic session. Extraneous lights should be eliminated to reduce possible disturbances in the patient's fixation. In keeping with the usual dictum, the *right* eye is photographed first. Therefore the camera base is displaced to the photographer's left and the fixation device is placed 2 or 3 in. in front of the patient's left eye. Final adjustment in position of the eye being photographed is secured by moving the fixation light before the opposite eye.

The one-eyed patient or the patient with loss of central vision in the opposite eye must concentrate on maintaining his fixation in the center of the camera barrel. This difficulty can be reduced by installation of an auxiliary fixation target into any model of the Zeiss camera. This creates a small black shadow on the final picture (Fig. 18-3). Its use, however, is limited to posterior polar photography, where it is particularly valuable in documenting fixation patterns. It is not a helpful stimulus or target for photography of the peripheral retina.

The patient should not be instructed to hold both eyes widely open until the photographer is completely ready to trip the shutter. The overly cooperative patient can develop epithelial drying by volitionally refraining from blinking during the preliminaries to actual film exposure.

Final focusing of camera

The lens cap, which is kept in place as much of the time as possible to minimize dust and finger smudges, is now removed.

The joy stick, located in the center of the instrument table top, is the most important control in positioning of the illuminating light ring. The joy stick should never be completely free nor forced into tight lock. With slight release, the entire system can be moved in any horizontal direction. Final vertical positioning is secured by manually rotating the large horizontal control knob in front of the joy stick. Fine focusing in depth to and from the patient is controlled by the coupled, large knobs on either side of the camera barrel.

For these adjustments the photographer must look around or to one side of the camera using his direct visualization of the patient's eye to control centering of the light ring—or bull's-eye—in the dilated pupil. The light ring is brought into sharp focus on the cornea over the pupil and then the joy stick partially snugged by rotation toward the locking position.

Final verification of uniform illumination and critical focusing is done through the camera eyepiece. If the desired field is not in focus, this is corrected by movement of the fixation device. Edge blurring in any one meridian suggests astigmatic distortion that may require correction by adjustment of the cross cylinder as controlled through the knobs on top of the camera. Crescents of light reflection (limbal catoptric image) at any edge of the field indicate that the illuminating ring is eccentrically displaced over the limbus at that area. Correction is made by tilting the joy stick to the opposite side if the bright crescent is lateral or by moving the camera vertically away from the crescent if it is apparent at the upper or lower edge of the field. If such bright reflection completely encircles the field, the camera is too close to the eye and must be withdrawn slightly. A diffuse gray haze over the entire field occurs when the camera is too far away from the eye. When illumination is proper and even, final snugging of the joy stick is completed. The photographer now makes final adjustment of the camera position to be certain that both the structures of interest and the cross hairs in the eyepiece are in crisp focus.

The patient is now asked to make a final blink to smooth his tear film and then to hold both eyes widely open. The shutter is tripped with the right hand, and then the film is wound or advanced for the next exposure.

Photographing the peripheral fundus

Focusing the extreme periphery often calls for ingenuity. Moderate displacement of the field can be achieved merely by rotating the eye, the camera, or both. A vertical arc adjustment affording 20 degrees of upward or downward camera angulation is available for the table-model Zeiss camera. Often it is necessary to angulate the patient's face for access to the periphery. Aperture No. 7 should still be used for these oblique positions, but often there will be meridional distortion when focusing beyond the equator. Trial and error use of the cross cylinder astigmatic correction system will usually improve focusing in the far periphery (Fig. 18-4).

At times the hand-held camera offers an advantage in photographing the far periph-

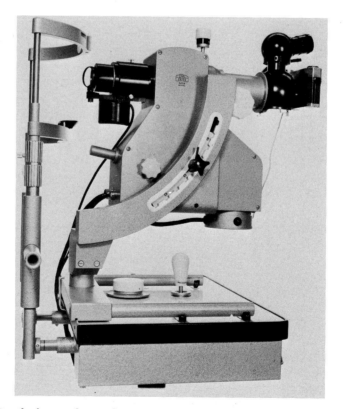

Fig. 18-4. Detail of vertical arc adjustment in left side mounting of new Carl Zeiss fundus camera. This affords 20 degrees of upward or downward angulation, in five-degree stops, from the horizontal position. (Allen Stereo Separator [1964] is shown attached to camera back for optic production of stereo-paired photographs.)

ery in the presence of spinal deformities or under anesthesia in the operating room.

EXTENT OF THE PHOTOGRAPHED FIELD

The Zeiss and most other cameras of this type encompass a field of about 30 degrees. This is displayed as a 22-mm. diameter disc on the film when no auxiliary magnification is used. The photographer should realize, however, that all of the light that will form the real aerial image emerges through a 2-mm. diameter spot in the center of the pupil and within the larger ring of illuminating light. The image as formed on the film is magnified about 2.5× to 10×.

FLUORESCEIN FUNDUS PHOTOGRAPHY (FLUORESCEIN ANGIOGRAPHY)

In 1961 the medical student H. R. Novotny and the budding young intern D. L. Alvis of Indiana University published their original and now classical report on "Photographing Fluorescence in Circulating Blood in the Human Retina" by the use of a sterile sodium fluorescein solution injected into an antecubital vein. Fluorescein is one of many compounds that absorbs light principally of one wavelength and subsequently emits part of this light as fluorescence at a longer wavelength. Novotny and Alvis' spectrofluorometric data on blood-fluorescein mixtures indicated that the wavelength of maximum absorption or activation is in the blue range of the visible spectrum at 490 mμ. The emanation maximum is in the green-yellow range at about 520 to 525 mμ.

Filters and films

For fluorescein fundus photography, two additional filters must be inserted in the camera. A blue gelatin filter (Wratten No. 47) is placed in the light path of the illuminating system to eliminate the longer wavelengths from both the electronic flash and the incandescent viewing lamp and yet to allow the maximum amount of appropriate, exciting light to reach the fundus. This

is called the *exciter filter*. The second filter is a yellowish color* (Wratten No. 15) and is placed directly in the camera back to cut out the reflected blue light and yet transmit the maximum amount of greenish yellow fluorescence to the film. This is called the *barrier filter*.

Of the many types and brands of film, Kodak TRI-X (ASA 400) is readily available, relatively inexpensive, and highly sensitive in the fluorescent wavelength. When properly developed it will yield fine detail. When immediate documentation and analysis are desired Polaroid type 107 can be used.

Timing and recycling

Because timing of the various phases of fundus fluorescence is of differential diagnostic importance, there is increasing need for rapid exposure rates. Cardiovascular physicians also have interest in measures of circulation times from antecubital injection to appearance in the eye. Because of the higher flash intensities needed, standard power packs are relatively slow in recycling and may require as much as 15 to 30 seconds for some instruments. This is far too slow for photographic recording of circulatory events in the fundus as indicated by dye passage.

Many modifications and adaptations of power supply have been evolved to meet the needs for rapid recycling, including motion picture recording. The Robert Bussey unit, essentially custom-made in Miami, Florida, will recycle the standard Carl Zeiss camera to one exposure per second. The Carl Zeiss Fundus Flash II will advance any Zeiss camera to 2 or 3 c.p.s. Dyonics† now produce a CineFlash system in three models for the Zeiss camera. Model 708 will recycle at rates up to 8 c.p.s., Model 730

---

*Formerly a greenish Wratten No. 58 was used as a barrier filter, but it allows more of the blue exciting light to reach the film and gives less contrast than can be achieved with the No. 15.

†Woburn, Massachusetts 01801; successor to ULE, Inc., 1963-1968, and also Iota-Cam Corp.

will recycle at 30 c.p.s., and Model 760 will recycle at 30 to 60 c.p.s.

Cooling of the power supply is a progressively more demanding task as the rate of recycling is advanced. These power units therefore have become table-height, caster-based consoles more suitable to special photographic laboratories than to private offices.

Dyonics also makes an Automatic Syringe Injector Control that both administers the dye and actuates the flash photography at preselected rates. A Data Box Clock Module is available from Dyonics to print the time on each film frame optically.

Many thousands of dollars can be invested in these elaborate refinements of fluorescein fundus studies, and high precision records may thereby be produced. The attentive clinician, however, can gain much fundamental information, particularly about the presence and localization of vascular leaks, the identification of hemangiomata, differentiation of "pseudo-optic neuritis" from true papilledema or malignant tumors from hematomata, and other similarly important distinctions merely by ophthalmoscopic observation of the fundus events as the dye passes through its various phases of circulation. It is, of course, necessary for the ophthalmoscope to be fitted with the appropriate exciter filter.

The dye

Though other contrast dyes have been used experimentally, sodium fluorescein has now been administered to thousands of patients in many areas of the world and is well understood as to both its optic properties and its very low incidence of toxic reactions.

A few variations in amounts and concentrations of dye have been employed. In Wills Eye Hospital and Research Institute thousands of studies have been done using a 5-ml. injection of 10% sodium fluorescein solution in an aqueous buffer.* This is a

minimum volume injection affording distinct arterial identification. Many others use a 5- or 10-ml. injection of 5% sodium fluorescein.* A following injection of sterile saline may or may not be given.

Transient nausea occurring 15 to 20 seconds after injection is reported in about 5% of patients. This seems particularly associated with rapid injection. Vomiting or sweating occurs in less than 0.5% of patients; hives and syncope each may occur in something less than 0.2% of patients. At least one case of localized thrombophlebitis has been noted, and one patient has had a repeat coronary occlusion during such study.

Patients should be advised of yellowish discoloration that will be noted in the urine for about 48 hours following injection. Inquiry should be made concerning dye, drug, or chemical sensitivity and also any history of marked allergy or anaphylaxis that might predispose to fluorescein reaction.

An emergency tray containing sterile syringes, epinephrine (Adrenalin), an antihistamine such as diphenhydramine hydrochloride (Benadryl), morphine sulfate, or similar preparations should always be available in the camera room.

Extravasation of the dye about the injection site will cause some pain and local reaction, but this subsides within a few days.

Phases of dye manifestation in the fundus

Appearance of the fluorescein dye either under direct visualization or by serial photographic record can reveal details of ocular pathology completely undetectable by other clinical means. Fluorescence may be *intravascular* (choroidal, arterial, venous), *transmitted* (through defects in normally opaque overlying structures, as is the case in early arterial fluorescence through angioid streaks), *staining or leakage* (as

---

*Smith, Miller and Patch, Inc., New Brunswick, New Jersey 08902.

*Fluorescite ampules, Moore/Kirk Laboratories, Inc., Hillside, New Jersey 07205.

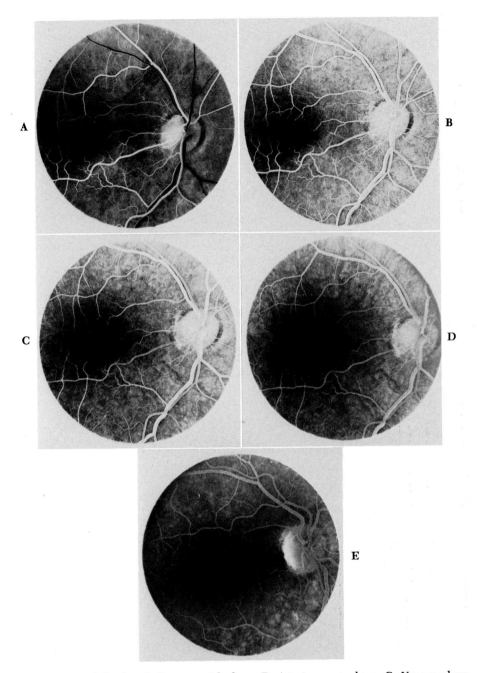

Fig. 18-5. Normal fundus. **A,** Late arterial phase. **B,** Arteriovenous phase. **C,** Venous phase. **D,** Late venous phase. **E,** Recirculation phase.

through localized vascular defects in central serous retinopathy or widespread vascular defects in diabetic retinopathy), or *pseudofluorescence* (artifactually apparent over nonpigmented areas of the fundus late or several hours after injection).

The time phases are, first, the very early or *choroidal* phase, which appears 8 to 10 seconds after injection as a diffuse mottling throughout the posterior pole, except for the macular area. Cilioretinal arteries, if present, are usually seen in this phase or in the early arterial phase, which follows. In the *early arterial phase* the retinal arteries are beginning to be outlined. Drusen, if present, light up in this phase and persist as bright dots of fluorscence as long as there is much circulating dye.

The arterial or *late arterial phase* (Fig. 18-5, *A*) shows all of the retinal arteries in bold contrast. This filling is usually completed in 1 or 2 seconds but may be delayed 5 to 20 seconds in central retinal artery occlusion. The *arteriovenous phase* (Fig. 18-5, *B*) shows filling of all the retinal veins, but the arteries are still visible though with reducing brightness. In the early part of this phase the veins may manifest lamellar variations in brightness, whereas later in the phase such findings occur in the arteries.

The next or *venous phase* (Fig. 18-5, *C*) is marked by fading of the arterial fluorescence. Diabetic neovascularization and disciform macular lesions of low-grade chorioretinal inflammatory origin begin to be apparent at this time. The *late venous phase* (Fig. 18-5, *D*) shows less arterial pattern and intense staining about disciform or apparently inflammatory macular lesions, which may persist for 15 to 30 minutes after injection.

The *recirculation phase* (Fig. 18-5, *E*) persists 10 to 12 minutes after the venous phase and presents even distribution of dye in all vascular components. The background or choroidal fluorescence also continues up to a total of about 25 or 30 minutes after injection.

Pseudofluorescence is a variously interpreted expression that should be reserved for luminescence after filling, which may persist for many hours against a nonpigmented or reflective background, such as an atrophic nerve head or a coloboma of the choroid and retina. This is caused by blue light excitation of fluorescein particles normally remaining in the vitreous and aqueous for a day or so after injection. Very little incident light returns through these particles except over white or high reflection areas.

Fundus photography is an excellent method of keeping accurate documentation of disease and objective evidence of response or progression. The addition of vital contrast studies with intravenous fluorescein gives new dimensions to identification of pathologic processes and places us a step closer to fundamental understanding of disease mechanisms. Without question, the use of intravenous fluorescein techniques has saved many eyes that might have been enucleated for choroidal hemorrhages or hemangiomata of the choroid. Similarly it has identified localized vascular leaks now suitable for photocoagulation therapy and has saved many such eyes from major visual loss.

Chapter 19

Diagnostic steps in dyslexia and reading retardation

"Reading retardation" and the unmodified term "dyslexia" are generic designations covering a host of etiologic mechanisms, both endogenous and exogenous, that play adverse roles in accomplishment of the reading task. Inability to read may further be a developmental defect associated with subtle disturbances in neurologic growth, or it may be an acquired defect from a clearly recognizable lesion of the parietotemporal lobe. In the latter case, the loss of a previously existing function should be termed "alexia."

Because the eye is the major sensory input route for the cortical process of symbol interpretation and association, it is understandable that parents and patients alike request ocular examination when faced with these problems, even though the eye itself rarely is the primarily offending organ. In order to organize proper diagnostic steps, the following classification (Keeney, 1968) will remind the examiner of the many mechanisms that can be involved.

All classifications in biology and medicine are provisional in character, by nature of the evolving science. Until every etiologic mechanism is identified and isolated, it will be helpful to continue some functional nosology.

Comprehensive classification of the dyslexias

A. Specific (primary) developmental dyslexia (strephosymbolia or dyssymbolia): inability or difficulty in the cortical process of symbol inter- pretation appearing in individuals of average to high performance I.Q. and with functionally adequate sensory input mechanisms; appears predominantly in males and has a dominant genetic inheritance

B. Symptomatic (secondary) dyslexia (secondary reading retardation)
   1. Secondary to organic brain pathology (brain damage, cerebral dysfunction, other encephalopathy, cerebral palsy, mental retardation, low I.Q., visual agnosia, anomia, soft neurologic stigmata)
      a. Genetically determined
      b. Posttraumatic (prenatal, natal, postnatal)
      c. Postinflammatory (intrauterine or extrauterine encephalitis, meningitis)
      d. Asphyxic (intrauterine, extrauterine)
      e. Prematurity
      f. Other specific brain lesion (aneurysm, meningioma, porencephalic cyst, others)
   2. Secondary to slow maturation (late bloomer, developmental delay)
   3. Secondary to emotional disturbances (hyperactivity, depression, anxiety)
   4. Secondary to uncontrolled seizure states
   5. Secondary to environmental disturbances (cultural deprivation, poor motivation, poor instruction)

C. Slow reading (handicap without symbolic confusion)
   1. Ocular impediment to sustained visual use (hyperopia, heterophoria, astigmatism, partial cataracts, retinal and macular abiotrophies)
   2. Auditory impairment
   3. Hypothyroid state

D. Alexia or acquired dyslexia: lesions usually in the region of the angular gyrus of the dominant hemisphere

E. Mixed types

DIAGNOSTIC STEPS
History

At least one additional question must always be asked in examination of the seemingly healthy child: "How is he doing in school?" Parents are occasionally reluctant to indicate that they are seeking consultation because of an inability to read, and they nearly always minimize or deny any reading difficulty in the father or older generations, though they will acknowledge it in the patient's siblings. Scholastic achievement in arithmetic as well as in reading and spelling should be delineated, because the dyslexic child will usually have more difficulty with reading than with arithmetic and most trouble of all with dictated spelling. It is a rare dyslexic patient, however, who has no trouble at all with arithmetic, and his difficulty is enhanced in higher grades of school when mathematic problems are posed in words.

Though predictor factors are being sought at the age of 5 (de Hirsch, 1966), dyslexia, of course, cannot be diagnosed until the patient is at an adequate age and culture for reading.

Ocular examination

The usual steps of preliminary inspection, preliminary examination, determination of acuity, refraction, and ocular motility, as well as fundus examination, must be done as in any case. In measuring acuity, the perceptive examiner can usually tell if the child is unable to identify letters or is unable to see them. This should be recorded. Usually reading is not possible without an underlying ability to handle the individual building blocks of words.

Optic defects (hyperopia, astigmatism, impairments of the media, and so on) have been shown to have no relation to symbol interpretation (Helveston, 1970), but they must be identified. If of significant magnitude, they may lead to ocular fatigue or asthenopia, which reduces the effective learning and attention span. Under these conditions they merit conventional therapy. Similarly, moderate degrees of heterophoria that may occasionally break into heterotropia can have a limiting effect on educational application and should be corrected where they are significant in their own right, particularly where difficulties in the reading-learning process coexist.

Although it is true that man reads with his brain and not with his eyes, patients presenting for evaluation of the visual system in relation to dyslexia or reading problems will be found to have a high incidence of modest or usually insignificant ocular irregularities. These include myopia, heterophoria, astigmatism, amblyopia, strabismus, nystagmus, poor lateralization, and others; but they appear to represent "soft neurologic signs" of associated disturbances rather than causative factors.

Graded reading

Graded reading paragraphs of some type (Durrell, 1960) should be included in the examination in order to (1) note directly the level and facility with which the patient attacks and accomplishes reading, (2) obtain a numerical reference point familiar to educators and psychologists, and (3) afford an index for comparison on subsequent examinations.

Paper and pencil tests

Constructional apraxia. Constructional apraxia, the inability to arrange geometric components, is a specific manifestation of parietotemporal lobe impairment, usually in the dominant hemisphere. Its presence is a rather objective measure of neurologic deficit with which symbol confusion can be expected. The patient is asked to draw a few simple figures on a fresh office form or unlined piece of paper. These may be limited to a bicycle, a person, or the face of a clock. Hesitancy in starting to draw these familiar objects, inability to relate two wheels into a bicycle, and poor distribution of numbers, especially crowding to one side or quadrant on the face of the clock, are positive findings. These may be augmented by asking the patient to write his own name at the top of the paper. The

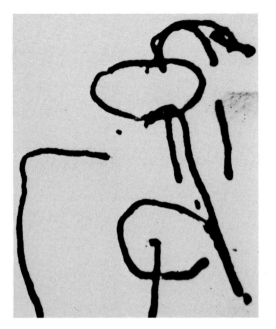

Fig. 19-1. Example of patient with acquired dyslexia, normal acuity, and right homonymous hemianopia attempting to draw a man. Disorganization of geometric units indicates constructional apraxia.

examiner must have some knowledge of the expected drawing skill of children, which may vary widely within normal limits at each age level.

Specific dyslexia, like poliomyelitis, appears in all degrees of severity. Significant amounts of this impairment are almost always associated with some constructional apraxia, and only the very mildest case may escape without it (Fig. 19-1).

Lateralization. Poor lateralization or right-left confusion is generally concomitant with constructional apraxia. Information about impairment of lateralization as well as constructional apraxia is obtained by asking the patient to draw a few simple arrows. The dyslexic patient will often be unable to arrange the barbs at the end of the shaft and to orient the arrow to right or left on request.

Dominance

Dominance is of interest in dyslexia primarily because there has been confusion about its interpretation and its importance.

In neurologic immaturity, ambidexterity, mixed dominance, or delayed right-left orientation are often apparent. Statistically, there is a slightly higher percentage of right-left orientation difficulty in the dyslexic population than in the comparable school-age population. This is now accepted to be accompanying rather than causative.

Hand and foot preference should be tested and noted, as should eye preference. Ocular lateralization, ocular preference, or so-called ocular dominance, however, should not be compared specifically with dominance or preference in the extremities. Because each eye is bilaterally represented in the cortex, rather than unilaterally as is true for the extremities, ocular "dominance" is primarily a peripheral quality (the better eye, the master eye, the sighting eye) easily subject to transient or prolonged alteration. Extremity dominance, conversely, has a central or hemispheric basis. Although current studies (Benton, 1970; Helveston, 1970; Rubin, 1970) fail to identify or implicate ocular dominance or preference with impairments of the reading-learning act, some test should be made for completeness in studying the patient.

There are more than two dozen tests relating to ocular dominance described in the literature. A simple sighting test—such as handing the youngster a paper with a tiny hole in it and asking him to look through it at a designated distant object, first with the paper at arm's distance and then instructing him to bring the paper close to his face as he continues to sight through the hole—is often sufficient. The child will ordinarily align the hole over the preferred eye. Other suggestions of eye dominance already ascertained are: (1) the eye with better vision is generally preferred, and (2) the eye that first breaks from near point of convergence testing is usually the nonpreferred eye.

Indications for related examinations

Most children presenting for ocular examination in relation to dyslexia have already had thorough and competent pediatric or general medical examinations. If such has been omitted, it should be done both as an appropriate periodic examination and to search for any subtle disturbances of consciousness (petit mal seizures, temper tantrums, grand mal), metabolic function (diabetes, hypothyroidism), neurologic impairment (porencephalic cysts, slight hemiparesis originating in the dominant hemisphere), or hearing aberrations (nerve deafness, chronic middle ear infections). Where uncertain or borderline diagnoses occur, there should be detailed consultation with the neurologist, otologist, or other indicated specialist.

The visual examiner and those in related medical fields are obligated to obtain for the educator the healthiest possible student with best visual function to facilitate his learning experience. Many a child with extremely limited vision, however, has progressed through school on schedule and with high academic attainments. It is important to show true interest, encouragement, and reward to the dyslexic child who faces a world of unintelligible symbols and written directions.

Though emotional or psychiatric factors rarely cause specific dyslexia, many children with this problem certainly become candidates for emotional disturbance, distractive behavior, and even delinquency. Psychiatric approaches are generally neither to diagnose nor to cure the dyslexia, but in the long-neglected, irrationally treated, or late case, psychiatric treatment may be truly needed.

Chapter 20

Ultrasonography

Ultrasonography is an exploration with narrow beams of acoustic energy at frequencies far above the limits of hearing for the purpose of identifying alterations in acoustic echoes that localize and quantitate tissues of varying density within the orbit. Ultrasonic waves, both as emanating from an original source and as returning echoes, travel at measurably different speeds through the various ocular tissues. Thus differences in ultrasonic velocity and energy ("time-amplitude" function) can be recorded and displayed on suitable oscilloscopic tubes as the waves strike interfaces of different acoustic density (refraction of ultrasonic waves at sites of acoustic mismatch) or as they pass through structures of varied tissue characteristics that affect acoustic impedance and thereby the velocity of such energy passing through them. The speed of sound through the lens is distinctly greater than through the vitreous, though all such figures are altered by temperature. Ultrasound passing through dense and irregular tissues such as neoplasms or organized blood clots yields sustained irregular echoes of generally high amplitude, whereas ultrasound passing through homogeneously filled, cyst-like lesions (such as mucoceles or serous retinal detachments) yields distinct high-amplitude echoes at the faces or surfaces of such lesions and relatively little disturbance within the fluid mass.

INDICATIONS

Ultrasound may be considered a diagnostic modality for soft tissue study, somewhat comparable to x-ray for bony tissue. Principal indications for diagnostic use are (1) evaluation of intraocular tissues obscured from visualization by opaque media such as corneal, lens, and vitreous opacities, (2) identification of solid or nonhomogeneous tissues from cystic or homogeneous masses, (3) determination of size, length, or thickness in ocular components, (4) investigation of retrobulbar soft tissue masses as in the presence of unilateral exophthalmos, and (5) identification, localization, and measurement of nonradiopaque foreign bodies.

EQUIPMENT
Components

Equipment for ultrasonic examination consists of three components: (1) a piezoelectric generating system supplying electric current to a transducer crystal such as barium titanate, which responds with high-frequency mechanical oscillations producing the ultrasound beam, (2) a piezoelectric receiving crystal onto which the returning ultrasonic echoes impinge and in turn generate electric potentials, and (3) an amplifier to convert these minute electric impulses into adequate magnitude for visible display on an oscilloscope. Significant echo displays may then be recorded by a Polaroid camera. Usually the same transducer crystal serves as generator and receiver because the ultrasonic energy is pulsed in brief bursts lasting about .000001 second, occurring about one thousand times a second. Thus the transducer crystal serves as a passive receiver for nearly a thousand

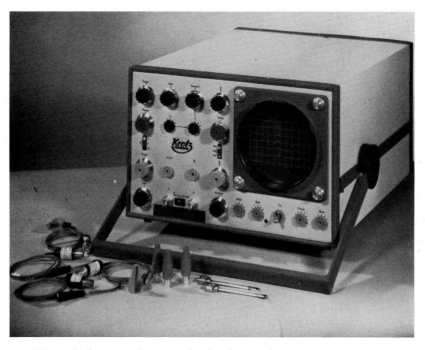

Fig. 20-1. Kretztechnik A-scan (time-amplitude ultrasound) equipment for ocular diagnosis. Variously shaped transducer tips are pictured in foreground before instrument. Oscilloscope screen in upper right hand corner contains linear measuring graticule.

times longer period each second than the time during which it is actively generating ultrasound.

Linear or A-scan (time-amplitude) ultrasound versus two-dimensional or B-scan (intensity-modulated) ultrasound

Without question the most practical, accurate, flexible, and economic ultrasound equipment is the unidirectional probe of A-scan. Like a flashlight in a large barn at night it is essentially a single beam and must be understandingly directed in a systematic exploration of the globe or retrobulbar orbit. It is certainly possible to miss significant masses, such as a small malignant melanoma under a large retinal detachment, unless the probe or scanning is done knowledgeably and methodically. On the other hand, false positive echoes essentially cannot occur with good equipment that has been checked and standardized, particularly when the operator is clearly aware of intensity levels and the gain or amplification characteristics of his equipment.

Two-dimensional or B-scan equipment is large, costly, and relatively inflexible; requires water-filled goggles or other unpleasant liquid coupling; and is available in only a few major laboratories. Though the photographic record of such an intensity-modulated display presents familiar similarity to an x-ray laminogram or planogram of the orbit, artifacts are often numerous. Components to assemble such equipment are available commercially.

Available linear or A-scan equipment

Several manufacturers produce ultrasonographic equipment specifically for ocular use. Component parts such as transducers,* generators,† amplifiers, and oscilloscopes can be purchased and assembled by acoustical or electronic engineers in most

---

*Valpey Corp., Holliston, Massachusetts 01746.
†Hewlett-Packard Corp., Palo Alto, California 94304.

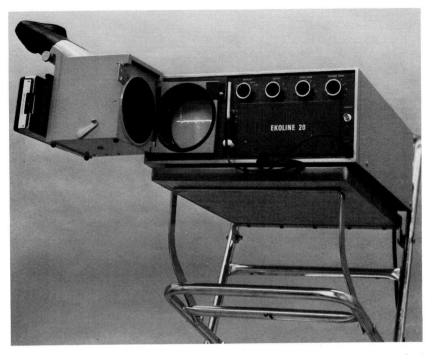

Fig. 20-2. Smith-Kline Ekoline 20 time-amplitude (A-scan) ultrasonic apparatus with 5-mm. diameter transducer in holder to right of oscilloscope. Polaroid camera is shown opened and turned away from oscilloscope.

medical centers. Kretztechnik of Zipf, Austria, produces two basic, high-resolution units for ocular and orbital use: the Kretz 7100 MA (Fig. 20-1) is widely useful and of high quality; the Kretz 7200 MA is more complex and affords coupling for semi-automatic linear and arc scanning with a simplified B display. Siemens Aktiengesellschaft of Erlangen, Germany, and Automation Industries, Inc., of Boulder, Colorado, also manufacture substantial equipment. Smith-Kline Instrument Company of Palo Alto, California, has had several years of experience with two models (Fig. 20-2) of A-scan ultrasonoscopes particularly applied to ophthalmic use. Their Ekoline 20, or larger instrument, is still compact enough to roll from examining room to operating room on a light aluminum carriage. A remote, 1-in. cathode ray tube is available with this instrument for a surgeon to watch immediately adjacent to the orbit during removal of foreign bodies. The smaller Ekoline 12 comes in a hand case

(30½ × 6 × 11 in.) and has a small oscilloscope display. Though portable, this instrument must also be treated with gentle caution and standardized frequently or daily against a Bronson glass plate.

In 1970 Kretztechnik introduced a very compact and light-weight portable Model 1001 MAB; this is battery operated and utilizes a small oscilloscope face. This portable A-scan instrument reduces a minimal investment in such equipment by about 50% and provides high-resolution linear echograms. It is about half the size of Ekoline 12, which is the smallest instrument in that line. It is not provided with energy attenuation scales, but it certainly makes basic instrumentation more available than ever before.

Many manufacturers produce specific equipment for continuous-wave Doppler effect examinations,* but all of these call

*Magnaflux Corp., MD Ultrasonic Doppler; Ames Co., Ultradop; Smith-Kline Instrument Co., Doptone.

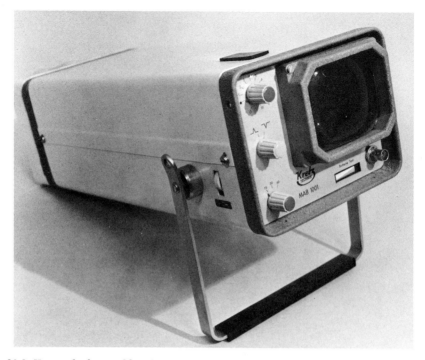

Fig. 20-3. Kretztechnik Portable Ultrasonoscope, Model MAB 1001. Scale display of 0 to 15, 0 to 30, or 0 to 60 mm. may be obtained by switch control.

for considerable care in quantitation of energy delivered.

PHYSICAL CHARACTERISTICS

Ultrasound is not heard, seen, or smelled. In the low energies used for ocular diagnosis it cannot be felt as heat or force and gives rise to no known tissue alterations. Thus its patient acceptability is high, and no special preparation or adaptation is required to begin the examination.

Pulsed versus continuous ultrasound. The use of repetitive short bursts of ultrasound allows the same transducer to also act as the echo receiver and reduces the potential for building up damaging levels of energy. Continuous ultrasound is used in Doppler effect studies (increasing frequency of sound waves as a moving source approaches the receiver, or decreasing frequency as the source recedes from the receiver) to qualitate blood surge in vessels such as the carotid and ophthalmic arteries. Uncertain, high, and potentially damaging

energy levels can be created at various tissue depths with continuous ultrasound. These problems may be intensified by large area or focusing transducer faces.

Frequencies. Five to twenty megacycles per second (megahertz) are commonly needed to obtain soft tissue penetration through the eye and into the orbit. Depth of penetration and identification of small differences in tissue density are facilitated by higher frequencies. To achieve penetration of high frequencies, however, energy levels must be increased.

Energy levels. Energy levels for diagnosis are generally in the range of microwatts per square centimeter per minute. Energies in the range of tenths of a watt per square centimeter per minute are potentially damaging. Higher energy levels have been selectively studied for therapeutic and destructive effects, including the production of corneal edema, cataracts, vitreous liquefaction, chorioretinal scars, and tissue necrosis.

Transducer (crystal) diameter. In ocular and orbital diagnosis narrow beams are more critically localizing, and therefore crystals about 5 mm. in diameter are commonly employed. This affords a light, easily held, and nonfrightening probe similar in size to a cigarette. Alignment of the probe for reception of the reflected and refracted echoes becomes more critical, however, as transducer diameter is reduced. A striking example is that of a spherical steel BB or lead shotgun pellet; this is easily seen on the poorest quality x-ray film, is of markedly different acoustic density in comparison to orbital soft tissues, and affords a gross "acoustic mismatch" at its surface. With a small-diameter transducer, however, the returning echo may easily be reflected beyond or wide of the crystal face if the sonic wave is not coincident or nearly coincident with a radius of the sphere (Fig. 20-12).

Coupling. Air is a highly effective insulator to ultrasound, and therefore fluid coupling between the transducer face and bulbar or lid tissue is essential for transmission of the ultrasound. Two to six percent methylcellulose is commonly used as a coupling medium. When the transducer probe is applied to the cornea, a topical anesthetic is instilled first.

FINDINGS

It must be remembered that sonic beams, like light beams, may be absorbed, transmitted, regularly reflected, irregularly reflected, refracted, or scattered by various interfaces and media in their pathway.

Normal results

The normal A-scan ultrasonogram is represented schematically by Fig. 20-4. The base line on the oscilloscope display has linear graduations to aid in measurement. When a sonic beam is undisturbed by variations in acoustic impedance, the display shows no deflection from the base line. When a transducer is fluid-coupled to an eye on its visual axis the first deflection is that of the anterior corneal surface. With equipment that greatly magnifies the length

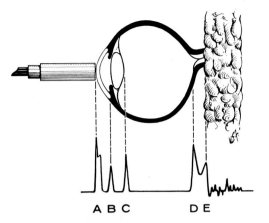

Fig. 20-4. Schematic representation of A-scan ultrasonogram made with transducer tip at left in direct fluid coupling to cornea. Opening deflection (opening bang) is shown at corneal surface, *A*. Reflection from anterior lens capsule is shown at *B* and posterior lens capsule is shown at *C*. The clear lens presents no echoes within its depths. Similarly, the clear vitreous presents no echoes. The posterior bulbar wall complex is represented by *D* and *E*. The retrobulbar fat at far right shows decreasing irregular spikes.

of the globe, it is possible to detect the posterior corneal surface and also stromal opacities. Normally the aqueous and vitreous are both acoustically homogeneous and therefore give rise to no echoes on the display. The lens, however, shows distinct echo deflections at its anterior and posterior surface; these should be of essentially equal amplitude if the beam is passing axially through the lens center. A large deflection is also created at the posterior bulbar wall or the vitreoretinal interface. Beyond the globe, irregularly decreasing echoes indicate the normal orbital fat pattern.

Lens echoes and refractive influence of the lens on the sonic beam can be avoided in aphakia or by placing the transducer beyond the lens equator (Fig. 20-5, lower tracing).

Altered results

Blood or inflammatory debris in the aqueous or vitreous give irregular, low-amplitude echoes (Fig. 20-6) that disappear at low intensities. Neoplasms, heavy exudates,

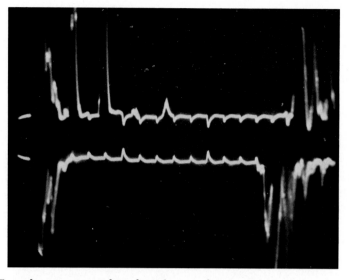

Fig. 20-5. Two ultrasonograms taken through a single eye. Upper tracing (positive deflection) is through the clear lens. Lower tracing (negative deflection) is taken obliquely across the eye. Example shows high myopia. Note 2-mm. scale marking along base line.

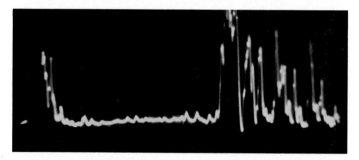

Fig. 20-6. Ultrasonogram showing low-amplitude disturbances in vitreous from scattered hemorrhage. Tracing is made peripheral to lens. Note normal retrobulbar fat pattern.

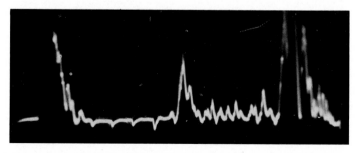

Fig. 20-7. Ultrasonogram showing solid tumor extending to midvitreous with sharply localized presenting face and irregular echoes throughout tumor mass to posterior bulbar wall. Echoes do not disappear when intensity is reduced. Histology later confirmed malignant melanoma.

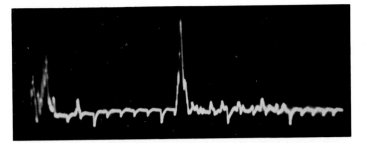

Fig. 20-8. Ultrasonogram of retrobulbar tumor showing dampening or reduction in the usual pattern of echoes from the retrobulbar fat caused by a homogeneous tumor mass.

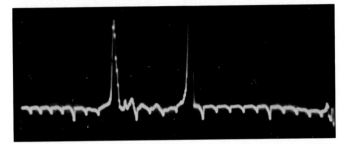

Fig. 20-9. Retrobulbar pattern of homogeneous or tumor-cyst type showing mass behind the posterior bulbar wall, obliteration of retrobulbar fat echoes, and sharp posterior limit to the lesion.

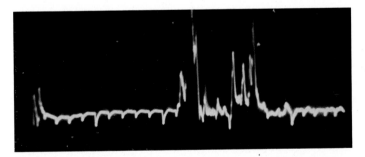

Fig. 20-10. Ultrasonogram showing solid retrobulbar tumor pattern with sharply localized posterior limit to the tumor mass.

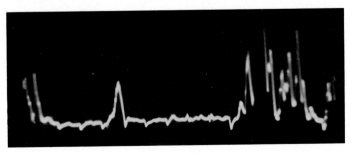

Fig. 20-11. Ultrasonogram showing intraocular foreign body slightly anterior to midvitreous. Sharp, localized echo spike is similar to that from surface of retina in serous detachment.

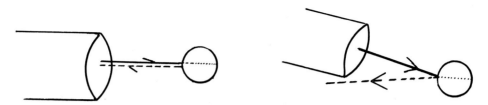

Fig. 20-12. Schematic illustration of difficulty in obtaining A-mode ultrasonic echo from a smooth spherical object such as a BB. Illustration at left shows the necessary near coincidence of sonic beam with the diameter of the BB in order for reflected echo to impinge on the 5-mm. transducer face. Illustration at right shows sonic beam striking surface obliquely so that echo returns beyond the diameter of transducer face.

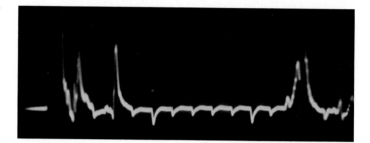

Fig. 20-13. A-mode ultrasonogram through the lens showing increased lens thickness (intumescence).

or old blood clots (Fig. 20-7) give sustained irregular echoes throughout, which persist even at low-intensity examination. Serous detachments of the retina show a sharp isolated spike resembling that of a foreign body; this can be verified from different axes corresponding to the extent and height of elevation.

Abnormal retrobulbar echoes are generally classifiable into (1) foreign body spikes of high amplitude, (2) dampening or reduction in the normal orbital fat pattern resulting from tumor displacement (Fig. 20-8), (3) homogeneous or tumor-cyst patterns with very little echo disturbance between distinct interface spikes (Fig. 20-9), and (4) nonhomogeneous tumor-cyst patterns with irregular echoes persisting at low intensities and sometimes delineated by a distinct posterior interface spike (Fig. 20-10). The deeper a lesion is in the orbit, the higher the frequency and energy requirements to detect it. Thus masses close to the apex may elude identification or be concealed by reverberation artifacts from the converging bony walls.

Foreign bodies generally afford distinct acoustic mismatch (Fig. 20-11) with identifying high-amplitude echoes. Though both radiopaque and radiolucent foreign bodies yield strong identifying and localizing echograms, the ultrasonic technique is especially indicated and uniquely valuable in the case of wood, glass, plastic, and similar materials that are difficult or often impossible to identify, even with the best of soft tissue x-ray techniques. Uniformly spherical foreign bodies such as BB's may be difficult to detect with A-scan ultrasound though quite conspicuous to x-ray (Fig. 20-12).

Oculometric results

Oculometry, and particularly axial length measurement, is helpful in diagnosing early phthisis (as in hypotony) or early buphthalmos (as in congenital glaucoma), though care must be taken not to press heavily or distort the globe with the probe. Measurement of presumably shrunken lenses and differentiation of normal lens thickness from intumescent lenses can be done with most A-scan equipment (Fig. 20-13). It is also possible to measure normally sized components of the eye that may be present in spite of other congenital anomalies such as microcornea, megalocornea, or posterior microglobus. Staphylomatous distensions of the globe can be localized and measured. In spite of current improvements in resolution capabilities of many instruments, it is still generally inaccurate or misleading to interpret echograms as valid in measurements of less than 0.1 mm. Thus the automatic read-out of spectacle prescriptions by ultrasonography requires further refinement in equipment and more accurate knowledge of the speed of sound through individual lenses and individual vitreous bodies.

CURRENT USE STATUS

Ultrasound is now a validated and valuable diagnostic adjunct, but it presents the limitation of requiring use by the physician or responsible examiner. It cannot be delegated to a technologist unfamiliar with the disease processes that may be affecting the globe or orbit. Wherever several eye physicians practice together, or in any hospital serving a small group of ophthalmologists, there certainly should be facilities for ultrasonic examination. It is essential that at least one physician in the group know the characteristics of the instrument and the technique of standardization, and he should be able to conduct valid and reproducible studies. B-scan equipment at present is suitable only for laboratory study and special investigations.

Chapter 21

Introduction to electrophysiologic diagnostic procedures

Several related but somewhat exotic test procedures have reached practicality through development of circuitry and amplification methods to capture or to record electric potentials associated with both sensory and motor ocular function. Much of this has been facilitated by the widespread use of electroencephalography and the polygraphs that record from such brain potentials. Indeed, the electroencephalogram (EEG) itself, when recording potentials from scalp leads over the occipital lobes and augmented by photic driving and visually evoked responses (VER), is a sensitive diagnostic aid to assess integrity of the visual pathways and the "perceptual" responses of the visual cortex.

Chapters 22 through 25 each deal with a specialized field of diagnostic study concerning the visual apparatus. Electroencephalography will be considered later in this chapter. The fields of electroencephalography, electroretinography, electrooculography, and electronystagmography all use similar polygraphs and ink-writing recorders with complete electric shielding and grounding of the room and equipment. These studies can be done in conjunction with existing electroencephalographic laboratories in most hospitals and medical centers.

The subject of electromyography (Breinin; Jampolsky; Miller; Bjork; Mertens) is less consonant because it requires different amplification and display equipment, involves

the somewhat unpleasant problem of inserting needle electrodes into extraocular muscles under no more than topical anesthesia, and is primarily a laboratory and investigative, rather than clinical, tool.

The major electrophysiologic diagnostic procedures for the visual apparatus are:

1. Electroencephalography (EEG): the recording of minute electric responses (30 to 100 μv) of the occipital cortex by means of small sets of electrodes inserted into the scalp
2. Electroretinography (ERG): the recording of light-evoked electric currents originating primarily from the rods, cones, and bipolar cells of the retina (pp. 245-255)
3. Electrooculography (EOG): the recording of changes in resting currents (standing corneoretinal potentials, CRP) that apparently arise in the pigment epithelium of the retina, initiated by excursions of the eye rather than by light (Testing is done in both the light-adapted and the dark-adapted states from skin electrodes affixed to the outer canthi [binocular] or to the inner and outer canthi [monocular].)
4. Electronystagmography (ENG): the recording of fluctuations in resting currents (CRP) occasioned by ocular excursions that may be spontaneous, induced, or modified by opticokinetic or labyrinthian stimuli (pp. 259-263)
5. Electromyography (EMG): the re-

cording of changes in electric potentials of ocular muscles at apparent rest under attempted movement or by stimulation of nerve supply. (Recording is done with needle electrodes inserted into the extraocular muscles; see pp. 264-265.)

ELECTROENCEPHALOGRAPHY

Electroencephalography, which dates from the discoveries of Berger in 1929, affords considerable data on the activity of the visual centers, particularly those occupying the large areas in the occipital poles. The normal alpha rhythm of cortical

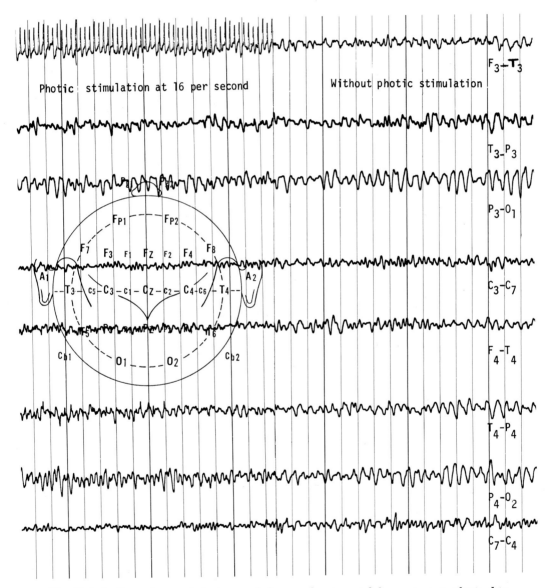

Fig. 21-1. Sections of normal electroencephalogram showing, at left, response to photic driving at 16 c.p.s. and, at right, response without photic stimulation. Responses appear predominantly in leads over occipital lobes. Designations at right indicate leads according to superimposed lead diagram at left.

discharges is 8 to 13 c.p.s. Their potential is about 30 to 50 μv* but tends to be less over the primary visual registration area (Brodmann's area 17) of the striate cortex and maximal over the visual association areas 18 and 19. This regular alpha rhythm is easily altered by visual attention or photic stimulation. With an intact visual pathway, the alpha rhythm of the striate cortex can be driven effectively with flashes of light at an intensity of about 80 foot candles; monochromatic light, particularly toward the blue end of the spectrum, appears more effective than white or red light. A maximum acceleration to about 30 to 35 c.p.s. can be achieved in leads from the striate cortex, but rates almost twice this high can be attained in leads from the optic nerve, geniculate body, and optic radiations. This is sometimes referred to as "flicker following."

Several other waves of visually evoked responses (VER) can be obtained singularly from the occipital cortex (Halliday, 1967; Dustman and Beck, 1967) at magnitudes of about 1 μv. Components of this VER wave, known as c^1 and c^2, seem related to photopic and scotopic mechanisms respectively and also to the state of attention. In the nonattentive state, the c^1 component seems to disappear. Latency periods

of six components of the VER vary between 30 and 200 msec. (Broughton and others, 1965).

In children with amblyopia, alterations in occipital alpha rhythm are found, and reduced effects of flicker driving may be seen. Where facilities exist for computer averaging* of the VER by an electronic toposcope, the c^1 wave generated from an amblyopic eye seems to be reduced, or the c^2 wave from the nonamblyopic eye is reduced in comparison to that of the amblyopic eye.

Thus electroencephalography with the conventional equipment found in most hospitals, medical centers, or neurologic services affords an objective, though crude, index of functioning in the visual cortex and gross measure of the integrity of the visual pathways from the retina to the occipital lobes (Fig. 21-1). A semiquantitative aspect is also available in demonstration of photic driving or flicker following. These tests give otherwise unobtainable evidence of intact visual pathways in infants, nonresponders, and unconscious patients. The vastly more complex equipment and procedures needed to study VER's (measured in microvolts rather than millivolts) hold great promise at the moment for objective study of visual fields, form recognition, and even quantitation of visual acuity.

---

*This represents attenuation of as much as 5,000 to 1 between cortex and scalp.

*Mnemotron-Cat-400.

Chapter 22

Electroretinography*

Arnold B. Popkin, M.D.

Electroretinography is the recording through electronic amplification of minute electric potentials in the range of 0.1 to 1 mv. generated by the retina in response to changes in light intensity. Stimuli may range from threshold values through increments of approximately 4 logarithmic units. Both light-adapted or photopic patterns of relatively low voltage and dark-adapted or scotopic patterns of higher voltage may be obtained. In addition an objective measurement of the Purkinje shift in maximal color or wavelength sensitivity can be recorded as the retina changes from the dark- to light-adapted state. This accounts for the change in spectral location of the sensation of maximum brightness in scotopic versus photopic vision.

Electroretinography, though subject to modern scientific study since the first of this century, has attained meaningful analysis only in the last few decades (Hartline, 1925; R. Grant, 1933; Riggs, 1941; Karpe, 1945; Henkes, 1949; A. Franceschetti, 1951; François, 1952) and has become a common, useful clinical technique only in the last few years (Jacobson, 1951; Schmoger, 1955; Sundmark, 1958; Rudemann, 1959). The United States had only a few electoretinographic laboratories in the 1950's but now almost every major eye department has such facilities. Current visual literature routinely refers to the electroretinogram (ERG) both as a diagnostic modality and more simply in terms of electroretinographic data in relation to case studies or other reports.

ELECTRORETINOGRAPHIC EQUIPMENT

Three components of equipment are required to record an ERG: (1) stimulus light, (2) active and neutral electrodes, and (3) amplifying and recording system. All three components are commercially available. Considerable variability in stimulus light is necessary for the ERG. Jacobson has stressed the wide availability and utility of standard electroencephalographic amplifiers, recorders, and shielded rooms in most general hospitals for adaptation to electroretinographic purposes.

Stimulators. The most usual stimulus is a gas discharge tube (electronic flash or stroboscope), which delivers a high-intensity discharge over a fixed period of milliseconds.* Intensity, wavelength, and frequency can be controlled by filters. A second common stimulus is an incandescent light behind a mechanical or electromagnetic shutter system to control the duration and frequency of stimulations. Ordinary strobe lights for photic driving of the EEG are easily adapted for this purpose. Stimu-

*This chapter was prepared with the assistance of the staff of the Electrophysiology Laboratory, Wills Eye Hospital and Research Institute, and with the particular help of Joel Porter, M.D., NINDS Trainee.

*Photo Stimulator, Grass Medical Instruments, Quincy, Massachusetts.

lus duration is commonly controlled at 10 to 100 msec.

Electrodes. The active or recording electrode is placed on the eye anteriorly, since posterior or retinal electrodes cannot practically be used in humans. These may be skin leads or may be fitted to contact lenses of either the corneal or scleral type.* Most require the use of contact fluid, such as 1% methylcellulose in saline. The Burian-Allen lens (1954) incorporates a retractor to keep the lids apart.† The contact lens manufactured by Obrig Laboratories‡ is simpler in design, and small sizes are made for infants and children. Any good contact lens technician can bond a silver wire lead to a narrow scleral flange contact lens for this purpose. An auxiliary filling tube through which additional fluid may be added is convenient. A large neutral or indifferent electrode is usually taped to the skin above the bridge of the nose after cleansing the skin and applying electrolyte jelly. This is not needed if a bipolar contact lens is used.

Recorder. Amplifying and recording the small electric potentials can be done in many ways. The simplest is the use of a standard electroencephalographic machine or Grass polygraph. The inkwriter gives an immediate record and is sufficiently detailed for most clinical purposes. Because of the inertia of the inkwriter, however, the wave forms are not recorded as critically as with a cathode ray oscilloscope, which has the disadvantage of requiring a photograph for permanent record. Computer recording and tape storage plus computerized averaging of responses facilitates the delineation of minute time-related responses that could not be detected on direct records.

ELECTRORETINOGRAPHIC WAVES AND THEIR ORIGIN

The size and shape of electroretinographic waves depend on both conditions

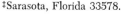

*Lo-Vac 1126, Medical Workshop, Groningen, The Netherlands.
†Manufactured by Hansen Laboratories, Iowa City, Iowa.
‡Sarasota, Florida 33578.

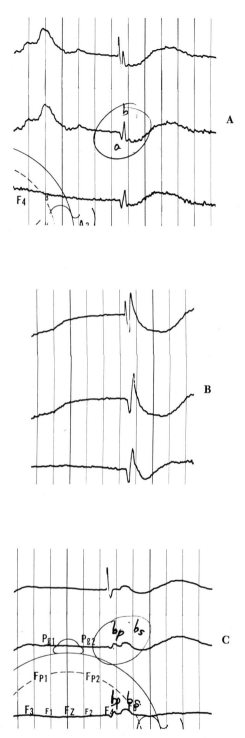

Fig. 22-1. Normal electroretinograms in 11-year-old female demonstrating **A**, photopic responses, **B**, scotopic responses, and **C**, scotopic b wave (b), elicited with use of red filter. Top tracings show stimulus artifact. Middle tracings are right eye, and bottom tracings are left eye.

of testing and health of the eye. Four waves may be seen. The first wave is a brief negative deflection called the *a wave;* the following wave is a longer lasting, greater amplitude positive deflection called the *b wave.* A slower, positive *c wave* and an off-effect or *d wave* may also be seen. There may be smaller wavelets superimposed on the b wave; these are oscillatory potentials. For most clinical studies, only the a and b waves are important (Fig. 22-1).

Both the a and b waves may appear double, and these then are designated a_1 and a_2 or b_1 or b_2. Since they probably represent photopic and scotopic function, they are sometimes called a_p and a_s and b_p and b_s. The b_p wave was originally called the *x wave* or b_x. The most common terms now are those with the photopic or scotopic subscripts.

Precise points of origin of these waves are still somewhat uncertain, but clarification has come from microelectrode studies at various depths in animal retinas, responses in the predominantly rod or cone retinas of certain species, alterations following use of drugs that selectively affect specific retinal areas, and correlating electroretinographic responses with known clinical entities.

The a wave probably originates in the outer segments of rods and cones. Bipolar cell activity is probably associated with the b wave, although the inner segments of the rods and cones may also contribute. The c wave is probably produced by the pigment epithelium. For simplification of understanding it is easiest to associate the a wave with the visual cells and the b wave with the bipolars. The ganglion cells and nerve fibers apparently do not contribute to the ERG. The ERG, however, apparently correlates with the beginning of a chain of electric activity ending in the occipital cortex. Some responses in the optic nerve or even farther back may occur before the electroretinographic potentials are recorded. The size, shape, and time relationships of the ERG depend on variations in stimulus parameters (intensity, duration, wavelength,

frequency), the condition of the eye (state of adaptation, pupil size, pathology), and extraneous nonretinal potentials (lid, bulbar, iris, and ciliary body motion).

The most important ocular variable is the state of adaptation. In the light-adapted state, all components of the normal ERG occur rapidly and are of low voltage. During the early phases of dark adaptation, the amplitude of the a and b waves increases rapidly. At first, this is especially true of a_p and b_p. The a_s and b_s can hardly be distinguished in the light-adapted state. As dark adaptation progresses, a_s and b_s increase and become larger than a_p and b_p. When dark adaptation is essentially complete, the a and b waves reach maximum size.

Variations in the stimulus cause greatly different ERG responses. The intensity of the light can change both the amplitude and form of the response. Generally, the amplitude of response increases in proportion to the logarithm of the intensity over a range of about 4 logarithmic units.

Stimuli of different wavelengths cause different shaped responses. For example, blue light tends to bring out the scotopic waves. A deep red stimulus causes a complex response with a double b wave. This apparently represents the photopic and scotopic b waves rather than a specific red response (Fig. 22-1, *C*).

The phenomenon of flicker fusion is useful in electroretinographic testing. In psychophysiologic tests, the critical flicker fusion frequency is that frequency at which a repetitive stimulus appears to be constant. With the ERG, it is that frequency at which responses are merged and no longer separable. The Grass polygraph can follow 40 to 60 stimuli per second. The cone system is known to be capable of responding separately at a much higher frequency than the rod system. With computer equipment, distinctly separate ERG's can be recorded at rates of over 100 per second. If the electroretinographic responses show fusion of repetitive stimuli at a low rate, this is evidence of cone dysfunction.

LIMITATIONS OF THE ERG

A major limitation of present techniques is in evaluating precise retinal areas and particularly macular function. The usual ERG is a mass response caused by spread of light by the media of the eye and interneuronal connections within the retina. Thus even if a narrow pencil of light is used as a stimulus and directed to the blind spot, the whole retina tends to respond. Research techniques using background saturation, however, may lead to a practical method for obtaining localized ERG's.

Another limitation of the ERG results from the fact that the rods greatly outnumber the cones. Some estimate that there are 120 million rods compared to 7 million cones in each retina. Though many important clinical disturbances affect the central vision or macular area, the ERG is imprecise in segregating these functions. In the visual mass response, rod activity overshadows that of the cones. Although the macular area contains almost entirely cones, there may be only about 350,000 cones there out of the total 7 million in the retina. Therefore a discrete macular lesion may entirely destroy these macular cones, but cone ERG responses might appear normal because of the mass response of the overwhelming number of extramacular cones.

However, photopic and scotopic tests, red light, and flicker fusion help separate the rod from the cone waves.

TECHNIQUE OF USE

Where ERG's are to be made in most general hospitals, major clinics, or group practice situations, the usual electrically shielded room for electroencephalography is quite adequate. Shielding may be generally satisfactory with copper wire screen or with thin solid copper plate or foil. The shielding, as well as all equipment, must be grounded through either cold water pipes or a separate ground stake going several feet into the earth. The room should easily accommodate a full-length stretcher with access to the patient. A ceiling lower than 8 ft. or a room length less than 10 ft. is often unpleasant and suggests a torture cell rather than a relaxed diagnostic setting.

Pupils should be fully dilated when possible with drops such as 1% Mydriacyl or 2.5% Neo-Synephrine, after inspection to ensure that the anterior chambers are at least of average depth. If the patient has had narrow-angle glaucoma or has a very shallow chamber, or if gonioscopy in uncertain cases shows a narrow filtration angle, then this aid to electroretinography must be omitted. The desirable use of these topical instillations tends to eliminate iris and ciliary muscle action potential as well as the alterations in stimulus intensity induced by changes in pupillary diameter.

Smoking should be omitted for at least 1 hour before examination. The face should be washed or cleansed of make-up and skin oils in the areas to be used for electrode contact.

The patient should be placed in a comfortable supine position on a padded couch or stretcher as he is given a clear accounting of what will transpire. If contact lens electrodes are used, a topical anesthetic such as proparacaine hydrochloride (Ophthaine) should be instilled. This is omitted if small skin electrodes are substituted for the active poles; they should be taped over a minute amount of electrolyte jelly at a point on the orbital rim below the cornea. The negative or indifferent electrode is taped to the skin above the glabella. The patient is instructed to leave both eyes open, to maintain steady fixation on an overhead point, and not to blink during the tests.

Routines may be quite simplified or complicated by use of many different stimuli and various adaptations. In all cases calibration should be established before and after each examination by recording a linear deflection of the pen equal to a known potential; ordinarily this should be about half of maximum response to be obtained. Preadaptation is achieved with a standard light source such as two 100-watt light bulbs behind a diffusing screen 5 ft. from the eyes for a period of 5 minutes. A light meter may be used to check consistency of this preadaptation light and to avoid unsuspected reduction caused by aging filaments.

Light-adapted responses can be elicited with the stroboscopic flash at maximum intensity. Individual flashes should be separated by at least 3 seconds. Brief bursts of flicker response should also be obtained. When satisfactory light-adapted tracings are recorded, all background and room light is extinguished. Dark adaptation responses are recorded at 1, 3, 5, 9, 15, and 25 minutes or other determined intervals. These brief test flashes even at high intensity do not alter the course of dark adaptation when presented at intervals of greater than 1 second. The patient may close his lids during the period of longer intervals between flashes.

When children are tested it is preferable to have a parent remain in the shielded room beside the child. Infants and very small children will require general or basal anesthesia. Attendants should not touch a patient during examination because this will create electric artifacts.

THE ERG IN PATIENTS WITH OCULAR ABNORMALITIES
Retinal degenerations (involutions)

The large group of retinal degenerations has been one of the most informative areas for use of the ERG. Aid is afforded in diagnosis, recording the functional course of the disease, finding carrier states in unaffected relatives, and providing a better understanding of the disease process. Conversely, correlating electroretinographic changes with the clinical findings has helped in understanding the ERG itself.

Primary pigmentary degeneration of the retina (retinitis pigmentosa). The ERG may be completely absent or of very low amplitude in retinitis pigmentosa. There may be only a small photopic ERG, with almost no scotopic response. This is evidence of widespread rod disease, which precedes the cone involvement with its late reduction of central acuity. This correlates with early impairments of dark adaptation and later night blindness (Fig. 22-2).

In some patients with loss of scotopic vision and early loss of the b wave, there may be no classical findings of bone corpuscle pigmentation. Narrowed vessels and waxy discs, however, help to establish the

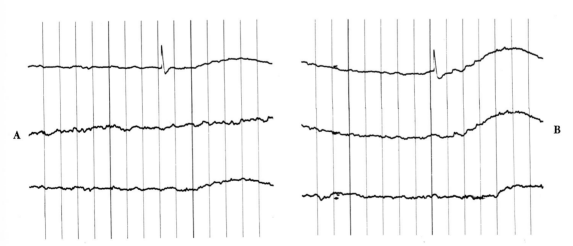

Fig. 22-2. Electroretinographic tracings showing **A**, essentially absent photopic responses and **B**, absent scotopic responses in 60-year-old Negro male with pigmentary degeneration of the retina. Top tracings show stimulus artifact; middle tracings are from right eye; bottom tracings are from left eye.

basic diagnosis of retinitis pigmentosa sine pigmento. In other cases, the pigment shows unusual form or distribution. The ERG may help to differentiate primary from secondary degenerations caused by syphilis, trauma, rubella, vaccinia, or febrile diseases. In the secondary degenerations, the ERG is normal or only slightly reduced in most cases. If the retina is severely affected, however, the ERG may be absent or very low, as in primary disease. If the ERG is near normal, the disease is probably secondary; if it is very abnormal, one cannot be certain.

The ERG is valuable in studying relatives of affected patients. The disease is commonly autosomal dominant, autosomal recessive, or sex-linked recessive, though isolated cases occur. Electroretinography may give early diagnosis in other members of the family, which can help in career planning and genetic counseling. Electroretinography and dark adaptometry are the most sensitive tests in retinitis pigmentosa.

Retinal abiotrophy. In cases of macular degenerations that are really only part of more widespread retinal disorders, as commonly found in children presenting pre-dominantly macular involution, the ERG may show severe changes similar to retinitis pigmentosa. This indicates widespread disease beyond its morphologic manifestations and consequently a poor prognosis. These disturbances are often associated with other systemic or ocular diseases. The finding of an abnormal ERG is evidence of retinal dysfunction that might go unsuspected in myotonic dystrophy, certain cases of Hurler's disease, and high myopia.

Retinitis punctata albescens. Retinitis punctata albescens, a rare form of involution, is characterized by great numbers of small white dot-like areas throughout the retina, with associated narrowing of retinal vessels and pigmentation. The full-blown disease often runs a progressive course with night blindness and contraction of the visual fields. A stationary type also occurs, usually evidenced by night blindness but with no tendency toward progression and therefore a better prognosis. It can be very difficult to distinguish the two types clinically. The ERG may be helpful here, but varying types of response have been recorded. In general, the ERG is severely reduced or absent in the advanced cases and relatively normal in the stationary form.

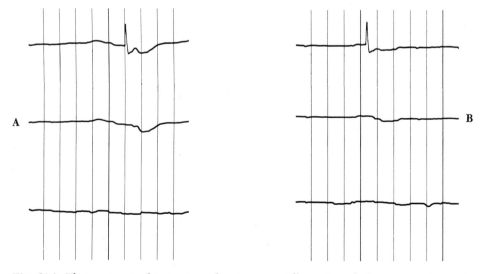

Fig. 22-3. Electroretinographic tracings showing essentially extinguished responses in a 69-year-old male with choroideremia. Top tracings show stimulus artifact. **A,** Tracings from right and left eye under photopic examination; **B,** under scotopic examination.

Following the patient with ERG's over a period of years may anticipate progression by revealing depression of the ERG before clinical evidence appears.

Choroideremia

Choroideremia is characterized by progressive atrophy of the choroid and pigment epithelium leading to night blindness and gross loss of field. It is a male, sex-linked manifestation, but the carrier females show milder fundus pigment abnormalities with mild or no loss of function. The ERG in choroideremia is usually absent (Fig. 22-3). The ERG is not necessary to establish the diagnosis in characteristic cases but may be helpful in atypical cases.

Circulatory diseases

Central retinal artery occlusion. The ERG usually shows a normal or larger than normal a wave with marked reduction of the b wave, especially b_s. This is the so-called negative ERG. Rarely a negative response is seen, with a large a and b_s wave. Electroretinographic findings correlate with the known retinal and choroidal circulation. Thus central retinal artery occlusion affects the inner retinal layers, usually down to the inner nuclear layer, and impairs bipolar cells more than the rods and cones, which derive their supply from the choroidal circulation. This explains retention of the a wave and reduction of the b wave. The amplitude of the b wave may be an indication of the degree of arterial obstruction; that is, a relatively normal b wave indicates only partial obstruction and better prognosis.

Central retinal vein occlusion. Electroretinographic findings are often similar to those of arterial occlusion, but the b wave is retained more often, probably indicating that partial occlusion is more common with the vein than with the artery. Depth of electroretinographic impairment may aid in prognosis, but correlation with the final visual result is not exact.

In branch vein occlusion, the ERG is usually normal or may show a slight reduction of the b wave. Occasionally a greater than normal b wave is seen. Such an ERG is called "supranormal" (Fig. 22-4).

Temporal (cranial) arteritis. A very large a wave, larger than in any other condition, and a slightly reduced b wave may be pathognomonic of temporal arteritis (Burian). The ERG is similar in both eyes, though

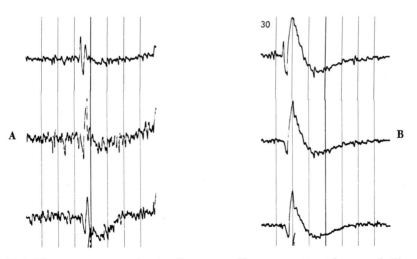

Fig. 22-4. Electroretinograms showing "supranormal" responses in right eye of 65-year-old patient with central retinal vein thrombosis. Top tracings show stimulus artifact; middle tracings are right eye. **A,** Photopic examination; **B,** scotopic examination.

only one eye is affected clinically. This is usually not seen if steroid therapy has been started.

Carotid artery disease. Ipsilateral diminished b waves are suggestive of carotid insufficiency (Wulfing, 1963; Krill, 1962). In bilateral disease, the ERG may be unequal on the two sides, probably reflecting the status of collateral circulation. Electroretinographic results must be correlated with other studies, such as ophthalmodynamometry and arteriography. The risks of arteriography should be avoided if other tests can give equally accurate information (pp. 213-218).

Systemic hypertension and arteriosclerosis. Mild degrees of interference with retinal vascular supply may cause an increase in the b wave, while more severe disturbance decreases the b wave. The increased response may result from greater irritability of neurons with mild degrees of anoxia.

Though not completely consistent, the ERG affords some index of the severity of the systemic disease and general prognosis.

Systemic diseases

Diabetes. In general, electroretinographic changes parallel the degree of retinal damage. After "glucose loading" by intravenous infusion of 500 ml. of 30% glucose, normal patients show no increase in retinal electric activity; however, long-standing diabetic patients show increased activity even if no retinopathy is visible ophthalmoscopically. Severe diabetic retinopathy is associated with an even greater increase in retinal electric activity. Henkes has coined the term "fundus diabeticus" to indicate the condition of patients with retinal dysfunction in the absence of ophthalmoscopic changes. Similarly fluorescein angiography often shows more widespread retinopathy than is revealed by ophthalmoscopy.

Thyroid disease. Generally the electroretinographic amplitude is found to parallel the thyroid status, being "supranormal" in hyperthyroidism and reduced in hypothyroidism. This returns to normal when either condition is effectually treated.

Myotonic dystrophy. Cataracts and ptosis are commonly found in myotonic dystrophy, and recent investigations have found decreased b waves in almost all patients with myotonic dystrophy, thus adding to understanding of the widespread nature of the disease.

Hurler's disease. Abnormal ERG's are found in many cases of Hurler's disease, which is primarily considered to present corneal opacity as the significant ocular finding.

Liver disease. Both acute or chronic hepatitis and cirrhosis of the liver cause elevated dark-adapted thresholds and reduced b waves. These changes are probably caused by abnormal vitamin A storage or metabolism but are not directly proportional to the degree of liver disease.

Drug toxicity

The ERG can be of value as an objective index both of degree and site of impairment from retinotoxic compounds.

Chloroquine. Chloroquine retinopathy, unlike the reversible corneal impairments caused by crystalline deposits, can cause severe permanent visual loss, and it is difficult to detect in early stages while potentially reversible. Usually the diagnosis is made morphologically or functionally after the characteristic macular pigmentation, or ring scotoma, is noted. In early stages, electroretinography and tests of dark adaptation may be equivocal; electroretinographic impairments are often very subtle until the disease is well established.

Thioridazine hydrochloride (Mellaril). Mellaril, a widely used tranquilizer, can also cause retinal damage after prolonged administration. Depressed ERG's have been found in some cases, but not enough patients have been studied.

Quinine. Quinine intoxication can cause severe visual loss. In the early and acute stage, the ERG is usually normal despite reduced vision, probably because initial damage is localized to the ganglion cells, which have no appreciable effect on the ERG.

Opaque media

In the presence of dense corneal opacities, pupillary occulusion, or cataract, the ERG gives an objective index of diffuse (mass) retinal function. Other tests of retinal function such as flicker fusion perimetry (pp. 197-198) and auto-ophthalmoscopic perimetry (p. 180), which are applicable when the fundus cannot be visualized, rely on subjective responses. The clinical ERG, however, does not give precise evidence of macular function per se.

Regardless of cataract density, a normal retina will yield a normal ERG. Comparison of ERG's before and after cataract extraction usually shows little or no difference. If the preoperative ERG is normal, there is no widespread retinal disease, but there still can be localized macular or focal disease or optic nerve pathology. If the preoperative ERG is diminished, one must expect some visual limitation after cataract extraction, particularly in the extent of peripheral vision.

Infants and children

The ERG can be objectively helpful in examination of children too young for subjective tests, such as acuity or fields, or when there is suggestion of decreased vision with normal or questionable fundi. In children with abnormal fundi, the ERG may yield information helpful in diagnosis, prognosis, and management. Children age 7 or over can usually be tested with topical anesthesia, as in adults, but younger children may require general or basal anesthesia or strong sedation that may alter their ERG (Goodman, Ripps, and Siegel, 1963).

Leber's congenital amaurosis. Congenital amaurosis is a defect in which vision is greatly diminished at birth or early in life. Nystagmus, photophobia, and also keratoglobus are common. The fundi may appear normal early in the disease, although pigmentation and vascular narrowing often

develop later. The ERG shows greatly reduced or absent photopic and scotopic responses. This proves the presence of widespread retinal dysfunction.

Congenital retinal dysfunction. Congenital retinal dysfunction is a term used by Karpe and Zetterstrom (1958) to describe children with decreased vision, normal fundi, and abnormal ERG's that later improve. This appears to be a developmental delay or retardation at the retinal level.

Congenital cone dysfunction syndromes. Congenital cone dysfunction may occur in complete or partial forms. When complete, the visual acuity is about 20/200 and there is nystagmus, photophobia, and total absence of color discrimination (achromatopsia). Partial forms show visual acuity of 20/40 to 20/100, minimal or no nystagmus and photophobia, and only a partial color vision defect. The fundi are usually normal but may show loss of foveal reflexes and macular abnormalities. This syndrome is frequently misdiagnosed as congenital nystagmus, particularly in children too young to test for color vision or if color vision tests are not done. The ERG is usually diagnostic, showing markedly decreased photopic responses, diminished flicker fusion frequency, and essentially normal scotopic responses (Fig. 22-5).

Albinism. Albinism is distinguished from true retinal degeneration or dysfunction by specific electroretinographic findings. Other ocular functions resemble the cone dysfunction syndrome, with nystagmus, photophobia, and decreased vision caused by macular hypoplasia. The ERG is normal or greater than normal because of increased reflection and scattering of light, in contrast to the various electroretinographic depressions in other types of pathology.

Night blindness. Detecting night blindness in children (as well as in adults) is an area in which the ERG may be very helpful. Progressive patterns, such as in retinitis pigmentosa, choroideremia, or retinitis punctata albescens, can at times be differentiated from stationary defects such

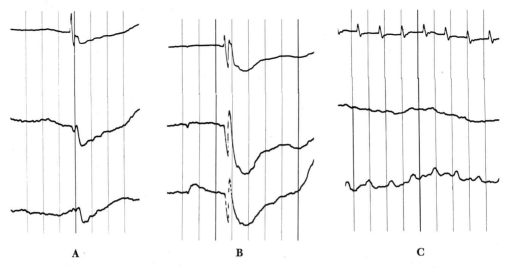

Fig. 22-5. Electroretinograms showing **A,** diminished photopic responses, **B,** less diminished scotopic responses, and **C,** reduced responses to flicker at 7 c.p.s. in 6-year-old Caucasian male with congenital cone dysfunction. Top tracings show stimulus artifacts.

as congenital night blindness. If the ERG is greatly decreased or absent, there is severe retinal degeneration, but if there is only modest decrease in scotopic responses, congenital night blindness is likely. Early cases of retinitis pigmentosa, however, may show similar findings, so that an absolute distinction cannot be made.

Other diseases. In optic nerve lesions, cortical or central blindness, and hysteria or malingering, the ERG is normal and may make unnecessary further and possibly hazardous tests, such as arteriography or pneumoencephalography.

In true retinal degenerations, the ERG may make the diagnosis before functional or ophthalmoscopic changes are noted. This will help in genetic counseling and education planning. The ERG may distinguish primary from secondary retinal changes (p. 250).

Neurology

Visually evoked responses. VER's recorded from scalp electrodes over the occiput following photic stimulation of the eyes are elaborations of electroretinographic and electroencephalographic techniques.

The two major aims of response studies are (1) to plot an "objective" visual field by stimulating localized retinal areas, and (2) to determine the exact location of lesions of the visual pathway anywhere from the retina to the occipital cortex. An objective visual field test would be very helpful in circumstances involving uncooperative or comatose patients and little children. Changes in the VER involve the shape, amplitude, and latency of the waves, which may differentiate the location of lesions causing similar field defects.

The VER in present laboratory conditions also seems able to detect macular or other localized conditions not identifiable with current ERG's. This is facilitated by the geographically large cortical area of projection associated with the macula. Amblyopia and migraine also seem to present changes in the laboratory VER that may soon become clinically useful.

Multiple sclerosis. Multiple sclerosis, a widespread disease of the nervous system with frequent ocular manifestations, has classically been thought to yield a normal ERG because the usual cause of decreased vision is damage to the optic nerve rather than to the retina. However, Gills (1966) has described abnormal ERG's in many multiple sclerosis patients. Some histopathology studies have found decreased cellularity of the inner nuclear layer, raising the possibility of retrograde transsynaptic degeneration.

Other ocular disorders

Glaucoma. Most investigators report a normal ERG in glaucoma except for acute congestive or very advanced stages. Glaucoma damage is primarily to the nerve fibers and ganglion cells, which do not contribute to the ERG. In some advanced cases, however, there is severe impairment of the retinal and choroidal circulation that diminishes or extinguishes the ERG.

In acute glaucoma there may be a temporary increase of the b wave similar to that in hypoxic states, such as hypertension or partial vascular occlusion.

Retinal detachment. In serous detachments, generally the higher the preoperative b wave amplitude, the better the final visual prognosis. The b wave in the "normal" fellow eye should be watched for reductions, which suggest a guarded outlook. Many other variables, however, affect the detached retina and make specific conclusions of limited validity. Nonetheless, patients with retinal detachment should have preoperative electroretinographic tests bilaterally, where these are available.

Siderosis. Early in the course of intraocular ferrous foreign bodies, both a and b waves are increased in amplitude. Later the b wave decreases, and finally the ERG becomes abolished in the late stages. These changes may be present before any subjective or objective manifestations of siderosis. The earliest changes represent a reversible stage, with return toward normal if the foreign body is removed successfully. Later stages are irreversible.

Myopia. The ERG is normal in the mild or usual type of myopia. In severe, progressive, or malignant myopia, however, the b wave is often decreased in proportion to the degree of retinal degeneration. The ERG may even be extinguished, which probably is evidence of other coexisting degeneration.

Harada's disease. Harada's disease is basically a posterior uveitis with exudative retinal detachment, and it is probably a part of the Vogt-Koyanagi syndrome. The ERG is greatly diminished early in the course of the disease because of retinal edema or detachment. The edema may be missed ophthalmoscopically, and the clinician is then faced with the problem of severe loss of vision without obvious cause. Associated neurologic symptoms and signs point to optic nerve or cerebral disease. A diminished ERG is definite evidence of widespread retinal involvement and helps make the correct diagnosis. The scotopic ERG is affected more than the photopic. The abnormal ERG usually returns toward normal as the detachment disappears, paralleling the return of vision.

Chapter 23

Electrooculography

Electrooculography is a diagnostic study of the integrity of the pigment epithelium of the retina as determined from changes in the standing corneoretinal potential of the eye. Such changes are elicited by voluntary rotation of the eyes through predetermined arcs in the dark-adapted and subsequently in the light-adapted states. Numerical values are expressed as a ratio or as the arithmetic quotient obtained from dividing the usually higher electric potential of the "light peak" by the usually lower electric potential of the "dark trough."

Twenty years of primarily investigative studies with the electrooculograph (Marg, 1951) have shown it to be a clinically sensitive diagnostic device to identify impairments in the retinal pigment epithelium. The ERG is less sensitive than the electrooculogram (EOG) in detecting such deep changes. On the other hand, EOG's in achromatic and nyctalopic patients may be identical to those from normal patients, whereas the ERG in the presence of such pathology will show marked reduction of electric activity. Like most electrophysiologic diagnosis procedures, however, a moderate amount of complex and fragile equipment is required. This is often best protected and operated in a special clinic where such devices are familiar to and cared for by specific technicians. Generally these devices are not expected in the offices of busy practitioners, and probably they should be located in hospitals or medical centers where they may be available to several users.

The EOG is based on a standing current or corneoretinal potential (CRP), which appears to flow through the eye in the direction of the visual axis, thus rendering the globe analogous to a rotatable dipole of positive charge at the cornea and negative charge at the maculopapular area. Because the pick-up electrodes are placed on the canthal skin, somewhat remote from the extraocular muscles, the EOG does not reflect action potentials of these muscles, which disturb the ERG. Electric potentials range between 15 and 30 mv. per degree of ocular rotation. The detecting and amplifying system must afford sufficient gain to display these signals on a recorder, such as the Grass polygraphs employed for electroencephalography.

In use, the patient should be seated comfortably with his occiput resting on a suitably positioned headrest (leaning slightly forward, for a chin and forehead support may be more fatiguing over the 20 or 25 minutes needed for testing). Two conspicuous fixation lights about 30 to 40 degrees apart are located equidistant to each side of the subject's sagittal plane. A screen, diffusing sphere, or other suitable bright illumination source is placed between them. Small, lightweight electrodes coated with conducting jelly are taped to the skin of the canthal regions with care not to drag or impede ocular rotations. The patient is instructed to perform horizontal rotations from one fixation light to the other at generally consistent speed (velocity of rotation is one of the variables that affects the electric potential). Heights of the vertical deflections on the recorder measure the amplitude of the standing potential.

The patient should gain familiarity with the test situation and then be permitted to dark-adapt for 12 minutes while repeating the ocular excursions at intervals of about 1 minute. A "dark trough" of minimal potential is usually reached between 8 and 12 minutes. The eye is then suddenly reilluminated and recording continued at 1-minute intervals for about another 12 minutes. A "light peak" of maximum potential is usually reached in 8 or 9 minutes.

Because absolute values are difficult to establish and are altered by several factors* in the test situation, more useful information is obtained from the "light peak/dark trough" ratio. Normal ratios are between 3 and 2. Ratios from 2 to 1.75 are borderline, and those between 1.75 and 1.5 are probably subnormal. Those lower than 1.5 are definitely pathologic, and a ratio of 1 shows no light response. (Sometimes these

---

*Preadaptation, light intensity, arc and speed of rotation, amplifying equipment, reduction in skin resistance with time, drowsiness, medications, and so forth.

figures are multiplied by 100 and expressed as percentages, which has the unfortunate connotation of suggesting that no light response is "100%.")

The same electric circuitry may be used for electronystagmography by recording the amplitude and frequency of potentials generated from the involuntary oscillations of the eyes (pp. 259-263).

Electrooculography is a functional diagnostic adjunct to verify or interpret morphologic disturbances in the pigment epithelium as seen ophthalmoscopically or with the aid of intravenous fluorescein studies. The EOG, in common with the ERG, tends to provide a diffuse response or to measure a diffuse disturbance, but unlike the ERG it derives primarily from the pigment epithelium and possibly metabolic activity in the outer limbs of the rods. The EOG does not reflect localized disturbances such as those confined to the macula. It does not reflect disturbances of the inner layers of the retina nor of the optic nerve. Thus the EOG is primarily valuable in early detection of abiotrophic processes, particularly those striking the pigment epithelium.

Chapter 24

Nystagmography

NYSTAGMOLOGY

There is no subject within ophthalmic, neurologic, or otologic literature wherein nomenclature is so varied and imprecise as in the field of nystagmology. Nystagmus itself should be defined as involuntary oscillations or tremors of the eyes independent of normal movements. It is usually bilateral but rarely may be unilateral or voluntary. For clarity of description, awareness of mechanism, and diagnostic thinking, the following seven components should be noted:

A. Onset
   1. Congenital and often hereditary: this is usually pendular and horizontal, though it may rarely be vertical or torsional
   2. Acquired
   3. Experimental (induced, opticokinetic)
B. Type or form of movements
   1. Pendular: this is characteristic of ocular nystagmus resulting from visual impairment of 20/100 or worse from birth or very early life
   2. Searching movements of blindisms: these are slow, irregular, inconstant, and not properly considered a true nystagmus
   3. Jerk nystagmus: this may be in any direction but typically has a slow component in one direction (which usually represents the pathologic mechanism) and a fast or recovery component in the opposite direction; it is classically seen in vestibular, central, and induced nystagmus
   4. Latent nystagmus: this is not manifest unless one eye is closed; it is characteristically a jerk nystagmus and is often associated with heterotropia
   5. Disjunctive and seesaw nystagmus: this is a rare manifestation in which the eyes oscillate toward and away from each other,

or one ascends while the other descends; it is possibly associated with pineal tumors
   6. Voluntary and fixation nystagmus: these are rare manifestations, usually of fine amplitude and very high frequency (fixation nystagmus is nonvoluntary aside from the fact that usually intent fixation on a nonmoving object is required for its development)
   7. Miscellaneous rare forms: these include periodic alternating nystagmus (generally a jerk nystagmus with changes in its laterality); opsoclonus (conjugate but chaotic and apparently random movements in a young child carrying a generally encouraging prognosis); retraction nystagmus (usually a serious midbrain lesion associated with difficulty in vertical gaze and sometimes related to pinealoma in children or vascular lesions in adults); downbeat nystagmus (associated with foramen magnum lesions and especially evoked in extremes of lateral gaze); and ocular flutter and bobbing (series of rapid movements during fixation or at times presenting spontaneously and usually associated with cerebellar lesions)
C. Direction (laterality): mechanistically this should specify the slow component as the pathologically incited phase, though much of the literature has previously named the fast component (recovery) as the direction of the nystagmus
D. Mechanism
   1. Physiologic, end point, or fatigue nystagmus or pseudonystagmus: this appears only in the extremes of ocular versions, particularly horizontal rotation, and is generally normal; it is obliterated by shifting the eyes a few degrees back toward the primary position
   2. Ocular: this is associated with visual impairments and poor fixation ability resulting from (1) congenital defects, such as albinism, cataracts, optic atrophy, or achromatopsia, or (2) acquired disturbances of

the visual mechanisms such as head-nodding (spasmus nutans) coming on at the age of 4 to 24 months or miner's nystagmus (allegedly associated with years of labor under poor lighting)

3. Vestibular or labyrinthine: this is the classical jerk nystagmus with or without conjugate deviation and past pointing; usually acquired; may be experimentally induced by galvanic, caloric, or pressure devices

4. Central or cerebellar: this is a jerk nystagmus frequently associated with cerebellar disease but which may also accompany disease of medulla, pons, or midbrain; it is accentuated when the eyes are closed or deviated to the side of the lesion; it may be abolished by ocular fixation when the eyes are open, and often this is effected in a particular position of gaze deviation

E. Speed (sometimes called "intensity"): this is expressed in degrees per second as read from the electronystagmographic tracing, or qualitatively described on direct observation as *slow, fast,* or *medium* speed

F. Amplitude (excursion): this is measured in degrees (Electronystagmographs should be adjusted so that a 20-degree eye movement equals a pen deflection of 20 mm. Clinically this is described as "coarse" when the amplitude is over 15 degrees, "fine" when it is less than 5 degrees, and "moderate" when it is between these extremes.)

G. Frequency (rate): this is expressed in oscillations (beats) per second, or qualitatively described on direct observation as *high* (rapid), *moderate,* or *low*

TECHNIQUE OF NYSTAGMOGRAPHY

JOSEPH U. TOGLIA, M.D.

Corneoretinal potential

The electronystagmogram (ENG) is based on recording of the standing corneoretinal potential (CRP). This shows, upon movement of the eyes, the transfer of a positive electric charge from the cornea to the nearest periorbital skin electrode. Its average strength varies from 400 to 800 mv. and is influenced by physiologic and extraphysiologic factors, among which are light and darkness, alertness and drowsiness, anoxia, acapnia, and medications. Schackel and Davis (1960) observed fluctuations as large as 400 mv. from day to day, and these could not be correlated with metabolic changes in the human body. Excitement of the patient significantly increases the strength of the CRP, even when the patient has been dark-adapted prior to testing. Some of the tests are performed in absolute darkness in order to avoid the inhibitory influence of fixation upon vestibular nystagmus. It is recommended that the patient be dark-adapted before electronystagmographic examinations are made.

Kitetsu (1966) has observed that the amplitude of the CRP in the course of dark adaption decreases to a minimum in about 13 minutes and thereafter gradually increases to return in 30 minutes to the original value. In the further course of light adaptation, the amplitude reaches a maximum in about 7 minutes, after which it gradually returns in about 14 minutes to the value observed at the beginning of light adaptation. These factors must be considered when interpreting electronystagmographic records.

Electrodes

Much attention has been devoted to the construction of special electrodes and devices to keep them in firm contact with the skin. Corneal electrodes are not generally recommended. The Beckman biopotential skin electrodes have generally eliminated the problems of stability and are very useful.

The arrangement of the electrodes varies. I use one electrode at the bridge of the nose and one at each lateral canthus for recording horizontal movements of each eye and a pair of vertical electrodes for each eye.

The electrodes are connected to the electroencephalographic amplifiers so that:

1. Upward and downward eye movements are recorded respectively as upward and downward pen deflections on the first two channels. The first channel (left vertical lead) is connected with the left eye, the second (right vertical lead) with the right eye.

2. Right and left horizontal eye movements are recorded correspondingly

as upward and downward pen deflections on both the third and fourth channels. The third channel (left horizontal lead) is connected with the left eye and the fourth (right horizontal lead) with the right.

3. Channel five (bitemporal lead) records horizontal gaze movements to the right as upward deflections and to the left as downward deflections, utilizing the bitemporal summation of both corneoretinal potentials.

Recording apparatus

Recording apparatus is selected not only on personal and economic choice but also in regard to specific applications. Otologists interested in labyrinthine function stress the velocities of each phase of nystagmus since they equate speed (degrees per second) of the slow phase to the speed of the endolymphatic flow. Modern apparatus, such as the Beckman Dynograph Type R,* has built-in

---

*Nystagmus Coupler, manufactured by Beckman Instruments, Inc., Bala Cynwyd, Pennsylvania. Electrooculographic equipment can be used for electronystagmography. Two-channel systems with recorders, skin electrodes, and Torok goggles are assembled by Instrumentation and Control Systems, Inc. (ICS), Addison, Illinois 60101.

electronic devices able to derive the speed of each phase. Ophthalmologists, like neurologists, are mainly interested in frequency (rate), amplitude, type, and form of the nystagmus and whether the nystagmus is monocular or binocular.

Some instruments use D.C. and others use A.C. With the D.C. type, the changes in voltage, recorded through the electrodes, are proportional to the angle of ocular deviation, and the position of the eyes is continuously recorded. With the A.C. type, the height of the pen deflection represents the speed and not the amplitude of the eye movements; the higher the spike, the higher the speed of the eye movements (Fig. 24-1).

I use a multichannel electronystagmograph but also use standard electroencephalographic equipment with complete satisfaction. The electroencephalograph is available in almost every hospital. It has suitable filters for eliminating high-frequency potentials, more channels than actually are needed, more than one paper speed, and more than one time constant. Modifications may be arranged so that a long time constant of 10 seconds is available if desired. The D.C. recording or a long time constant of 10 seconds is advisable for continuously

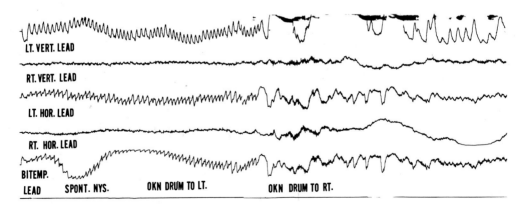

LT. VERT. LEAD

RT. VERT. LEAD

LT. HOR. LEAD

RT. HOR. LEAD

BITEMP.
LEAD   SPONT. NYS.   OKN DRUM TO LT.   OKN DRUM TO RT.

Fig. 24-1. Nystagmogram of patient with prosthesis in right orbit following surgical removal of the globe. Vision in the left eye is reduced to poor light projection with resultant pendular nystagmus. No electric activities can be seen on the right. Rotation of opticokinetic drum to left does not change pendular nystagmus. Rotation to the right, however, converts the pendular nystagmus to an irregular nystagmus with slow component to the left and rapid recovery movement to the right.

and simultaneously recording the ocular position and the nystagmus. Position information is important because gaze deviation toward the slow phase decreases the nystagmus, whereas deviation toward the fast phase increases the nystagmus (Alexander's law). Convergence and vertical deviation of the eyes also influence the nystagmus to a great extent.

To record eye movements of each eye in both horizontal and vertical planes, at least a four-channel apparatus is needed, and thus the electroencephalograph, available in almost every hospital, remains the first choice. A recording should be obtained using a time constant of 10 seconds (Fig. 24-2).

Photoelectric pickups

Torok's (1951) or Pfaltz's (1956) techniques use a photoelectric cell placed immediately in front of one eye to pick up variations of reflected infrared light focused astride the corneoscleral margin so that it falls partly on the sclera and partly on the iris. During nystagmus, reflections of the infrared beam from the sclera increase and decrease rhythmically. Since the reflection coefficient of light is greater for the white sclera than the darker iris, the total reflected light increases and decreases proportionally with the eye movements. This avoids skin electrodes.

Antonuccio and Galletti (1965) modified the photoelectric technique, eliminating the effect of light and fixation by using a photoresistor. All photoelectric techniques eliminate the problems relative to the variations of CRP, position of electrodes, electric discharges of muscle, cutaneous sweating, and so on. However, the greatest disadvantage of photoelectronystagmography is again that the recording is limited to only one or two channels.

Calibration

Calibration spikes of 10 or 20 mm. are obtained by asking the patient to look alternately at two points marked on the wall or ceiling so as to give a rotational angle of 20 degrees. Two small red lights that alternately flash with a preset frequency, varying from 20 to 100 flashes per minute, give calibration by stimulating the patient automatically to move his eyes between the flashing lights. The lights must be at least 3 meters from the patient to avoid convergence unless one eye only is used. Calibration is one of the most important technical aspects if quantitative anlysis is desired. Unfortunately the CRP is subject to many influences, some of which are difficult to control, so quantitative analysis remains dubious. Calibrations must be repeated frequently during the examination (Fig. 24-3).

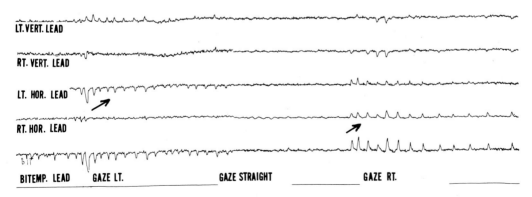

Fig. 24-2. Electronystagmogram showing marked horizontal jerk type nystagmus predominantly appearing in the abducted eye during extremes of horizontal gaze rotation. Two top tracings show very little vertical activity. Bottom tracing, representing bitemporal leads, shows position of the two eyes first in gaze left and then in gaze right. Patient has multiple sclerosis.

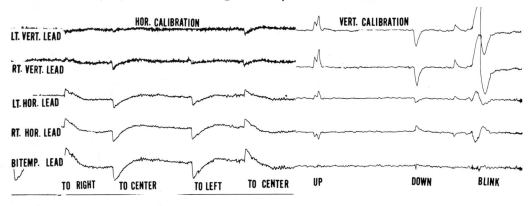

Fig. 24-3. Electronystagmogram in normal subject showing calibration at 10 degrees horizontal and vertical gaze deflections.

Use

In use, the patient is placed supine on a table with the head elevated 30 degrees. The face is carefully cleaned with alcohol to remove all make-up and facial oils. Small electrodes covered with electrolyte jelly are then taped to the outer canthi and one (ground or indifferent) electrode is taped to the glabella. For vertical tracings, active electrodes are placed immediately below the center of the brow and on the center of the inferior orbital rim. A paper movement speed of 2.5, 5.0, or 10 mm. per second is convenient for calculating frequency and speed in degrees per second. After calibration, the eyes are closed to eliminate visual fixation, which is a very powerful suppressor of vestibular nystagmus. A spontaneous horizontal nystagmus of under 5 or 6 degrees per second may be found in 20% to 25% of the population when the lids are closed.

Caloric induction of nystagmus

For induced vestibular nystagmus of the horizontal canal alone, it is necessary to elevate the head to 30 degrees before caloric stimulation through either external auditory canal. Two constant-temperature water baths (30° and 44° C.) should be maintained for consistency of cold and hot responses. Irrigating techniques have generally been standardized at 30 seconds for the 30° C. water, with the trace beginning exactly 60 seconds after commencement of

irrigation and continuing an additional 30 seconds. A similar routine is then repeated in the opposite ear 5 minutes after the onset of irrigation in the first ear. Subsequently, at 5-minute intervals the two external auditory canals are irrigated with water at 44° C.

From the 30-second tracing, representative 10-second segments of paper are cut and mounted. By measuring the lengths of the fast components in this 10-second segment, adding them, and dividing the sum by 10, the average speed in degrees per second is obtained. When a base line spontaneous nystagmus is present, its amplitude or speed must be subtracted in calculation of the related induced responses.

To diagnose relative impairment of one vestibular mechanism, at least a 20% differential should be quantitated between responses evoked from right and left stimuli before significance can be inferred. In questionable vestibular deficiency, confirmatory irrigation may be done with 30 ml. of ice water.

A competent technician should obtain good nystagmograms and complete induction tests in 30 minutes. The results can be analyzed in a few seconds. Spontaneous nystagmus is often not seen when the eyes are open but is revealed on closing the lids. Normally caloric testing evokes essentially similar nystagmus from either side and by hot or cold stimulus. The normal rhythmic frequency of response varies between 20

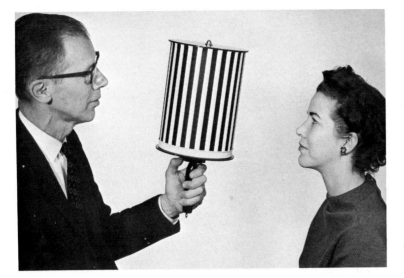

Fig. 24-4. Vertically striped drum, which can be rotated slowly to right or left in front of patient for voluntary or involuntary visual fixation and analysis of opticokinetic nystagmus to or away from the side of suspect visual pathway lesions.

and 25 beats per 10-second period. A hyperactive response (increased frequency) with caloric stimulation indicates active endorgan function of the labyrinth, but it may also represent impairment of brainstem inhibition. Nonfunctioning of a vestibular mechanism (incorrectly called "canal paresis") is illustrated by good responses to both cold and hot on one side but no response from irrigations of the opposite canal; this is typical of acoustic neuroma. Directional preponderance from irrigation with cold on one side and hot on the other indicates a disorder somewhere in the vestibular system. Irregular rhythm (dysrhythmia) is commonly associated with brainstem abnormalities. If nystagmus from caloric stimulation with the eyes open and fixed is greater than with the eyes closed, there is failure of fixation suppression and presumptive evidence of central nervous system lesion. Opening the eyes in darkness tends to reduce the speed of spontaneous nystagmus but not to alter its form or direction.

Simple observation of the character and components of nystagmus in a patient affords immediate information concerning the eyes and local disease as well as the labyrinthian mechanism and the central nervous system. The most revealing items and the ones that must always be recorded are the history and onset (in the patient as well as his family), the type or form of movement, and the direction (when a fast component is present). These facts, plus the details of ocular examination, usually reveal the mechanism. A test for latent nystagmus is automatically performed whenever one eye is covered, but the observer must note such an event and recall the unfailing impairment of monocular visual performance when it is elicited.

Induced or opticokinetic nystagmus obtained with a drum or tape elicits further diagnostic data regarding the depth or site of lesion. This is well included as a special office examination. The electronic studies of nystagmus, or the reverse studies of electrooculography obtainable with the same equipment, are generally clinical or laboratory procedures requiring considerable equipment and environmental controls. The clinician, however, must be aware of their value and the conditions calling for their use.

Chapter 25

Electromyography

Electromyography is the recording of action potentials or integrated voltage discharges of the several related muscle fibers that constitute an individual motor unit. The group of muscle fibers and their motor end plates, which are innervated by a single nerve fiber, discharge synchronously but at various frequencies and amplitudes which depend on the resting or activity state of the muscles and the presence or absence of pathologic alterations. Discharges normally appear as diphasic spikes and are amplified for visual display on a cathode ray oscilloscope or for auditory display through a loudspeaker.

Although human electromyographic studies have been critically made for about two decades (Bjork, 1952; Adler, 1953; Breinin, 1955), the technique is largely a laboratory or research tool and is highly vulnerable to errors and artifacts of instrumentation, techniques, and interpretation. The examiner must be intimately aware of the range of fluctuations and variations within his equipment as well as the alterations generated or imposed by various muscular activities of the patient. Both subtle physiologic movements and overt changes in position of the head, the eyes, and the inserted recording needles can produce gross alterations in the recordings. The examiner must accomplish numerous, repeated observations at any sitting, with critical preparation to discard incompatible recordings and to insist upon more than a few consistent recordings before attempting any interpretations.

Technique with the patient calls for full cooperation, an electrically shielded room, and adequate stretcher space for the patient to recline comfortably. Topical anesthesia is used. General, local block, or infiltration anesthesia grossly impairs or extinguishes electrical activity and hence cannot be used. This precludes testing in most preadolescent patients. Needles are 28- to 30-gauge coaxial type with a separately insulated electrode fixed within the center of the lumen. The outer surface is insulated so that contact is limited to the very tip.

A lid speculum may be used to facilitate placement of the needle electrodes but must be removed during recording. The needles are inserted through the bulbar conjunctiva and into the long axis of the extraocular muscles proximal to their tendinous portions. It is advantageous to have the needles and the recording apparatus connected to auditory signaling during insertion. Thus the examiner's undivided visual attention can be maintained on the insertional path while he attains guidance assistance from changes in the sound of the auditory monitoring.

Just as ocular muscles differ histologically and pharmacologically from skeletal muscles, there is also difference in their electrical activity. The amplitude of discharge is low, measuring 5 to 100 mv. in the resting position and 400 to 600 mv. during rotational or contraction efforts. The duration of the diphasic discharge of a single spike is short, measuring

1 to 5 msec. whether the muscle is "at rest" or in active contracture. The frequency of discharge is high, measuring 100 to 200 per second during rest and increasing by several hundred during activity.

In the so-called position of rest, all extraocular muscles are found to be firing in generally similar patterns. This is in contradistinction to skeletal muscles at rest, which show essentially no electrical activity. Sherrington's law of reciprocal innervation and Herring's law of equal bilateral innervation are corroborated by increased frequency and amplitude of activity in the agonists and correlated drops in the antagonists. *Complete* electrical silence in the absence of disease, however, is rare except under deep anesthesia, deep sleep, and extremes of opposite gaze.

Areas of electromyographic usefulness beyond strictly research applications are in the identification of lower motor neuron basis for an extraocular muscle paralysis, diagnosis of local muscular dystrophies, establishment of stage or therapeutic responsiveness in myasthenia gravis, identification of inflammatory lesions in the muscles, and possibly the differentiation of central or gaze lesions by their disturbances of agonist-antagonist relationships. The electrodes, however, record only from the motor units with which they are in direct contact, and therefore it is not accurate to generalize widely from such a given point to an entire muscle.

Additional readings

Ocular examination

Apt, L.: Diagnostic procedures in pediatric oph-thalmology, Boston, 1964, Little, Brown & Co.

Berliner, M. L.: Biomicroscopy of the eye, New York, 1966, Hafner Publishing Co.

Blodi, F., Allen, L., and Frazier, O.: Stereoscopic manual of the ocular fundus in local and sys-temic disease, ed. 2, St. Louis, 1970, The C. V. Mosby Co.

Draeger, J.: Tonometry, New York, 1966, Hafner Publishing Co.

Duke-Elder, W. S.: System of ophthalmology, vol. VII, St. Louis, 1962, The C. V. Mosby Co., pp. 231-458.

Evans, R. M.: Introduction to color, New York, 1948, John Wiley & Sons, Inc.

Gitter, K. A., Keeney, A. H., Sarin, L. K., and Meyer, D.: Ophthalmic ultrasound, St. Louis, 1969, The C. V. Mosby Co.

Gloster, J.: Tonometry and tonography, Boston, 1965, Little, Brown & Co.

Gorin, G., and Posner, A.: Slit lamp gonioscopy, ed. 3, Baltimore, 1967, The Williams & Wilkins Co.

Haessler, F. H.: Eye signs in general disease, Springfield, Illinois, 1960, Charles C Thomas, Publisher.

Hruby, K.: Slit lamp examination of vitreous and retina, Baltimore, 1967, The Williams & Wilkins Co.

Huber, A.: Eye symptoms in brain tumors, trans-lated by S. Van Wiin, St. Louis, 1961, The C. V. Mosby Co.

Johnson, W.: People in quandries, New York, 1946, Harper & Row, Publishers.

Kalmus, H.: Diagnosis and genetics of defective color vision, Elmsford, New York, 1965, Perga-mon Press.

Keeney, A. H., and Keeney, V. T.: Dyslexia: diag-nosis and treatment of reading disorders, St. Louis, 1968, The C. V. Mosby Co.

Kestenbaum, A.: Clinical methods of neuro-oph-thalmologic examination, ed. 2, New York, 1961, Grune and Stratton, Inc.

Korzybski, A.: Manhood of humanity, ed. 2, Gar-den City, New York, 1950, Country Life Press.

Korzybski, A.: Science and sanity, ed. 3, Garden City, New York, 1950, Country Life Press.

Lee, I. J.: Language habits in human affairs, New York, 1941, Harper & Row, Publishers, p. 44.

Nover, A.: The ocular fundus: methods of exam-ination, Philadelphia, 1966, Lea & Febiger.

Sloane, A. E.: Visual function is not a number (editorial), Arch. Ophthal. **68:**440, 1962.

Smith, J. L.: Optokinetic nystagmus: its use in topical neuro-ophthalmologic diagnosis, Spring-field, Illinois, 1963, Charles C Thomas, Publisher.

Thiel, R.: Atlas of diseases of the eye: typical ocular diseases, differential diagnosis, and histo-pathology, New York, 1963, Elsevier Publish-ing Co.

Von Noorden, G. K., and Maumenee, A. E.: Atlas of strabismus, St. Louis, 1967, The C. V. Mosby Co.

Neurologic aspects of examination

Bender, M. B.: The approach to diagnosis in mod-ern neurology, New York, 1967, Grune and Stratton, Inc.

Bickerstoff, E. R.: Neurological examination in clinical practice, ed. 2, Philadelphia, 1968, F. A. Davis Co.

Krayenbuhl, H., and Yesargil, M. G.: Cerebral angiography, ed. 2, Philadelphia, 1968, J. B. Lippincott Co.

Van Allen, M. W.: Pictorial manual of neurologic tests, Chicago, 1969, Year Book Medical Pub-lishers, Inc.

Identification and classification of ocular disturbances

Geeraets, W. J.: Ocular syndromes, ed. 2, Phila-delphia, 1969, Lea & Febiger.

Scheppart-Kimmijser, J., Colenbrender, J. A., and Franken, S.: Coding systems for disorders of the eye, White Plains, New York, 1968, Phiebig Publishing Co.

Thornton, F. T.: Ophthalmic eponyms and encyclo-pedia of named signs, syndromes, and diseases, Birmingham, 1967, Aesculapius Publishing Co.

Index